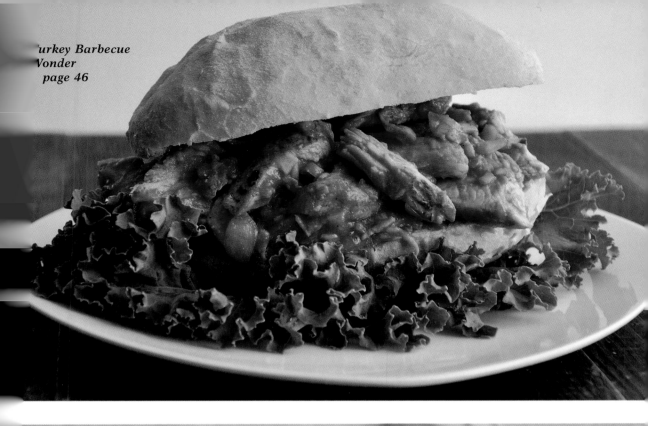

Turkey Barbecue
Wonder
  page 46

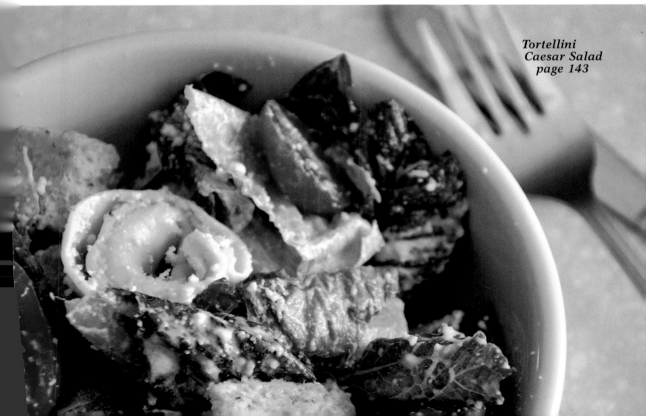

Tortellini
Caesar Salad
page 143

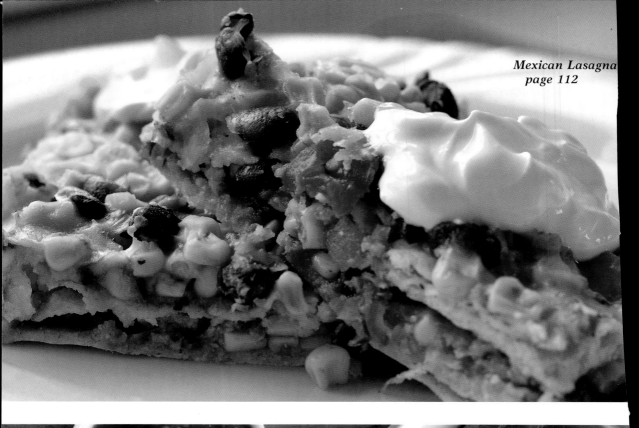

Mexican Lasagna
page 112

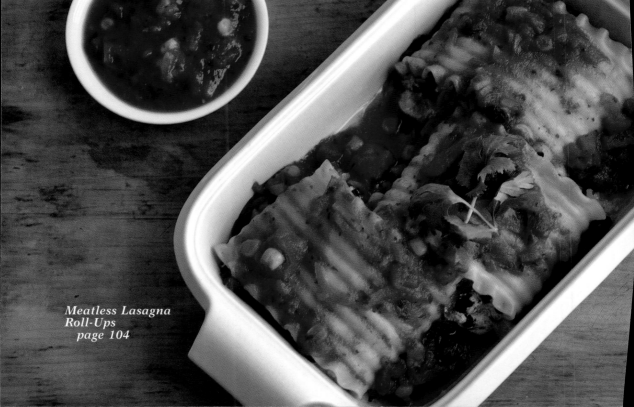

Meatless Lasagna
Roll-Ups
page 104

FIX-IT and ENJOY-IT!®

CHURCH SUPPERS
DIABETIC
COOKBOOK

***500** Great Stove-Top and Oven Recipes –*
for Everyone!

Suggested Healthy Serving Sizes for People with Diabetes

These serving sizes are here to help you determine simple, healthy portion sizes in general. These serving sizes are not intended to be used for all of the recipes in this cookbook.

Appetizer dips: 1-2 Tbsp.

Beans and legumes, cooked: ½ cup

Beverages: 1 cup

Desserts: ½ cup, ⅛ pie

Fruit: ½ cup

Frozen desserts: ½ cup

Grains and pasta side dishes: ½ cup

Main-dish sauces (for pasta, etc.): ½ cup

Meat, poultry and seafood, cooked: 3-4 ounces, about the size of a deck of cards

One-dish meals (meat, poultry, seafood, meatless), cooked: 1-1½ cups

Salad dressings, barbecue sauce: 2 Tbsp.

Salads: ½ cup fruit, grain, or bean salads; 1½ to 2 cups lettuce salads

Sauces: 2 Tbsp.

Soup: ¾-1 cup (as a side dish or appetizer); 1-1½ cups (as a main dish)

Vegetables, cooked: ½ cup

Table of Contents

Yes, a Church Suppers Cookbook for Anyone with Diabetes!

When our kids were in college, they perfected a scouting system to discover which churches were having a carry-in meal each Sunday. Then they and their friends would systematically, and apparently without shame, show up at the church serving food that day, join the line in the fellowship hall, and enjoy the taste of home-plus.

Church suppers are an American institution. Some are held once a month or once a season. Others happen weekly over the dinner hour and during the week. Some go on at noon on Sundays, right after church.

In certain communities, everyone contributes food to a specified menu. Elsewhere, each person or household who comes brings a dish of their choice for the buffet.

But if you have diabetes, you likely stand back and watch others filling their plates—or join in guiltily.

The recipes in this book are for anyone who's concerned about their calorie and carbohydrate intake. But we especially wanted to make it possible for persons with diabetes to enjoy a church supper. So take these dishes to your church's next fellowship meal—or to any potluck. Or create a church supper or potluck menu from the recipes in this collection.

And don't forget to prepare and eat these dishes at home—whenever you want to!

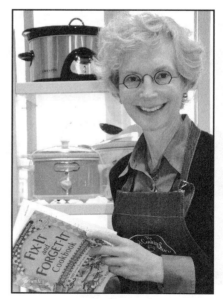

Phyllis Pellman Good

2

Managing Diabetes Day-to-Day

The American Diabetes Association joined us in this *Cookbook*, using their know-how to adapt the recipes and analyze them so they fit into nutritional meal plans. Each recipe is accompanied by Exchange Lists/Food Choices and its Basic Nutritional Values. Persons with diabetes need this information so they can manage their calories and their carb, fat, and sodium counts.

When eating, you'll want to flip often to pages 5–7, "Learning Portion Control," until you've learned to recognize appropriate food amounts at a glance.

How We Calculated the Recipes' Nutritional Analyses

The nutritional analysis for each recipe includes all ingredients except those labeled "optional," those listed as "to taste," or those calling for a "dash."

If an ingredient is listed with a second choice, the first choice was used in the analysis.

If a range is given for the amount of an ingredient, the first number was used.

Foods listed as "serve with" at the end of a recipe, or accompanying foods listed without an amount, were not included in the recipe's analysis.

In recipes calling for cooked rice, pasta, or other grains, the analysis is based on the starch being prepared without added salt or fat, unless indicated otherwise in the recipe.

The analyses were done assuming that meats were trimmed of all visible fat, and that skin was removed from poultry.

A Church Supper for Everyone!

I suggest when you make a dish from this *Cookbook* for your next church supper or potluck, that you also prepare a simple tent sign. (Fold an index card, or another rectangle of stiff paper, in half so that it will stand up straight.) Write on the card— "Safe to eat if you have diabetes!" And give the "Exchange List Values" for the dish on the sign, too. Then welcome *everyone* to the table!

Phyllis Pellman Good

Tips for Healthier, Happier Eating

How to Plan Healthy Meals

Healthy meal planning is an important part of diabetes care. If you have diabetes, you should have a meal plan specifying what, when, and how much you should eat. Work with a registered dietitian to create a meal plan that is right for you. A typical meal plan covers your meals and snacks and includes a variety of foods. Here are some popular meal-planning tools:

1. **An exchange list** is a list of foods that are grouped together because they share similar carbohydrate, protein, and fat content. Any food on an exchange list may be substituted for any other food on the same list. A meal plan that uses exchange lists will tell you the number of exchanges (or food choices) you can eat at each meal or snack. You then choose the foods that add up to those exchanges.

2. **Carbohydrate counting** is useful because carbohydrates are the main nutrient in food that affects blood glucose. When you count carbohydrates, you simply count up the carbohydrates in the foods you eat, which helps you manage your blood glucose levels. To find the carbohydrate content of a food, check the Nutrition Facts label on foods or ask your dietitian for help. Carbohydrate counting is especially helpful for people with diabetes who take insulin to help manage their blood glucose.

3. **The Create Your Plate method** helps people with diabetes put together meals with evenly distributed carbohydrate content and correct portion sizes. This is one of the easiest meal-planning options because it does not require any special tools—all you need is a plate. Fill half of

4

your plate with nonstarchy vegetables, such as spinach, carrots, cabbage, green beans, or broccoli. Fill one-quarter of the plate with starchy foods, such as rice, pasta, beans, or peas. Fill the final quarter of your plate with meat or a meat substitute, such as cheese with less than 3 grams of fat per ounce, cottage cheese, or egg substitute. For a balanced meal, add a serving of low-fat or nonfat milk and a serving of fruit.

No matter which tool you use to plan your meals, having a meal plan in place can help you manage your blood glucose levels, improve your cholesterol levels, and maintain a healthy blood pressure and a healthy weight. When you're able to do that, you're helping to control—or avoid—diabetes.

Learning Portion Control

Portion control is an important part of healthier eating. Weighing and measuring your foods helps you familiarize yourself with reasonable portions and can make a difference of several hundred calories each day. You want to frequently weigh and measure your foods when you begin following a healthy eating plan. The more you practice weighing and measuring, the easier it will become to accurately estimate portion sizes.

You'll want to have certain portion-control tools on hand when you're weighing and measuring your foods. Remember, the teaspoons and tablespoons in your silverware set won't give you exact measurements. Here's what goes into your portion-control toolbox:

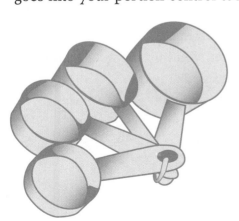

- Measuring spoons for ½ teaspoon, 1 teaspoon, ½ tablespoon, and 1 tablespoon
- A see-through 1-cup measuring cup with markings at ¼, ⅓, ½, ⅔, and ¾ cup
- Measuring cups for dry ingredients, including ¼, ⅓, ½, and 1 cup.

You may already have most of these in your kitchen. Keep them on your counter—you are more likely to use these tools if you can see them. Get an inexpensive food scale ($5–15) for foods that are measured in ounces, such as fresh produce, baked goods, meats, and cheese.

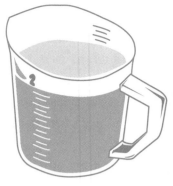

When you're weighing meat, poultry, and seafood, keep in mind that you will need more than 3 ounces of raw meat to produce a 3-ounce portion of cooked meat. For example, it takes 4 ounces of raw, boneless meat—or 5 ounces of raw meat with the bone—to produce 3 cooked ounces. About 4½ ounces of raw chicken (with the bone and skin) yields 3 ounces cooked.

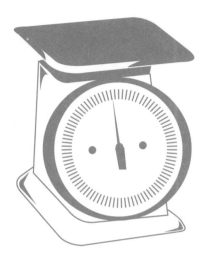

Remember to remove the skin from the chicken before eating it.

There are other easy ways to control your portions at home in addition to weighing and measuring:

- Eat on smaller plates and bowls so that small portions look normal, not skimpy.
- Use a measuring cup to serve food to easily determine how much you're serving and eating.
- Measure your drinking glasses and bowls, so you know how much you're drinking or eating when you fill them.
- Avoid serving your meals family-style because leaving large serving dishes on the table can lead to second helpings and overeating.
- Keep portion sizes in mind while shopping. When you buy meat, fish, or poultry, purchase only what you need for your meal.

When you're away from home, your eyes and hands become your portion-control tools. You can use your hand to estimate teaspoons, tablespoons, ounces, and cups. The tip of your thumb is about 1 teaspoon; your whole thumb equals roughly 1 tablespoon. Two fingers lengthwise are about an ounce, and

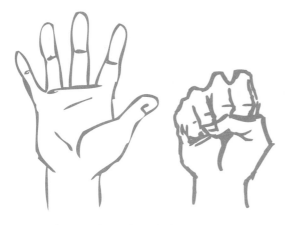

3 ounces is about the size of a palm. You can use your fist to measure in cups. A tight fist is about half a cup, whereas a loose fist or cupped hand is closer to a cup.

These guidelines are true for most women's hands, but some men's hands are much larger.

The palm of a man's hand is often the equivalent of about 5 ounces. Check the size of your hand in relation to various portions.

Remember that the more you weigh and measure your foods at home, the easier it will be to estimate portions on the road.

Controlling your portions when you eat at a restaurant can be difficult. Try to stay away from menu items with portion descriptors that are large, such as "giant," "supreme," "extra-large," "double," "triple," "king-size," and "super." Don't fall for deals in which the "value" is to serve you more food so that you can save money. Avoid all-you-can-eat restaurants and buffets.

You can split, share, or mix and match menu items to get what you want to eat in the correct portions. If you know that the portions you'll be served will be too large, ask for a take-home container when you place your order and put half of your food away before you start eating.

Gradually, as you become better at portion control, you can weigh and measure your foods less frequently. If you feel like you are correctly estimating your portions, just weigh and measure once a week, or even once a month, to check that your portions are still accurate. A good habit to get into is to "calibrate" your portion control memory at least once a month, so you don't start overestimating your portion sizes. Always weigh and measure new foods and foods that you tend to overestimate.

Frequently Asked Questions about Diabetes and Food

1. *Do people with diabetes have to eat a special diet?*

No, they should eat the same foods that are healthy for everyone—whole grains, vegetables, fruit, and small portions of lean meat. Like everyone else, people with diabetes should eat breakfast, lunch, and dinner and not put off eating until dinnertime. By then, you are ravenous and will eat too much. This sends blood sugar levels soaring in people with diabetes, and doesn't allow them to feel hungry for breakfast the next morning.

2. *Can people with diabetes eat sugar?*

Yes, they can. Sugar is just another carbohydrate to the body. All carbohydrates, whether they come from dessert, breads, or carrots, raise blood sugar. An equal serving of brownie and of baked potato raise your blood sugar the same amount. If you know that a rise in blood sugar is coming, it is wise to focus on the size of the serving.

The question of "how much sugar is too much?" has to be answered by each one of us. No one who wants to be healthy eats a lot of sugar.

3. *What natural substances are good sugar substitutes? Are artificial sweeteners safe for people with diabetes?*

Honey, agave nectar, maple syrup, brown sugar, and white sugar all contain about the same amount of calories and have a similar effect on your blood glucose levels. All of these sweeteners are a source of carbohydrates and *will* raise blood glucose quickly.

If you have diabetes, you can use these sweeteners sparingly if you work them into your meal plan. Be aware of portion sizes and the carbohydrate content of each sweetener:

- 1 tablespoon honey = about 64 calories, 17 grams of carbohydrate
- 1 tablespoon brown sugar = about 52 calories, 13 grams of carbohydrate
- 1 tablespoon white sugar = about 48 calories, 13 grams of carbohydrate
- 1 tablespoon agave nectar = about 45 calories, 12 grams of carbohydrate
- 1 tablespoon maple syrup = about 52 calories, 13 grams of carbohydrate
- 1 packet of artificial sweetener = about 4 calories, <1 gram of carbohydrate

Artificial sweeteners are a low-calorie, low-carb option. Because they are chemically modified to be sweeter than regular sugar, only a small amount is needed to sweeten foods and drinks. There are several different artificial sweeteners available under various brand names: stevia, aspartame, acesulfame-K, saccharin, or sucralose. These are safe for people with diabetes when used in moderate amounts.

4. *How many grams of carbohydrates should someone with diabetes eat per day? How many at each meal?*

This is a very common question. About 45–60 grams of carbohydrates per meal is a good *starting point* when you are carb-counting. If you follow that recommendation, you will be eating a total of 135–180 grams of carbohydrates per day. However, some people may need more, and some may need less. Talk with your health care team to create an individualized meal plan to help you meet your health goals.

5. *What types of fruit can I eat? Is canned or fresh fruit better for people with diabetes?*

You can eat any type of fruit if you work it into your meal plan. Fruits are loaded with vitamins, minerals, and fiber. Fresh, canned, or frozen fruit without added sugars are all good options. You get a similar amount of nutrients from each. When you buy canned fruit, be sure the fruit has been canned in water or juice—not in syrup.

Fruit is nutritious, but it is not a "free food." The following portions have about 15 grams of carbohydrates:

- 1 small piece of whole fruit such as a small apple, small orange, or kiwifruit
- ½ cup of frozen or canned fruit
- ¾–1 cup of fresh berries or melon
- ⅓–½ cup 100% no-sugar-added fruit juice
- 2 tablespoons of dried fruit

6. Besides meat, what can I eat to make sure I get enough protein?

There are many protein sources. Proteins that are low in saturated and trans fats are the best options. Choose lean sources of protein like these:

- Eggs, egg whites, and egg substitutes
- Vegetarian proteins: beans, soy products, veggie burgers, nuts, and seeds
- Low-fat or nonfat dairy products
- Fish and shellfish
- Poultry without the skin
- Cheeses with 3 grams of fat or less per ounce
- When you do eat meat, choose lean cuts

People with diabetes can follow a vegetarian or vegan diet. Plant-based diets that include some animal products like eggs and milk can be a healthy option. However, animal products are not necessary. A mix of soy products, vegetables, fruits, beans, and whole grains provides plenty of protein and nutrients.

7. Why should I eat whole grains instead of refined grains?

Even a food made with 100% whole-wheat flour will raise your blood glucose levels. All grains—whole or not—affect blood glucose because they contain carbohydrates. However, you shouldn't completely avoid starchy foods. People with diabetes need some carbohydrates in their diet.

Whole grains are a healthy starch option because they contain fiber, vitamins, and minerals. Choose whole-wheat or whole-grain foods over those made with refined grains, but watch your portion sizes.

8. *Can people with diabetes eat potatoes and sweet potatoes?*

Yes! Starchy vegetables are healthy sources of carbohydrates. They also provide you with important nutrients like potassium, fiber, and vitamin C. You can include them in your meal plan as part of a balanced meal. Just pay attention to portion sizes and avoid unhealthy toppings. If you are carb counting, remember that there are about 15 grams of carbohydrates in:

- ½ cup of mashed potatoes
- ½ cup of boiled potatoes
- ¼ of a large baked potato with the skin

9. *Without salt and fat, food tastes bland. What can I do?*

When you are preparing healthy foods, try to limit added fats and extra salt. Look for recipes that use herbs (fresh or dried) and spices for flavor instead. There are many spice blends available in the baking aisle at the grocery store—choose salt-free blends. Other healthy ways to flavor your foods include:

- Squeezing lemon or lime juice on vegetables, fish, rice, or pasta
- Using onion and garlic to flavor dishes
- Baking meats with sugar-free barbecue sauce or any low-fat marinade
- Adding low-fat, low-calorie condiments, such as mustard, salsa, balsamic vinegar, or hot sauce

10. *Are gluten-free products okay for people with diabetes to eat?*

About 1% of the total population has celiac disease, which is an allergy to gluten—a protein found in wheat, rye, and barley. About 10% of people with type 1 diabetes also have celiac disease. People with celiac disease or gluten intolerance should follow a gluten-free diet.

However, unless you have one of these conditions, following a gluten-free diet is unnecessary and can make meal planning more difficult. Gluten-free products may contain more grams of carbohydrates per serving than regular products. For example, gluten-free bread can have twice as many grams of carbohydrates as whole-wheat bread. You can use gluten-free products and recipes, but just be sure to check the carbohydrate content and calories.

A Word About Brands and Sugar Substitutes

These are products we used to make these church supper recipes appropriate for people with diabetes. Use this information as you shop for ingredients or if you need to substitute something (be aware that substitutions alter the nutritional analysis that follows the recipe). The following brand names are presented as examples but do not constitute an endorsement. They may be a helpful starting point when you are shopping for groceries.

1. lower sodium marinara, pasta, and spaghetti sauce such as Amy's
2. lower sodium, lower fat condensed soup such as Campbell's Healthy Request
3. reduced fat cheeses, 75% less fat, sharp cheddar cheese such as Cabot
4. low fat mayonnaise dressing or light mayonnaise such as Hellmann's, known as Best Foods west of the Rockies
5. tub margarine, trans-fat free such as Smart Balance
6. lean Italian turkey sweet sausage such as Jennie-O
7. 7%-fat ground turkey such as Jennie-O
8. 50%-reduced-fat pork sausage such as Jimmy Dean's Light Pork Sausage
9. lower sodium chicken stuffing mix such as Stove-Top

Basically there are two types of sweeteners available to replace granulated sugar, brown sugar, honey, corn syrup, etc. in recipes:

1. **Sugar blends** (made with granulated sugar, non-nutritive sweeteners, and ingredients that add bulk).

    1 cup sugar in a recipe is replaced with ½ cup of the blend. These products are specifically designed for baking, where sugar has a major role in baked characteristics such as browning, volume, texture, and moisture retention. The blends can also be used in beverages and on cereals. Examples are:

		CALORIES	CARB (G)	INGREDIENTS
Sugar	1 cup	775	200	
Splenda Blend for Baking	½ cup	385	96	Sugar, sucralose
Splenda Brown Sugar Blend	½ cup	370	92	Brown sugar, sucralose
Domino Light Sugar Blend	½ cup	327	82	Cane sugar, stevia
Truvia Baking Blend, Stevia and Sugar Blend	½ cup	96	24	Maltodextrin, Stevia extract, erythritol

2. Granulated replacements for sugar. 1 cup sugar in a recipe is replaced by 1 cup sweetener. These products are designed to be used in recipes that use sugar for sweetness. Examples are:

		CALORIES	CARB (G)	INGREDIENTS
Sugar	1 cup	775	200	
Splenda granulated	1 cup	90	23	Maltodextrin, sucralose
Stevia in the Raw, cup for cup Bakers Bag	1 cup	90	23	Maltodextrin, stevia extract
Equal Classic Spoonful	1 cup	95	23	Maltodextrin, aspartame
Sugar Twin granulated white	1 cup	52	13	Maltodextrin, sodium saccharin, calcium chloride
Sugar Twin granulated brown	1 cup	52	13	Maltodextrin, sodium saccharin, calcium chloride, caramel color

For this list and additional updated information about brands and ingredients that are appropriate for people with diabetes, go to our website www.Fix-ItandForget-It.com/diabeticsubstitutes

Carrying-in-the-Food Tips

1. Choose a dish that you can make almost completely in advance. (Almost completely? Well, so that all you need to do is add the almonds and the dressing to the green salad or the crushed nachos to the top of the casserole.)

2. Make a dish that will travel well. (A 4-layer cake with wobbly decorations on top? Probably not. A frozen dessert? Only if it's a 10-minute drive or less to the destination, with a freezer immediately available when you get there.)

3. Prepare a dish that won't self-destruct if it sits and waits. (Skip a soufflé or a designed dusting of confectioners sugar on a warm volcano cake.)

4. If you have a winner of a dish, double or triple it, depending on the size of the group. But make sure it's a recipe that survives that kind of expansion – and that you have adequately-sized containers to prepare and then transport it.

5. If kids are attending the potluck, keep them in mind when you decide what to make. Finger foods are especially easy for kids to handle.

6. If you made the dish last year and people loved it, make it again this year. Good chance someone's hoping you'll show up with that same amazing Chicken Chili Bake. The idea is not to show your versatility as a cook, but to bring the dish that always gets eaten up after the first pass-through.

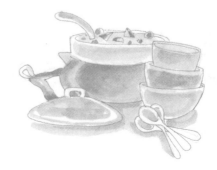

7. Label your container and its lid.

8. Take your own serving spoon. (The host probably doesn't have an infinite supply). Label it, too.

9. If you don't have time to cook, put together a cheese board.

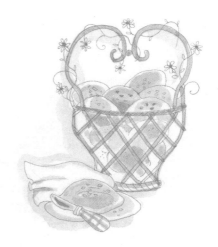

Eight or fewer people eating? Choose two or three cheeses, about one pound of each. You can go mild and creamy, paired with hard and bitey.

For eight to twelve people, select about 4 different cheeses, again a variety of textures and flavors.

Add some cut-up fruit that's not too juicy (apples, grapes, dates, dried apricots), breadsticks, or crackers, maybe some mustards for dipping.

Have a separate knife for each kind of cheese.

Hosting Tips

1. Clear the fridge so people can park the food they've brought in it until it's time to eat.

2. Be prepared to offer serving spoons for anyone who forgets to bring their own.

3. Remember any vegetarians in your group, and make sure there's food that they can eat and enjoy.

4. Offer simple tent signs (rectangles of stiff paper folded in half that will stand up straight) and pens for contributors to write the names of the dishes they brought. Place them in front of the dishes so guests know what they're looking at.

5. Plan in advance where you'll line up the dishes of food – and in what order. (Should the Salads go before the Hot Dishes, or after, and so on.)

6. Set up a drink station at a location away from the buffet table to prevent traffic jams.

7. Put out several trash receptacles that are easy for the guests to find. Have a back-up supply of trash bags so you can empty them throughout the event if they get full.

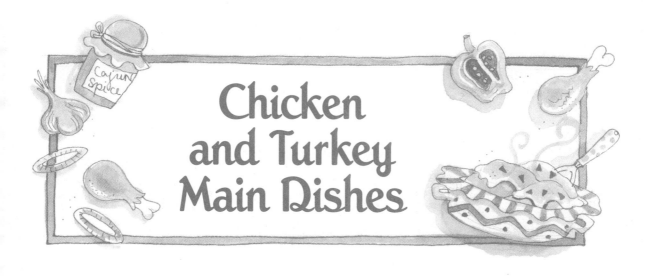

Chicken and Turkey Main Dishes

Oven Barbecued Chicken

Carol Eberly
Harrisonburg, VA

Makes 12 servings,
1 thigh per serving

Prep. Time: 10 minutes
Baking Time: 1¼ hours

3 Tbsp. ketchup
2 Tbsp. Worcestershire
 sauce
2 Tbsp. vinegar
2 Tbsp. light soy sauce
3 Tbsp. brown sugar
1 tsp. spicy brown mustard
1 tsp. salt
1 tsp. pepper
12 boneless, skinless chicken
 thighs, 2 lbs. total

1. In a mixing bowl, combine ketchup, Worcestershire sauce, vinegar, soy sauce, brown sugar, mustard, salt, and pepper. Blend well.

2. Lay chicken pieces in one layer in well-greased baking dish.

3. Pour sauce over top.

4. Bake at 350° for 40 minutes.

5. Turn pieces over. Bake 35 more minutes.

Tip:

You can use chicken legs or chicken breasts, too. Check the legs after they've baked for a total of 50 minutes to be sure they're not drying out. Check breasts after they've baked for a total of 30 minutes to be sure they're not becoming dry.

Exchange List Values
- Carbohydrate 0.5
- Lean Meat 2.0

Basic Nutritional Values
- Calories 130
 (Calories from Fat 55)
- Total Fat 6 gm
 (Saturated Fat 1.5 gm,
 Trans Fat 0.0 gm,
 Polyunsat Fat 1.3 gm,
 Monounsat Fat 2.1 gm)
- Cholesterol 50 mg
- Sodium 410 mg
- Potassium 170 gm
- Total Carb 5 gm
- Dietary Fiber 0 gm
- Sugars 5 gm
- Protein 13 gm
- Phosphorus 100 gm

We usually have carry-in fellowship meals and everyone is involved in the preparation. People seem to have specialties — Paul brings pasta dishes, Lee brings breads and Don makes shoo-fly pies. We feel like one big family when we eat together.

Ruby Lehman, Towson, MD

Oven-Fried Chicken Legs

Hazel N. Hassan
Goshen, IN

Makes 12 servings, 1 leg (thigh and drumstick) per serving

Prep. Time: 25 minutes
Baking Time: 1 hour

1 cup bread crumbs
¼ tsp. salt, *or less*
1 tsp. paprika
1 tsp. poultry seasoning
½ tsp. onion salt
¼ tsp. pepper
2 Tbsp. canola oil
12 chicken legs, skin removed

1. Mix bread crumbs, seasoning and oil.
2. Rinse chicken legs under running water and roll each leg in crumb mixture, shaking off excess.
3. Place legs in two rows in greased 9×13 baking pan, alternating thick and thin side of legs.
4. Bake at 350° for 1 hour. Remove from oven and place in clean, hot casserole dish. Wrap well in newspaper for transporting to church.

Warm Memories

I first made this dish for the benefit of the children, and was amused to see adults put one leg on child's plate and take one for themselves.

Exchange List Values
• Starch 0.5   • Fat 0.5
• Lean Meat 4.0

Basic Nutritional Values
• Calories 240   • Sodium 255 mg
  (Calories from Fat 100) • Potassium 255 gm
• Total Fat 11 gm   • Total Carb 7 gm
  (Saturated Fat 2.5 gm, • Dietary Fiber 0 gm
  Trans Fat 0.0 gm,   • Sugars 1 gm
  Polyunsat Fat 2.7 gm,   • Protein 27 gm
  Monounsat Fat 4.5 gm)   • Phosphorus 190 gm
• Cholesterol 90 mg

Oven-Fried Chicken Thighs

Eleanor Larson
Glen Lyon, PA

Makes 8 servings, 1 thigh per serving

Prep. Time: 20 minutes
Baking Time: 1 hour

8 boneless, skinless chicken thighs, each about 4 oz. in weight
½ cup flour
¼ tsp. paprika
½ tsp. salt
butter-flavored cooking spray

1. Grease a 9×13 baking dish well.
2. Combine flour, paprika and salt in plastic bag.
3. Drop chicken into bag, one piece at a time. Shake to coat well. Discard leftover flour mixture.
4. Place coated pieces of chicken in baking dish.
5. Spray chicken with 4 sprays of cooking spray.
6. Bake at 375° for 30 minutes.
7. Turn each piece over.
8. Spray chicken with 4 sprays of cooking spray.
9. Return to oven. Bake an additional 30 minutes.

Exchange List Values
• Lean Meat 3.0   • Fat 1.0

Basic Nutritional Values
• Calories 180   • Sodium 165 mg
  (Calories from Fat 80) • Potassium 185 gm
• Total Fat 9 gm   • Total Carb 4 gm
  (Saturated Fat 2.3 gm, • Dietary Fiber 0 gm
  Trans Fat 0.0 gm,   • Sugars 0 gm
  Polyunsat Fat 1.9 gm,   • Protein 20 gm
  Monounsat Fat 3.3 gm)   • Phosphorus 145 gm
• Cholesterol 70 mg

Herbed Chicken

Dale Peterson
Rapid City, SD

Makes 4 servings

Prep. Time: 20 minutes
Baking Time: 50–55 minutes

2 Tbsp. canola oil
½ cup flour
½ cup fine dry bread crumbs
1 tsp. paprika
¾ tsp. salt
¼ tsp. pepper
¼ tsp. ground thyme
3½-lb. chicken, skin removed, cut into 2 breast halves and 2 legs, wings and back reserved for another use
butter-flavored cooking spray

1. Put oil in 9×13 baking dish.
2. Mix flour, bread crumbs, paprika, salt, pepper, and thyme in plastic bag.
3. Put chicken pieces

in bag, one at a time, and shake. Discard leftover flour mixture.

4. Place chicken in baking dish. Spray with 4 sprays of cooking spray. Bake at 375° for 30 minutes.

5. Reduce heat to 350°. Turn each piece of chicken over.

6. Bake 20–25 minutes more, or until thermometer inserted in center of chicken registers 165°.

Exchange List Values
- Starch 1.0
- Fat 1.0
- Lean Meat 5.0

Basic Nutritional Values
- Calories 355
  (Calories from Fat 135)
- Total Fat 15 gm
  (Saturated Fat 2.6 gm,
  Trans Fat 0.0 gm,
  Polyunsat Fat 3.8 gm,
  Monounsat Fat 7.2 gm)
- Cholesterol 105 mg
- Sodium 495 mg
- Potassium 330 gm
- Total Carb 17 gm
- Dietary Fiber 1 gm
- Sugars 1 gm
- Protein 36 gm
- Phosphorus 270 gm

Barbecued Chicken Thighs

Ida H. Goering
Dayton, VA

*Makes 20 servings,
1 thigh per serving*

Prep. Time: 10 minutes
Chilling Time: 3–6 hours
Grilling Time: 15–20 minutes

**20 boneless, skinless
  chicken thighs, 3 oz. each**
½ cup oil
1 cup vinegar
¼ cup ketchup

2 tsp. salt
½ tsp. poultry seasoning
½ tsp. black pepper

1. Place chicken on a single layer, if possible, in a nonmetallic dish.

2. Combine oil, vinegar, ketchup, salt, poultry seasoning, and pepper. Mix well.

3. Pour sauce over chicken pieces.

4. Marinate 3–6 hours in the fridge. Discard up to half the marinade.

5. Grill chicken thighs over medium heat until done, about 15–20 minutes.

Tips:

I like this recipe because I can make it ahead of time and either keep it hot until ready to serve at the potluck. Or I can easily heat it up by placing it in a microwave-safe dish, covering it tightly, and mic-ing it over medium heat until heated through, but not cooked again.

Exchange List Values
- Lean Meat 2.0
- Fat 1.0

Basic Nutritional Values
- Calories 160
  (Calories from Fat 90)
- Total Fat 10 gm
  (Saturated Fat 2.0 gm,
  Trans Fat 0.0 gm,
  Polyunsat Fat 2.6 gm,
  Monounsat Fat 5.0 gm)
- Cholesterol 55 mg
- Sodium 250 mg
- Potassium 150 gm
- Total Carb 1 gm
- Dietary Fiber 0 gm
- Sugars 1 gm
- Protein 15 gm
- Phosphorus 105 gm

Crunchy Chicken

Joette Droz
Kalona, IA

*Makes 4 servings,
2 thighs per serving*

Prep. Time: 20 minutes
Baking Time: 30–45 minutes

**8 boneless skinless chicken
  thighs, about 1 lb.**
½ cup egg substitute
**1⅓ cups stuffing mix for
  chicken, crushed fine**
¼ cup Parmesan cheese

1. Cover baking sheet with foil.

2. Spread chicken thighs with egg substitute. Place on foil-covered baking sheet,

3. Empty stuffing mix into a pie plate.

4. Roll each piece of chicken in dry stuffing mixture. Return to baking sheet.

5. Bake at 375° for 30–45 minutes.

Exchange List Values
- Starch 1.0
- Fat 1.0
- Lean Meat 3.0

Basic Nutritional Values
- Calories 260
  (Calories from Fat 80)
- Total Fat 9 gm
  (Saturated Fat 2.5 gm,
  Trans Fat 0.0 gm,
  Polyunsat Fat 1.9 gm,
  Monounsat Fat 3.2 gm)
- Cholesterol 75 mg
- Sodium 480 mg
- Potassium 285 gm
- Total Carb 17 gm
- Dietary Fiber 1 gm
- Sugars 3 gm
- Protein 26 gm
- Phosphorus 175 gm

Encore Dijon Chicken

Dorothy VanDeest
Memphis, TN

*Makes 6 servings,
1 breast half per serving*

*Prep. Time: 5–10 minutes
Baking Time: 20 minutes*

½ tsp. Italian seasoning
4 Tbsp. Dijon mustard
2 Tbsp. vegetable oil
1 tsp. garlic powder, *or*
 refrigerated minced garlic
6 boneless chicken breast
 halves, about 6-oz. each
 in weight

1. Grease a 9×13 baking dish.
2. Mix Italian seasoning, mustard, oil, and garlic in either a large bowl or plastic bag.
3. Add chicken pieces, one at a time. Dredge or shake to coat each piece.
4. Lay in baking dish.
5. Bake at 375° for 20 minutes, or until thermometer inserted in center of each piece registers 165°.

Exchange List Values
• Lean Meat 5.0

Basic Nutritional Values
• Calories 245
 (Calories from Fat 80)
• Total Fat 9 gm
 (Saturated Fat 1.5 gm,
 Trans Fat 0.0 gm,
 Polyunsat Fat 2.3 gm,
 Monounsat Fat 4.6 gm)
• Cholesterol 100 mg
• Sodium 325 mg
• Potassium 315 gm
• Total Carb 2 gm
• Dietary Fiber 0 gm
• Sugars 1 gm
• Protein 37 gm
• Phosphorus 275 gm

Baked Chicken

Mary Smucker
Goshen, IN

Makes 8 servings

*Prep. Time: 30 minutes
Cooking/Baking Time: 2 hours*

3-lb. chicken, cut in pieces
2½ Tbsp. canola oil,
 divided
1 small onion, chopped
3 tsp. curry powder
1 apple, diced
14½-oz. can lower-fat,
 lower-sodium cream of
 mushroom soup
12-oz. can fat-free
 evaporated milk
salt, pepper and paprika

1. Skin chicken and remove fat. Brown chicken in 2 Tbsp. canola oil. Place chicken pieces in casserole dish.
2. Sauté onion and curry powder in ½ Tbsp. canola oil.
3. Mix onion and curry powder with rest of ingredients. Pour over chicken.
4. Bake at 350° for 1½ hours.

Exchange List Values
• Carbohydrate 1.0 • Fat 0.5
• Lean Meat 3.0

Basic Nutritional Values
• Calories 220
 (Calories from Fat 80)
• Total Fat 9 gm
 (Saturated Fat 1.7 gm,
 Trans Fat 0.0 gm,
 Polyunsat Fat 2.5 gm,
 Monounsat Fat 4.5 gm)
• Cholesterol 50 mg
• Sodium 235 mg
• Potassium 590 gm
• Total Carb 13 gm
• Dietary Fiber 1 gm
• Sugars 9 gm
• Protein 20 gm
• Phosphorus 220 gm

Golden Chicken Breasts

Lorna Rodes
Port Republic, VA

*Makes 8 servings,
one breast half per serving*

*Prep. Time: 15 minutes
Baking Time: 45–55 minutes*

2 Tbsp. freshly grated
 Parmesan cheese
¼ cup grated 75%-less fat
 cheddar cheese
¼ cup snack cracker crumbs
½ tsp. dried thyme
2 tsp. dried basil
½ tsp. salt
¼ tsp. pepper
½ cup egg substitute
8 boneless, skinless
 chicken breast halves,
 5 oz. each
butter-flavored cooking
 spray

1. Grease a 9×13 baking dish.
2. In a shallow bowl, combine Parmesan cheese, cheddar cheese, cracker crumbs, thyme, basil, salt, and pepper.
3. Pour egg substitute into another shallow bowl.
4. Roll each chicken breast in egg substitute. Sprinkle each breast half with about 1 Tbsp. crumb mixture.
5. Place coated chicken breasts in baking dish.
6. Spray chicken with 4 sprays of cooking spray.
7. Bake at 350° for 45 minutes, or until thermometer

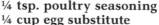

inserted into center of chicken registers 165°.

Exchange List Values
• Lean Meat 4.0

Basic Nutritional Values
• Calories 190
  (Calories from Fat 40)
• Total Fat 4.5 gm
  (Saturated Fat 1.5 gm,
  Trans Fat 0.0 gm,
  Polyunsat Fat 1.0 gm,
  Monounsat Fat 1.6 gm)
• Cholesterol 85 mg
• Sodium 305 mg
• Potassium 280 gm
• Total Carb 2 gm
• Dietary Fiber 0 gm
• Sugars 0 gm
• Protein 33 gm
• Phosphorus 250 gm

Crispy Chicken

Kitty Hilliard
Punxsutawney, PA

*Makes 4 servings,
1 breast half per serving*

Prep. Time: 10 minutes
Baking Time: 20–25 minutes

2 Tbsp. flour
1½ cups crisp rice cereal,
  coarsely crushed
½ tsp. salt
¼ tsp. dried thyme

¼ tsp. poultry seasoning
¼ cup egg substitute
4 boneless, skinless
  chicken breast halves,
  each about 5 oz.
butter-flavor cooking spray

1. Grease a 7×11 baking dish.
2. In a shallow bowl, combine flour, cereal, salt, thyme, and poultry seasoning.
3. Place egg substitute in another shallow bowl.
4. Dip chicken in egg substitute, then into cereal mixture. Discard any remaining cereal mixture.
5. Place in greased 11×7 baking pan.
6. Spray lightly with cooking spray, 2 sprays total.
7. Bake at 400° for 20–25 minutes, or until thermometer inserted in center registers 165°.

Exchange List Values
• Starch 0.5   • Lean Meat 4.0

Basic Nutritional Values
• Calories 205
  (Calories from Fat 30)
• Total Fat 4 gm
  (Saturated Fat 1.0 gm,
  Trans Fat 0.0 gm,
  Polyunsat Fat 0.8 gm,
  Monounsat Fat 1.3 gm)
• Cholesterol 80 mg
• Sodium 390 mg
• Potassium 280 gm
• Total Carb 9 gm
• Dietary Fiber 0 gm
• Sugars 1 gm
• Protein 32 gm
• Phosphorus 230 gm

Cranberry Chicken

Judi Manos
West Islip, NY

Makes 8 servings

Prep. Time: 10 minutes
Baking Time: 50 minutes

4 lbs. skinless, bone-in
  chicken pieces; your
  choice of breast halves
  or thighs
7 oz. (half of a 14-oz. can)
  whole cranberry sauce
1 cup fat-free Catalina
  dressing
1 recipe salt-free onion
  soup mix (see page 271)

1. Place chicken in single layer in two well-greased 9×13 baking dishes.
2. In mixing bowl, blend together cranberry sauce, Catalina dressing, and onion soup mix.
3. Pour over chicken pieces.
4. Bake 50 minutes, or until chicken is done. Thermometer inserted in center of meat should register 165°.

Exchange List Values
• Carbohydrate 1.0   • Lean Meat 5.0

Basic Nutritional Values
• Calories 295
  (Calories from Fat 70)
• Total Fat 8 gm
  (Saturated Fat 2.3 gm,
  Trans Fat 0.0 gm,
  Polyunsat Fat 1.9 gm,
  Monounsat Fat 3.1 gm)
• Cholesterol 105 mg
• Sodium 275 mg
• Potassium 595 gm
• Total Carb 17 gm
• Dietary Fiber 1 gm
• Sugars 12 gm
• Protein 33 gm
• Phosphorus 255 gm

Subtly Wonderful Grilled Chicken

Joyce Zuercher, Hesston, KS

Makes 8 servings

Prep. Time: 5 minutes
Standing/Marinating Time:
2 hours
Grilling Time: 10–15 minutes

4 skinless boneless chicken breast halves, 5 oz. each
4 skinless boneless chicken thighs, 5 oz. each
½ cup oil
½ cup lemon juice, *or* vinegar of your choice
¼ cup water
2 tsp. salt
¼ tsp. pepper
1 Tbsp. sugar
1 tsp. paprika
1 Tbsp. minced onion

1. Place chicken in single layer in nonmetallic bowl.
2. Measure remaining ingredients into bowl, and mix well.
3. Let sauce stand 1 hour to allow flavors to blend.
4. Pour sauce over chicken in pan. Cover. Marinate chicken 1 hour in fridge.
5. Brush pieces with sauce before grilling, or dip pieces in sauce.
6. Grill according to pieces used, brushing on more sauce while grilling.
7. Turn pieces over during grilling, allowing about 5–10 minutes total for breasts and 10–15 minutes total for legs and/or thighs.

Exchange List Values
- Lean Meat 4.0   • Fat 1.0

Basic Nutritional Values
- Calories 245   • Sodium 370 mg
  (Calories from Fat 125) • Potassium 250 gm
- Total Fat 14 gm   • Total Carb 2 gm
  (Saturated Fat 2.4 gm, • Dietary Fiber 0 gm
  Trans Fat 0.0 gm,   • Sugars 1 gm
  Polyunsat Fat 3.5 gm, • Protein 27 gm
  Monounsat Fat 6.9 gm) • Phosphorus 200 gm
- Cholesterol 85 mg

Grilled Chicken Breasts

Gloria Mumbauer
Singers Glen, VA

Thelma F. Good
Harrisonburg, VA

Makes 2½–2¾ cups marinade;
12 chicken breast halves,
1 breast half per serving

Prep. Time: 5 minutes
Marinating Time: 6–8 hours or
overnight
Grilling Time: 15–18 minutes

12 boneless skinless chicken breast halves, 5 oz. each
¾ cup vegetable oil
¾ cup light soy sauce
¼ cup Worcestershire sauce
2 tsp. prepared mustard
1 tsp. black pepper
½ cup apple cider vinegar
2 garlic cloves, minced, *or* 1½ tsp. garlic powder
⅓ cup lemon juice

1. Place chicken breasts in a single layer in a nonmetallic dish.
2. In a bowl, mix together oil, soy sauce, Worcestershire sauce, mustard, black pepper, vinegar, garlic, and lemon juice.
3. When well blended, pour over chicken.
4. Cover. Marinate 6–8 hours or overnight. Turn chicken over about half-way through, if it's not the middle of the night and you're able to, to coat both sides.
5. Remove from marinade. Grill over medium heat until cooked through, about 15–18 minutes. Do not overcook or meat will dry out!

Tips:
To serve at a potluck, slice grilled chicken into strips about ¾" wide so lots of people get a taste. Do not expect to bring any of this chicken home from a potluck!
Thelma Good
Harrisonburg, VA

Warm Memories:
Our children are delighted when this recipe is on our menu at home. They love to slice it over a big salad for a delicious meal that is both healthy and tasty!
Thelma Good
Harrisonburg, VA

Exchange List Values
- Lean Meat 4.0

Basic Nutritional Values
- Calories 210   • Sodium 275 mg
  (Calories from Fat 70) • Potassium 280 gm
- Total Fat 8 gm   • Total Carb 1 gm
  (Saturated Fat 1.3 gm, • Dietary Fiber 0 gm
  Trans Fat 0.0 gm,   • Sugars 0 gm
  Polyunsat Fat 2.0 gm, • Protein 31 gm
  Monounsat Fat 4.1 gm) • Phosphorus 230 gm
- Cholesterol 80 mg

Super Easy Chicken

Lauren Eberhard
Seneca, IL

3 oz. per serving

Prep. Time: 10 minutes
Cooking Time: 5–6 minutes each

1 4-oz. chicken breast
  for each person you're
  serving
1 tsp. Mrs. Dash Garlic
  and Herb flavoring,
  or any flavor you like,
  divided
2 tsp. olive oil
cooking spray

1. Pound each chicken breast to ½" thickness.
2. Use the following instructions for each breast.
3. Heat oil in skillet over medium-high heat.
4. Sprinkle breast with ½ tsp. Mrs. Dash on 1 side.
5. Spray seasoned side with a little cooking spray.
6. Place seasoned side of chicken down. Sauté until golden, about 3–4 minutes.
7. While this side is cooking, season the up side as you did previously.
8. Turn chicken over. Continue sautéeing until done, about 2 more minutes. This happens fast, so be careful not to overcook the pieces!
9. As each piece finishes, place on oven-proof platter, covered with foil. Keep covered platter in oven set at 250° until ready to serve.

Tip:
I make extra breasts when I'm in the swing so I have them on hand to cut up for salads and soups.

Exchange List Values
• Lean Meat 3.0   • Fat 1.5

Basic Nutritional Values
• Calories 215   • Sodium 55 mg
  (Calories from Fat 110) • Potassium 215 gm
• Total Fat 12 gm   • Total Carb 1 gm
  (Saturated Fat 1.5 gm,   • Dietary Fiber 0 gm
  Trans Fat 0.0 gm,   • Sugars 0 gm
  Polyunsat Fat 3.2 gm,   • Protein 24 gm
  Monounsat Fat 7.0 gm)   • Phosphorus 175 gm
• Cholesterol 65 mg

Cola Chicken

Esther S. Martin
Ephrata, PA

Makes 4 servings,
1 breast half per serving

Prep. Time: 5 minutes
Cooking Time: 1 hour

12-oz. can diet cola
¾ cup no-salt-added ketchup
¼ c. water
½ tsp. seasoned salt
4 boneless, skinless,
  chicken breast halves, 5
  oz. each in weight

1. In a large skillet, mix cola and ketchup until smooth.
2. Bring to a boil.
3. Add chicken breasts and submerge in sauce.
4. Cover skillet. Reduce heat, simmering for about 45 minutes, or until chicken is almost tender.
5. Remove cover. Increase heat until liquid boils.
6. Continue cooking until sauce thickens and chicken is cooked but not dried out. (Thermometer inserted into center of pieces should register 165°.)

Good Go-Alongs:
We like the sauce from this dish better than gravy on mashed potatoes.

Exchange List Values
• Carbohydrate 1.0   • Lean Meat 4.0

Basic Nutritional Values
• Calories 220   • Sodium 275 mg
  (Calories from Fat 30)   • Potassium 465 gm
• Total Fat 4 gm   • Total Carb 15 gm
  (Saturated Fat 1.0 gm,   • Dietary Fiber 1 gm
  Trans Fat 0.0 gm,   • Sugars 12 gm
  Polyunsat Fat 0.8 gm,   • Protein 30 gm
  Monounsat Fat 1.2 gm)   • Phosphorus 245 gm
• Cholesterol 80 mg

Learn how to use spices. I'm still learning and it's amazing how the right spice can make a good dish great!
Ann Good, Perry, NY

Lemony Chicken

Cynthia Morris
Grottoes, VA

Makes 8 servings,
3¼"×4½" rectangle per serving

Prep. Time: 20 minutes
Baking Time: 45–60 minutes

1 cup fat-free sour cream
10¾-oz. can lower-sodium, lower-fat cream soup, your choice of flavor
2 Tbsp. lemon juice
6 boneless, skinless chicken breasts halves, 5 oz. each, cubed
4-oz. can mushrooms, drained
1 cup 75%-less fat shredded cheddar cheese
1 cup crushed wheat thins crackers, *divided*

1. In large mixing bowl, blend together sour cream, soup, and lemon juice.
2. When smooth, stir in cubed chicken breasts, mushrooms, cheese, and half of crushed crackers.
3. Pour into well-greased 9×13 baking pan.
4. Sprinkle with remaining crackers.
5. Bake at 350° for 45–60 minutes, or until chicken is cooked through and no pink remains in meat.

Variation:
You can also use already-cooked chicken in this dish. When doing so, reduce baking time to 30–40 minutes, or until heated through.

Exchange List Values
• Carbohydrate 1.0 • Lean Meat 4.0

Basic Nutritional Values
• Calories 250
(Calories from Fat 65)
• Total Fat 7 gm
(Saturated Fat 2.0 gm,
Trans Fat 0.0 gm,
Polyunsat Fat 1.9 gm,
Monounsat Fat 1.7 gm)
• Cholesterol 70 mg
• Sodium 455 mg
• Potassium 530 gm
• Total Carb 17 gm
• Dietary Fiber 1 gm
• Sugars 4 gm
• Protein 30 gm
• Phosphorus 310 gm

Creamy Baked Chicken Breasts

Naomi Ressler, Harrisonburg, VA
Jan Rankin, Millersville, PA
Joyce Kaut, Rochester, NY
Anna Musser, Manheim, PA

Makes 8 servings,
1 breast half per serving

Prep. Time: 15–20 minutes
Baking Time: 45–55 minutes

8 boneless, skinless chicken breast halves, each 5 oz. in weight

8 slices ultra-thin Swiss cheese, *optional*
10¾-oz. can lower-fat, lower-sodium cream of chicken soup
¼ cup dry white wine, *or* water
2 cups herb-seasoned stuffing mix
cooking spray

1. Arrange chicken in lightly greased 9×13 baking dish.
2. Top with optional cheese slices.
3. In a mixing bowl, combine soup and wine until smooth.
4. Spoon evenly over chicken and cheese.
5. Sprinkle with stuffing mix.
6. Spray lightly with 4 sprays of cooking spray.
7. Bake at 350° for 45–55 minutes, or until chicken is tender in the middle.

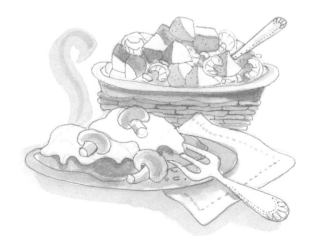

Exchange List Values
- Carbohydrate 1.0
- Lean Meat 4.0

Basic Nutritional Values
- Calories 225
  (Calories from Fat 40)
- Total Fat 4.5 gm
  (Saturated Fat 1.1 gm,
  Trans Fat 0.0 gm,
  Polyunsat Fat 1.1 gm,
  Monounsat Fat 1.5 gm)
- Cholesterol 80 mg
- Sodium 375 mg
- Potassium 450 gm
- Total Carb 12 gm
- Dietary Fiber 1 gm
- Sugars 1 gm
- Protein 31 gm
- Phosphorus 245 gm

Chicken Parmesan

Jessalyn Wantland
Napoleon, OH

Makes 4 servings,
1 breast half per serving

Prep. Time: 10 minutes
Baking Time: 45 minutes

4 boneless, skinless
chicken breast halves,
about 5 oz. each
1 egg, beaten
½ cup Italian-seasoned
bread crumbs
12 oz. low-sodium, fat-free
pasta sauce with basil
¾ cup shredded Parmesan
cheese

1. Grease 7×11 baking dish.
2. Place egg in shallow bowl.
3. Place bread crumbs in another shallow bowl.
4. Dip each piece of chicken in egg, and then in bread crumbs.
5. Place coated chicken in baking dish.
6. Bake at 400° for 30 minutes.
7. Spoon pasta sauce over chicken.
8. Top evenly with cheese.
9. Bake another 15 minutes, or until heated through and cheese is melted.

Exchange List Values
- Starch 1.0
- Lean Meat 5.0

Basic Nutritional Values
- Calories 280
  (Calories from Fat 55)
- Total Fat 6 gm
  (Saturated Fat 2.4 gm,
  Trans Fat 0.0 gm,
  Polyunsat Fat 0.9 gm,
  Monounsat Fat 2.0 gm)
- Cholesterol 85 mg
- Sodium 450 mg
- Potassium 575 gm
- Total Carb 17 gm
- Dietary Fiber 1 gm
- Sugars 6 gm
- Protein 37 gm
- Phosphorus 320 gm

Chicken Cacciatore

Donna Lantgen
Arvada, CO

Makes 6 servings,
1 breast half per serving

Prep. Time: 10 minutes
Cooking/Baking Time: 65–90
minutes, depending on
thickness of chicken

6 boneless skinless chicken
breast halves, each
about 5 oz. in weight
1 medium green bell
pepper, chopped
1 medium onion, chopped
15½-oz. can tomatoes,
chopped, *or* 2 cups fresh
tomatoes, diced and
peeled
1 Tbsp. Italian seasoning
mozzarella, *or* Parmesan
cheese, shredded

1. Place chicken in well greased 9×13 baking pan.
2. In mixing bowl, stir together green pepper, onion, tomatoes, and seasoning.
3. Spoon vegetables evenly over chicken.
4. Cover. Bake at 350° for 45 minutes.
5. With a sharp knife make 2–3 vertical slashes in thickest part of each chicken breast. (Do not cut the whole way through.) Baste with pan juices.
6. Cover. Return to oven and continue baking 15 more minutes, or until thermometer inserted in center of chicken registers 165°.
7. Top chicken with cheese.
8. Return to oven for 5–10 minutes, or until cheese melts.

Exchange List Values
- Vegetable 1.0
- Lean Meat 4.0

Basic Nutritional Values
- Calories 185
  (Calories from Fat 30)
- Total Fat 4 gm
  (Saturated Fat 1.0 gm,
  Trans Fat 0.0 gm,
  Polyunsat Fat 0.8 gm,
  Monounsat Fat 1.2 gm)
- Cholesterol 80 mg
- Sodium 175 mg
- Potassium 465 gm
- Total Carb 7 gm
- Dietary Fiber 2 gm
- Sugars 3 gm
- Protein 31 gm
- Phosphorus 245 gm

Easy Chicken Cordon Bleu

Sharon Miller
Holmesville, OH

*Makes 8 servings,
half a roll-up per serving*

Prep. Time: 35 minutes
Cooking Time: 45–60 minutes

**4 large boneless, skinless
  chicken breast halves,
  each about 8 oz. in
  weight**
**½ cup Italian-seasoned dry
  bread crumbs**
**2 slices ultra-thin Swiss
  cheese, cut in half**
**2 oz. lean lower-sodium
  deli ham**
8 sturdy toothpicks

1. Grease a 9×13 baking
dish.
2. Pound each chicken
breast to about ¼-½" thickness.
3. Place bread crumbs in
shallow bowl.
4. Dredge each chicken
piece in bread crumbs,
coating each side.
5. Lay slice of Swiss cheese
and slice of ham on each
chicken breast.
6. Tightly roll up each
layered breast.
7. Holding roll firmly,
re-roll in crumbs.
8. Stick 2 toothpicks
through each roll to maintain
its shape.
9. Place in baking dish.
Cover with foil.
10. Bake at 350° for 30

minutes.
11. Remove foil. Bake an
additional 15 minutes.
12. Cut each roll in half
before serving.

Tip:
If the cheese is too
"exposed" instead of being
enclosed in the bundle, it
melts outside the bundle.

Exchange List Values
- Starch 0.5
- Lean Meat 3.0

Basic Nutritional Values
- Calories 170
  (Calories from Fat 35)
- Total Fat 4 gm
  (Saturated Fat 1.3 gm,
  Trans Fat 0.0 gm,
  Polyunsat Fat 0.7 gm,
  Monounsat Fat 1.3 gm)
- Cholesterol 70 mg
- Sodium 225 mg
- Potassium 240 gm
- Total Carb 5 gm
- Dietary Fiber 0 gm
- Sugars 0 gm
- Protein 27 gm
- Phosphorus 215 gm

Japanese Chicken

Marjorie Nolt
Denver, PA

Erma Martin
East Earl, PA

Mary Jane Musser
Manheim, PA

*Makes 6 servings,
about 4 oz. meat plus
about 2 oz. sauce per serving*

Prep. Time: 20 minutes
Baking Time: 45 minutes

**2 lbs. chicken, skinless
  and boneless breasts *or*
  thighs cut in half**
⅓ cup flour
¼ tsp. garlic salt
¼ tsp. seasoned salt

¼ tsp. paprika
**½ cup Splenda Blend for
  Baking**
½ cup rice vinegar
3 Tbsp. light soy sauce
½ cup water

1. In a shallow bowl, mix
together flour, garlic salt,
seasoned salt, and paprika.
Roll chicken in flour mixture.
2. Brown on both sides in
a skillet. Put in 9×13 baking
pan.
3. Boil together Splenda,
vinegar, soy sauce, and water
until Splenda melts. Pour over
chicken.
4. Bake uncovered at 350°
for 45 minutes. Serve with
rice if desired.

Exchange List Values
- Starch 0.5
- Carbohydrate 1.0
- Lean Meat 4.0

Basic Nutritional Values
- Calories 290
  (Calories from Fat 65)
- Total Fat 7 gm
  (Saturated Fat 2.1 gm,
  Trans Fat 0.0 gm,
  Polyunsat Fat 1.7 gm,
  Monounsat Fat 2.8 gm)
- Cholesterol 90 mg
- Sodium 475 mg
- Potassium 285 gm
- Total Carb 23 gm
- Dietary Fiber 0 gm
- Sugars 17 gm
- Protein 31 gm
- Phosphorus 230 gm

Chicken Recuerdos de Tucson

Joanna Harrison
Lafayette, CO

Makes 6 servings,
1 leg and thigh per serving

Prep. Time: 15 minutes
Cooking Time: 30–40 minutes

6 chicken legs with thigh included, skin removed
1 Tbsp. olive oil
1 medium onion, chopped coarsely
3 cloves garlic, minced
1 tsp. cumin, ground
2–3 green chilies, chopped, according to your taste preference
1 green bell pepper, chopped
1–2 zucchini, sliced
1 cup tomatoes, chopped
2 cups frozen corn
2 tsp. dried oregano
1 tsp. dried basil
2 cups lower-sodium, non-fat chicken broth
chopped cilantro for garnish

1. Brown chicken in olive oil in Dutch oven or large stockpot. Remove chicken to platter. Reserve pan drippings.
2. Gently sauté onion and garlic until wilted.
3. Stir in cumin, green chilies, green pepper, and zucchini. Sauté until peppers wilt.
4. Add tomatoes, corn, oregano, basil, and broth.
5. Return chicken to pot.
6. Cover. Simmer 30–40 minutes, or until chicken is tender to the bone.
7. Garnish with cilantro and serve.

Pastel de Choclo

Mary Hochstedler
Kokomo, IN

Makes 20 servings,
a 2⅗"×4½" rectangle per serving

Prep. Time: 25 minutes
Cooking/Baking Time: 1½ hours

10 ears fresh corn
2 tsp. salt
1 Tbsp. fresh basil
3 Tbsp. sugar
3-lb. chicken
1 lb. 93%-fat-free ground beef
2 onions, diced
¾ cup raisins
½ tsp. salt
½ tsp. pepper
¼ tsp. cumin
¼ tsp. cayenne pepper
¼ tsp. dried oregano
¼ tsp. paprika
1 cup lower-sodium fat-free chicken broth
10–12 olives
2 hard-boiled eggs, sliced
¼ cup Splenda Brown Sugar Blend

1. Cut corn from ears. Run through blender with 1 Tbsp. salt, basil and 3 Tbsp. sugar. Set aside.
2. Cook chicken until tender. Cool, skin, and bone chicken. Discard fat. Chop chicken.
3. Brown ground beef and onions. Drain excess fat. Add chicken, raisins, seasonings and chicken broth. Set aside.
4. Using two 9×13 baking pans layer ¼ of corn mixture into each pan. Cover with chicken and ground beef mixture. Top with remaining corn.
5. Garnish with olives and hard-boiled eggs. Press down into corn mixture to prevent drying out. Sprinkle with Splenda.
6. Bake at 350° for 40–45 minutes or until bubbly and browned on top.

Magra's Chicken & Rice

Carolyn Spohn
Shawnee, KS

Makes 8 servings,
3 oz. chicken plus about ¾ cup rice

Prep. Time: 20 minutes
Baking Time: 40–60 minutes

1–2 tsp. olive oil
2–3 medium carrots, chopped
1 medium onion, chopped
1 rib celery, chopped
2 cloves garlic, chopped
¼ tsp. crumbled dried
  rosemary
1½ cups uncooked
  long-grain rice
3 cups lower-sodium,
  fat-free chicken broth
1 lb. boneless skinless
  chicken thighs
1 lb. boneless skinless
  chicken breasts

1. Sauté carrots, onion, and celery in olive oil in skillet until softened and lightly browned.
2. Add garlic and sauté 1 minute. Do not brown garlic.
3. Add rosemary and mix well with vegetables.
4. Add uncooked rice to pan with vegetables and stir well to coat rice and evenly mix it with the vegetables.
5. Pour mixture into large, well-greased roaster.
6. Pour chicken broth over rice until it just covers rice.
7. Add chicken pieces on top of rice, pushing down into rice-vegetable mix.

8. Cover. Bake at 350° for approximately 40–60 minutes, or until rice and chicken are nearly cooked but not dry.
9. Remove cover and bake a few more minutes, or until chicken browns slightly.

Tip:
You may need to use more or less broth to cover rice.

Exchange List Values
- Starch 2.0
- Lean Meat 3.0

Basic Nutritional Values
- Calories 295
  (Calories from Fat 55)
- Total Fat 6 gm
  (Saturated Fat 1.7 gm,
  Trans Fat 0.0 gm,
  Polyunsat Fat 1.4 gm,
  Monounsat Fat 2.5 gm)
- Cholesterol 70 mg
- Sodium 270 mg
- Potassium 385 gm
- Total Carb 32 gm
- Dietary Fiber 1 gm
- Sugars 2 gm
- Protein 26 gm
- Phosphorus 225 gm

Lemon-Chicken Oven Bake

Judi Manos
West Islip, NY

Makes 4 servings

Prep. Time: 10–15 minutes
Baking Time: 50 minutes

¼ cup Zesty Italian
  Dressing
½ cup fat-free, lower-
  sodium chicken broth
1 Tbsp. honey
1½ lbs. bone-in chicken
  legs and thighs, skin
  removed
1 lb. new potatoes,
  quartered

5 cloves garlic, peeled
1 lemon, cut in half, and
  then each half into 4
  wedges
1 tsp. dried rosemary,
  optional

1. In a mixing bowl, blend together dressing, broth, and honey.
2. Arrange chicken, potatoes, and garlic in well-greased 9×13 baking dish.
3. Drizzle with dressing mixture.
4. Situate lemons among the chicken and potatoes.
5. Bake at 400° for 45–50 minutes, or until chicken is done and potatoes are tender. (Temperature probe inserted into center of chicken should register 165°.)
6. Serve lemons as garnish if you wish.

Exchange List Values
- Starch 1.0
- Carbohydrate 0.5
- Lean Meat 3.0
- Fat 1.0

Basic Nutritional Values
- Calories 285
  (Calories from Fat 90)
- Total Fat 10 gm
  (Saturated Fat 2.1 gm,
  Trans Fat 0.0 gm,
  Polyunsat Fat 2.9 gm,
  Monounsat Fat 3.1 gm)
- Cholesterol 75 mg
- Sodium 290 mg
- Potassium 670 gm
- Total Carb 25 gm
- Dietary Fiber 2 gm
- Sugars 6 gm
- Protein 24 gm
- Phosphorus 215 gm

Chicken Baked with Red Onions, Potatoes, and Rosemary

Kristine Stalter
Iowa City, IA

Makes 8 servings

Prep. Time: 10–15 minutes
Baking Time: 45–60 minutes

2 red onions, each cut into 10 wedges
1¼ lbs. new potatoes, unpeeled and cut into chunks
2 garlic bulbs, separated into cloves, unpeeled
salt
pepper
3 tsp. extra-virgin olive oil
2 Tbsp. balsamic vinegar
approximately 5 sprigs rosemary
8 chicken thighs, skin removed

1. Spread onions, potatoes, and garlic in single layer over bottom of large roasting pan so that they will crisp and brown.
2. Season with salt and pepper.
3. Pour over the oil and balsamic vinegar and add rosemary, leaving some sprigs whole and stripping the leaves off the rest.
4. Toss vegetables and seasonings together.
5. Tuck chicken pieces among vegetables.
6. Bake at 400° for 45–60 minutes, or until chicken and vegetables are cooked through.
7. Transfer to a big platter, or take to the table in the roasting pan.

Warm Memories:
    A neighbor and friend shared this simple recipe with me when my family and I were on sabbatical in the UK.

Exchange List Values
- Starch 1.0
- Fat 1.5
- Lean Meat 2.0

Basic Nutritional Values
- Calories 235
  (Calories from Fat 100)
- Total Fat 11 gm
  (Saturated Fat 2.3 gm,
  Trans Fat 0.0 gm,
  Polyunsat Fat 1.9 gm,
  Monounsat Fat 5.9 gm)
- Cholesterol 50 mg
- Sodium 55 mg
- Potassium 485 gm
- Total Carb 18 gm
- Dietary Fiber 2 gm
- Sugars 3 gm
- Protein 16 gm
- Phosphorus 155 gm

Chicken a la King

Makes 12 servings,
about ½ cup per serving

Prep. Time: 30 minutes
Cooking Time: 30 minutes

4-oz. can mushrooms, drained
½ cup chopped green pepper
4 Tbsp. trans-fat-free tub margarine
½ cup flour
1 tsp. salt
¼ tsp. pepper
2 cups lower-sodium, fat-free chicken broth
2 cups fat-free half-and-half
2 cups diced, cooked chicken
½ cup chopped pimento

1. Sauté mushrooms and green pepper in butter.
2. Blend in flour and seasonings. Cook over low heat, stirring until mixture is smooth and bubbly. Remove from heat.
3. Slowly add broth and cream. Return to heat and bring to a boil over low heat, stirring constantly. Boil 1 minute.
4. Add chicken and pimento.
5. Continue cooking until chicken is heated through. Serve over baked potatoes.

Exchange List Values
- Carbohydrate 0.5
- Fat 1.0
- Lean Meat 1.0

Basic Nutritional Values
- Calories 125
  (Calories from Fat 45)
- Total Fat 5 gm
  (Saturated Fat 1.4 gm,
  Trans Fat 0.0 gm,
  Polyunsat Fat 1.7 gm,
  Monounsat Fat 1.7 gm)
- Cholesterol 25 mg
- Sodium 425 mg
- Potassium 220 gm
- Total Carb 9 gm
- Dietary Fiber 1 gm
- Sugars 3 gm
- Protein 9 gm
- Phosphorus 125 gm

Keep canned or frozen cooked chicken on hand — you can make a casserole in a short time.
Elena Yoder, Albuquerque, NM

One-Dish Chicken and Gravy

Martha Ann Auker
Landisburg, PA

Makes 8 servings

Prep. Time: 10 minutes
Baking Time: 50 minutes

3½ lb. frying chicken,
  skin removed, cut into 2
  breast halves and then
  halved again, 2 thighs, 2
  drumsticks, 2 wings
  (save chicken back for
  another purpose)
¼ cup flour
2 Tbsp. canola oil
1 Tbsp. minced onion
1 cup fat-free half-and-half
10¾-oz. can lower-sodium,
  lower-fat cream of
  mushroom soup
¼ tsp. salt
¼ tsp. pepper
dash of paprika

1. Pour oil in 9×13 baking
pan. Swirl oil to cover bottom
of pan.
2. Roll chicken in flour, one
piece at a time. Place in oiled
baking pan.
3. Bake uncovered at 425°
for 30 minutes.
4. While chicken is baking,
mix onion, half-and-half,
soup, salt, and pepper
together in mixing bowl.
5. Pour over chicken.
6. Sprinkle with paprika.
7. Cover with foil. Reduce
heat to 325° and bake 20
more minutes.

Tip:
  This is good served with
rice.

Exchange List Values
- Carbohydrate 0.5   • Fat 0.5
- Lean Meat 3.0

Basic Nutritional Values
- Calories 200
  (Calories from Fat 70)
- Total Fat 8 gm
  (Saturated Fat 1.7 gm,
  Trans Fat 0.0 gm,
  Polyunsat Fat 2.2 gm,
  Monounsat Fat 3.9 gm)
- Cholesterol 60 mg
- Sodium 285 mg
- Potassium 470 gm
- Total Carb 9 gm
- Dietary Fiber 0 gm
- Sugars 2 gm
- Protein 20 gm
- Phosphorus 190 gm

Easy Chicken Enchiladas

Lois Peterson
Huron, SD

Makes 6 servings,
1 enchilada per serving

Prep. Time: 35–45 minutes
Baking Time: 40 minutes

10¾-oz. can lower-sodium,
  lower-fat cream of
  chicken soup
½ cup fat-free sour cream
¼ cup picante sauce
¾ cup no-salt-added
  tomato sauce
2 tsp. chili powder
2 cups cooked chicken,
  chopped
1 oz. reduced-fat pepper
  Jack cheese
6 6" flour, *or* whole wheat,
  tortillas
1 large tomato, chopped
1 green onion, sliced

1. Stir soup, sour cream,
picante sauce, tomato sauce
and chili powder in a medium
bowl.
2. In a large bowl, combine
1 cup sauce mixture, chicken,
and cheese.
3. Grease 9×13 baking
dish.
4. Divide mixture among
tortillas.
5. Roll up each tortilla.
Place in baking dish, seam
side down.
6. Pour remaining sauce
mixture over filled tortillas.
7. Cover. Bake at 350° for
40 minutes or until enchiladas are hot and bubbling.
8. Top with chopped
tomato and onion and serve.

Exchange List Values
- Starch 1.0   • Lean Meat 2.0
- Carbohydrate 0.5   • Fat 1.0
- Vegetable 1.0

Basic Nutritional Values
- Calories 260
  (Calories from Fat 70)
- Total Fat 8 gm
  (Saturated Fat 2.5 gm,
  Trans Fat 0.0 gm,
  Polyunsat Fat 1.8 gm,
  Monounsat Fat 3.0 gm)
- Cholesterol 50 mg
- Sodium 565 mg
- Potassium 650 gm
- Total Carb 28 gm
- Dietary Fiber 3 gm
- Sugars 4 gm
- Protein 19 gm
- Phosphorus 200 gm

To tell if chicken is done, pierce the thickest piece with a fork. If the juice runs clear, it's done.

Carolyn Spohn, Shawnee, KS

Tex-Mex Chicken Casserole

Ruth C. Hancock
Earlsboro, OK

Makes 6 servings,
a 4"×2⅔" rectangle per serving

Prep. Time: 45 minutes
Baking Time: 35 minutes

2 cups shredded cooked chicken
2 cups coarsely crushed baked low-fat tortilla chips
15-oz. can pinto beans, rinsed and drained
1 cup frozen corn kernels
⅔ cup fat-free sour cream
½-1 tsp. chili powder, according to your taste preference
1½ cups low-sodium salsa, *divided*
1 cup 75%-less-fat shredded cheese, *divided*

1. Combine chicken, chips, beans, corn, sour cream, and chili powder in mixing bowl.
2. Grease 2-quart baking dish or 8×8 baking pan.
3. Layer half of chicken mixture into baking dish.
4. Top with half of salsa.
5. Top with half of cheese. Repeat layers.
6. Cover with foil.
7. Bake at 350° for 25 minutes.
8. Uncover and bake 10 minutes more.

Exchange List Values
• Starch 2.0   • Lean Meat 3.0
• Vegetable 1.0

Basic Nutritional Values
• Calories 310
  (Calories from Fat 55)
• Total Fat 6 gm
  (Saturated Fat 2.3 gm,
  Trans Fat 0.0 gm,
  Polyunsat Fat 1.3 gm,
  Monounsat Fat 1.8 gm)
• Cholesterol 50 mg
• Sodium 595 mg
• Potassium 635 gm
• Total Carb 37 gm
• Dietary Fiber 6 gm
• Sugars 4 gm
• Protein 28 gm
• Phosphorus 355 gm

Creamy Chicken Enchiladas

Cheryl Martin
Turin, NY

Makes 10 servings,
1 enchilada per serving

Prep. Time: 30 minutes
Baking Time: 30–40 minutes

2 10¾-oz. cans lower-sodium, lower-fat cream of chicken soup
8 oz. fat-free sour cream
¼ tsp. cumin
¼ tsp. dried oregano
3 cups slivered, cooked chicken
4-oz. can chopped green chilies
1 tsp. chili powder
1 cup shredded 75%-less fat cheddar cheese, *divided*
10 6" flour tortillas

1. In large mixing bowl, combine soup with sour cream, cumin, and oregano to make sauce.
2. In another bowl combine 1 cup sauce with chicken, green chilies, chili powder, and 1 cup shredded cheese.
3. Fill each tortilla with equal portion of chicken mixture.
4. Roll up tortillas. Arrange in greased 9×13 glass baking dish.
5. Spoon remaining sauce over tortillas.
6. Sprinkle with remaining cheese.
7. Bake at 350° for 30–40 minutes, or until enchiladas are heated through and sauce is bubbly.

Tips:
1. You can make this ahead, and then refrigerate or freeze it until ready to bake. If frozen, thaw before baking.
2. Barbecued chicken adds a tasty, bacon-like flavor to the dish.
3. I like to use an ice cream scoop to divide the filling mixture equally between the tortillas.

Exchange List Values
• Starch 1.0   • Lean Meat 3.0
• Carbohydrate 0.5

Basic Nutritional Values
• Calories 240
  (Calories from Fat 55)
• Total Fat 6 gm
  (Saturated Fat 1.9 gm,
  Trans Fat 0.0 gm,
  Polyunsat Fat 1.3 gm,
  Monounsat Fat 2.2 gm)
• Cholesterol 45 mg
• Sodium 565 mg
• Potassium 505 gm
• Total Carb 25 gm
• Dietary Fiber 1 gm
• Sugars 2 gm
• Protein 21 gm
• Phosphorus 225 gm

Cheesy Mexican Chicken

Lori Newswanger
Lancaster, PA

Makes 8 servings,
3¼"×4½" rectangle per serving

Prep. Time: 15 minutes
Baking Time: 35–45 minutes

2 lbs. boneless, skinless
chicken breasts
10¾-oz. can lower-fat,
lower-sodium cream of
chicken soup
1¾ cups shredded
75%-less-fat cheddar
cheese, *divided*
½ cup fat-free milk
7 tsp. salt-free taco
seasoning (see page 271)
3 cups baked low-fat corn
chips, *or* tortilla chips,
coarsely crushed

1. Grease 9×13 baking dish.
2. Slice chicken in 1"-wide strips. Spread chicken in baking dish.
3. Combine soup, 1¼ cups cheese, milk, and taco seasoning in mixing bowl. Spoon over chicken.
4. Top with chips.
5. Cover dish.
6. Bake at 375° for 30–40 minutes, or until chicken is cooked through and no pink remains. (Fish out a piece from middle of dish and check.)
7. Remove cover. Top with remaining ½ cup cheese.
8. Bake uncovered until cheese is melted, about 5 minutes.

Tip:
Serve over rice.

Exchange List Values
- Starch 1.0
- Carbohydrate 0.5
- Lean Meat 4.0

Basic Nutritional Values
- Calories 275
  (Calories from Fat 55)
- Total Fat 6 gm
  (Saturated Fat 2.4 gm,
  Trans Fat 0.0 gm,
  Polyunsat Fat 1.3 gm,
  Monounsat Fat 1.8 gm)
- Cholesterol 75 mg
- Sodium 495 mg
- Potassium 505 gm
- Total Carb 20 gm
- Dietary Fiber 2 gm
- Sugars 1 gm
- Protein 35 gm
- Phosphorus 380 gm

White Chicken Chili Casserole

Zoë Rohrer
Lancaster, PA

Makes 8 servings,
a 3"×4" rectangle per serving

Prep. Time: 15 minutes
Baking Time: 35 minutes
Standing Time: 10 minutes

1 small onion, diced
1 clove garlic, minced
2 ribs celery, diced
1 green bell pepper, diced
1–2 tsp. oil
4 cups cooked white beans
1 cup lower-sodium, fat-
free chicken broth
1 cup fat-free sour cream
¼ tsp. salt
1 tsp. ground cumin
½ tsp. black pepper
10¾-oz. can lower-
sodium, fat-free cream
of chicken, *or* cream of
celery soup
2 cups cooked chopped
chicken
4 8" whole wheat tortillas,
divided
2 cups 75%-less-fat
shredded cheddar
cheese, *divided*

1. In a large skillet, sauté onions, garlic, celery, and green pepper in a bit of oil until soft.
2. Add beans, broth, sour cream, salt, cumin, pepper, and soup. Bring to a boil while stirring.
3. Remove from heat. Stir in chicken.
4. Spread ⅓ of chicken mixture in bottom of well-greased 9×13 baking dish.
5. Top with 2 tortillas, cutting them to fit the pan.
6. Spread on half of remaining chicken mixture.
7. Top with half the cheese.
8. Follow with remaining 2 tortillas, a layer of remaining chicken, and a layer of remaining cheese.
9. Bake for 30–35 minutes, or until bubbly.
10. Let stand 10 minutes before serving.

Good Go-Alongs:
Great served with salsa

Exchange List Values
- Starch 2.0
- Carbohydrate 0.5
- Lean Meat 3.0

Basic Nutritional Values
- Calories 340
  (Calories from Fat 55)
- Total Fat 6 gm
  (Saturated Fat 2.4 gm,
  Trans Fat 0.0 gm,
  Polyunsat Fat 1.2 gm,
  Monounsat Fat 1.8 gm)
- Cholesterol 40 mg
- Sodium 600 mg
- Potassium 905 gm
- Total Carb 43 gm
- Dietary Fiber 7 gm
- Sugars 4 gm
- Protein 29 gm
- Phosphorus 370 gm

Chicken Spinach Casserole

Laverne Nafziger
Goshen, IN

Makes 6 servings

Prep. Time: 15–20 minutes
Baking Time: 35–40 minutes

¾ cup fat-free mayonnaise
¾ cup fat-free plain yogurt
½ cup fat-free sour cream
1 cup shredded 75%-less-fat cheddar cheese
1 tsp. minced garlic
1½ cups cooked and diced chicken
10-oz. pkg. frozen chopped spinach, thawed and squeezed dry
½ cup crushed soda crackers
⅓ cup freshly grated Parmesan cheese

1. In a good-sized mixing bowl, blend together mayonnaise, yogurt, sour cream, cheddar cheese, and garlic.
2. Stir in chicken and spinach.
3. Spoon into buttered 6½×8½ baking dish.
4. In mixing bowl, stir together cracker crumbs and Parmesan cheese.
5. Sprinkle over top.
6. Bake at 350° for 35–40 minutes, or until topping is lightly browned and mixture is bubbly.

Exchange List Values
• Carbohydrate 1.0
• Lean Meat 3.0

Basic Nutritional Values
• Calories 190
 (Calories from Fat 55)
• Total Fat 6 gm
 (Saturated Fat 2.5 gm,
 Trans Fat 0.0 gm,
 Polyunsat Fat 0.7 gm,
 Monounsat Fat 1.4 gm)
• Cholesterol 35 mg
• Sodium 600 mg
• Potassium 315 gm
• Total Carb 16 gm
• Dietary Fiber 2 gm
• Sugars 5 gm
• Protein 19 gm
• Phosphorus 265 gm

Broccoli Chicken Casserole

Joette Droz
Kalona, IA

Makes 6 servings,
3½" square per serving

Prep. Time: 35 minutes
Baking Time: 1 hour

10¾-oz. can lower-sodium, lower-fat cream of chicken soup
5 oz. (half the can) lower-sodium, lower-fat cream of chicken soup
⅓ cup light mayonnaise
2 cups garlic croutons, slightly crushed
2 cups cooked chopped chicken
10-oz. pkg. frozen chopped broccoli, thawed and drained
8-oz. can sliced water chestnuts, drained
4-oz. can sliced mushrooms, drained

1. Mix soup and mayonnaise together in large mixing bowl until smooth.
2. Stir in croutons, chicken, broccoli, water chestnuts, and mushrooms. Mix well.
3. Spread in well-greased 7×11 baking pan.
4. Cover with foil.
5. Bake at 350° for 45 minutes.
6. Uncover. Continue baking for 15 minutes.

Exchange List Values
• Starch 0.5
• Carbohydrate 0.5
• Vegetable 1.0
• Lean Meat 2.0
• Fat 1.0

Basic Nutritional Values
• Calories 235
 (Calories from Fat 80)
• Total Fat 9 gm
 (Saturated Fat 1.9 gm,
 Trans Fat 0.0 gm,
 Polyunsat Fat 3.4 gm,
 Monounsat Fat 2.7 gm)
• Cholesterol 50 mg
• Sodium 555 mg
• Potassium 625 gm
• Total Carb 21 gm
• Dietary Fiber 3 gm
• Sugars 3 gm
• Protein 18 gm
• Phosphorus 165 gm

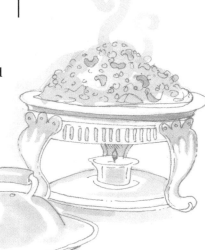

Chicken Corn Casserole

Lois Niebauer
Pedricktown, NJ

Makes 6 servings,
3" square per serving

Prep. Time: 30 minutes
Baking Time: 45 minutes

2 cups diced cooked
chicken
1½ cups frozen corn
½ cup shredded 75%-less-
fat cheddar cheese
3 Tbsp. chopped pimentos
½ cup canned French-fried
onions, *divided*
2 Tbsp. oil
¼ cup flour
10¾-oz. can chicken broth
¼-½ tsp. salt
¼ tsp. pepper

1. Combine chicken, corn,
cheese, pimentos, and ¾ can
fried onions in mixing bowl.
2. Combine oil, flour,
chicken broth, and seasonings
in small saucepan.
3. Cook over low to medium
heat, stirring until thickened.
4. Add thickened sauce to
other ingredients and mix
thoroughly.
5. Place in well-greased
7×11 baking dish.
6. Sprinkle reserved onion
over top.
7. Bake at 325° for 45
minutes.

Tip:
You can make this ahead
through Step 6 and freeze

until you need it. You can
put it in the oven frozen; just
bake longer until bubbly,
about 1–1¼ hours.

Exchange List Values
- Starch 1.0
- Fat 1.5
- Lean Meat 2.0

Basic Nutritional Values
- Calories 235
  (Calories from Fat 110)
- Total Fat 12 gm
  (Saturated Fat 2.5 gm,
  Trans Fat 0.0 gm,
  Polyunsat Fat 2.7 gm,
  Monounsat Fat 5.1 gm)
- Cholesterol 45 mg
- Sodium 390 mg
- Potassium 270 gm
- Total Carb 14 gm
- Dietary Fiber 1 gm
- Sugars 1 gm
- Protein 19 gm
- Phosphorus 175 gm

Chicken and Broccoli Bake

Jan Rankin
Millersville, PA

Makes 12 servings, 3" square

Prep. Time: 15 minutes
Baking Time: 30 minutes

2 10¾-oz. cans lower-
sodium, lower-fat cream
of chicken soup
2½ cups fat-free milk,
divided
16-oz. bag frozen
chopped broccoli,
thawed and
drained
3 cups cooked
and chopped
chicken breast
2 cups reduced-
fat buttermilk
baking mix

1. Mix soup, and 1 cup
milk together in large mixing
bowl until smooth.
2. Stir in broccoli and
chicken.
3. Pour into well-greased
9×13 baking dish.
4. Mix together 1½ cups
milk and baking mix in
mixing bowl.
5. Spoon evenly over top of
chicken-broccoli mixture.
6. Bake at 450° for 30
minutes.

Exchange List Values
- Starch 1.0
- Lean Meat 2.0
- Carbohydrate 0.5

Basic Nutritional Values
- Calories 180
  (Calories from Fat 30)
- Total Fat 4 gm
  (Saturated Fat 0.7 gm,
  Trans Fat 0.0 gm,
  Polyunsat Fat 1.0 gm,
  Monounsat Fat 1.4 gm)
- Cholesterol 35 mg
- Sodium 445 mg
- Potassium 485 gm
- Total Carb 22 gm
- Dietary Fiber 2 gm
- Sugars 5 gm
- Protein 16 gm
- Phosphorus 280 gm

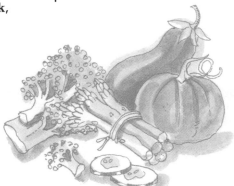

Yogurt Chicken Curry

Laverne Nafziger
Goshen, IN

*Makes 12 servings,
about ¾ cup per serving*

Prep. Time: 20 minutes
**Marinating Time: 8 hours, or
overnight**
Cooking Time: 2 hours

2½ lbs. boneless, skinless
  chicken breasts, cut into
  1" cubes
2 lbs. plain nonfat yogurt
4 heaping tsp. curry powder
2 heaping tsp. turmeric
1 heaping tsp. ground
  coriander
2 Tbsp. vegetable oil
1 large onion, chopped
5 garlic cloves, chopped
1" ginger root grated *or*
  finely chopped
½ tsp. salt
1 cup fat-free sour cream
1 medium potato, grated
1 cup cilantro, chopped,
  optional

1. Mix chicken, yogurt,
curry powder, turmeric, and
coriander in large nonmetallic
bowl. Marinate 8 hours or
overnight.
2. Sauté onions, garlic, and
ginger in oil in large stockpot
2–5 minutes until lightly
brown.
3. Add chicken-yogurt
mixture, salt, sour cream, and
grated raw potato.
4. Cover. Simmer gently for
2 hours.

5. Just before serving, stir
in cilantro if you wish.

Tip:
  Serve over cooked rice.

Exchange List Values
- Carbohydrate 1.0 • Lean Meat 3.0

Basic Nutritional Values
- Calories 205
  (Calories from Fat 45)
- Total Fat 5 gm
  (Saturated Fat 1.0 gm,
  Trans Fat 0.0 gm,
  Polyunsat Fat 1.2 gm,
  Monounsat Fat 2.3 gm)
- Cholesterol 55 mg
- Sodium 215 mg
- Potassium 425 gm
- Total Carb 14 gm
- Dietary Fiber 1 gm
- Sugars 7 gm
- Protein 25 gm
- Phosphorus 270 gm

Chicken Biriyani

Laverne Nafziger
Hopedale, IL

*Makes 9 servings,
about 1¼ cups per serving*

Prep. Time: 30 minutes
Cooking Time: 2 hours

3 lb. whole chicken, cut in
  pieces, skin removed
1 clove garlic
1" piece fresh ginger root
1 small green chili
1 large onion, diced
4 whole cardamom pods
6 whole cloves
3 bay leaves
2–3 Tbsp. chopped fresh
  cilantro

1 tsp. turmeric powder
¼ cup cooking oil
salt to taste
2 cups uncooked rice
4¾ cups reserved chicken
  broth, *or* water
2 large tomatoes, chopped

1. Cover chicken pieces
with water in a pot. Bring
to simmer and cook over
low until chicken is cooked
through, 30–60 minutes.
2. Debone chicken and cut/
shred into bite-sized pieces.
Reserve broth.
3. Combine garlic, ginger
root and chili into a paste in
blender.
4. In large pan sauté onion
and spices in oil. Add all
remaining ingredients and
cook until rice is tender.
5. Discard whole spices.
Serve.

Exchange List Values
- Starch 2.0 • Lean Meat 2.0
- Vegetable 1.0 • Fat 1.0

Basic Nutritional Values
- Calories 325
  (Calories from Fat 90)
- Total Fat 10 gm
  (Saturated Fat 1.6 gm,
  Trans Fat 0.0 gm,
  Polyunsat Fat 2.7 gm,
  Monounsat Fat 5.2 gm)
- Cholesterol 45 mg
- Sodium 90 mg
- Potassium 440 gm
- Total Carb 38 gm
- Dietary Fiber 2 gm
- Sugars 3 gm
- Protein 19 gm
- Phosphorus 180 gm

*Use low-fat ingredients, such as low-fat yogurt
or milk, in recipes whenever possible.*

Chicken Curry

Tina Hartman
Lancaster, PA

*Makes 8 servings,
about 3–4 oz. per serving*

Prep. Time: 20 minutes
Cooking Time: 10–15 minutes

3 Tbsp. tub margarine, no
   trans-fat
¼ cup minced onion
1½ tsp. curry powder
3 Tbsp. flour
¾ tsp. salt
¾ tsp. sugar
⅛ tsp. ground ginger
1 cup lower-sodium, fat-
   free chicken broth
1 cup fat-free milk
2 cups diced, cooked
   chicken
½ tsp. lemon juice

1. In good-sized skillet,
melt margarine over low heat.
2. Sauté onions and curry
in margarine.
3. Blend in flour and
seasonings.
4. Cook over low heat
until mixture is smooth and
bubbly. (This removes the raw
flour taste.)
5. Remove from heat.
6. Stir in chicken broth
and milk.
7. Return to heat. Bring to
a boil, stirring constantly.
8. Boil one more minute,
continuing to stir.
9. Remove from heat. Stir
in chicken and lemon juice.
10. Serve over cooked
rice, and with toppings for
individuals to choose.

Tips:
   This is a wonderful family
or large gathering meal
because of the toppings. You
can use any toppings you
can imagine. We once had 22
different topping options! We
almost always serve this at our
extended family gatherings.

Good Go-Alongs:
   Experiment by topping
this recipe with Mandarin
oranges, cashews, coconut,
peaches, bananas, olives,
celery, tomatoes, onions,
cheese individually or mixed
as you prefer.

Exchange List Values
- Carbohydrate 0.5 • Fat 1.0
- Lean Meat 1.0

Basic Nutritional Values
- Calories 125   • Sodium 360 mg
  (Calories from Fat 55) • Potassium 175 gm
- Total Fat 6 gm   • Total Carb 5 gm
  (Saturated Fat 1.4 gm, • Dietary Fiber 0 gm
  Trans Fat 0.0 gm, • Sugars 2 gm
  Polyunsat Fat 1.9 gm, • Protein 12 gm
  Monounsat Fat 2.0 gm) • Phosphorus 110 gm
- Cholesterol 30 mg

Chopstick Chicken

Mary Ann Lefever
Lancaster, PA

*Makes 10 servings,
about 6 oz. per serving*

Prep. Time: 20 minutes
Baking Time: 40 minutes

10¾-oz. can lower-sodium,
   lower-fat cream of
   mushroom soup

10¾-oz. can lower-sodium,
   lower-fat cream of
   chicken soup
5-oz. can chow mein
   noodles, *divided*
2 cups chopped celery
1 cup chopped onions
3 cups cooked chicken, cut
   into bite-size pieces
11-oz. can mandarin
   oranges, drained
½ cup cashews, salted *or*
   unsalted
1 Tbsp. parsley

1. Mix together soups, half
the noodles, celery, onion,
and chicken in a large mixing
bowl.
2. Place in greased cas-
serole dish.
3. Bake at 350° for 20
minutes.
4. Stir in cashews.
5. Return to oven. Bake 20
more minutes, or until bubbly
and heated through.
6. Remove from oven. Top
with oranges and sprinkle
with parsley just before
serving.

Exchange List Values
- Carbohydrate 1.0 • Fat 1.5
- Lean Meat 2.0

Basic Nutritional Values
- Calories 245   • Sodium 370 mg
  (Calories from Fat 110) • Potassium 595 gm
- Total Fat 12 gm   • Total Carb 19 gm
  (Saturated Fat 2.4 gm, • Dietary Fiber 2 gm
  Trans Fat 0.0 gm, • Sugars 4 gm
  Polyunsat Fat 4.2 gm, • Protein 16 gm
  Monounsat Fat 4.3 gm) • Phosphorus 165 gm
- Cholesterol 40 mg

Korean Fried Rice

Kum Smith
Morton, IL

*Makes 6 servings,
about 1 cup per serving*

Prep. Time: 20 minutes
Soaking Time: 5 minutes
Cooking Time: 45 minutes

1 cup long-grain rice
1½ cups water
2⅔ Tbsp. canola oil, *divided*
1 medium white onion, finely chopped
2 large mushrooms, finely chopped
1 medium green pepper, finely chopped, *or* 1 cup peas
1 carrot, finely chopped
1 lb. chicken breast
salt and pepper to taste

1. Soak rice in water for 5 minutes. Cover and bring to boil. Cook over medium high heat for 5 minutes. Cover and simmer for 15–20 minutes.
2. Meanwhile, heat 1 tsp. shortening in skillet and sauté one vegetable at a time. Clean skillet after each vegetable. Set each vegetable aside.
3. Fry chicken in 1 tsp. oil also and season to taste. Set aside.
4. Stir fry cooked rice in 1 Tbsp. oil until light brown. Add salt and pepper to taste.
5. Combine all ingredients in large skillet and cook until heated.

Exchange List Values
- Starch 1.5
- Vegetable 1.0
- Lean Meat 2.0
- Fat 1.0

Basic Nutritional Values
- Calories 285 (Calories from Fat 70)
- Total Fat 8 gm (Saturated Fat 1.1 gm, Trans Fat 0.0 gm, Polyunsat Fat 2.3 gm, Monounsat Fat 4.7 gm)
- Cholesterol 45 mg
- Sodium 50 mg
- Potassium 300 gm
- Total Carb 31 gm
- Dietary Fiber 2 gm
- Sugars 2 gm
- Protein 19 gm
- Phosphorus 180 gm

Chicken Fried Rice

*Makes 8 servings,
about ¾ cup per serving*

Prep. Time: 20 minutes
Cooking Time: 15 minutes

1 oz. dried mushrooms
4 eggs, beaten
4 tsp. canola oil, *divided*
7 oz. diced lean, low-sodium ham
3½ oz. green onions, sliced
4 cups steamed rice
½ can bamboo shoots, sliced
4 Tbsp. green beans, *or* more
7 oz. diced cooked chicken
salt and pepper to taste

1. Boil mushrooms in water to cover for 3–5 minutes until softened. Drain water and slice mushrooms.
2. Stir fry eggs in 1 tsp. oil. Add ham and cook until heated through. Set aside.
3. Stir fry onion in 3 tsp. oil.
4. Add rice, mushrooms, bamboo shoots, green beans, chicken, eggs and ham. Stir fry at least 5 minutes. Salt and pepper to taste before serving.

Exchange List Values
- Starch 1.5
- Vegetable 1.0
- Lean Meat 2.0
- Fat 0.5

Basic Nutritional Values
- Calories 260 (Calories from Fat 70)
- Total Fat 8 gm (Saturated Fat 2.0 gm, Trans Fat 0.0 gm, Polyunsat Fat 1.8 gm, Monounsat Fat 3.7 gm)
- Cholesterol 130 mg
- Sodium 300 mg
- Potassium 290 gm
- Total Carb 27 gm
- Dietary Fiber 1 gm
- Sugars 1 gm
- Protein 18 gm
- Phosphorus 200 gm

What is good for people with diabetes to eat is good for everybody to eat. No need to label some dishes on the church supper table as "diabetic."

Chicken Spectacular

Rebecca Meyerkorth, Wamego, KS
Melissa Wenger, Orrville, OH

Makes 12 servings,
3" square per serving

Prep. Time: 30 minutes
Baking Time: 30 minutes
Standing Time: 5 minutes

½ lb. uncooked wild rice
3 cups cooked chicken, diced
10¾-oz. can lower-sodium, lower-fat cream of celery soup
1 medium jar chopped pimentos, drained
1 medium onion, chopped
15-oz. can green beans, French-cut style, drained
1 cup low-fat mayonnaise
½ tsp. Worcestershire sauce
¼ tsp. pepper
½ tsp. dried parsley
¼ tsp. dried sage
¼ tsp. dried rosemary
¼ tsp. dried thyme
8-oz. can sliced water chestnuts, drained
1 cup grated reduced-fat cheddar cheese

1. Prepare rice according to package directions.
2. In large bowl, mix together prepared rice, chicken, soup, pimentos, onion, beans, mayonnaise, Worcestershire sauce, pepper, parsley, sage, rosemary, thyme and water chestnuts.
3. Pour into greased 9×13 baking dish.

4. Bake at 350° for 30 minutes, or until bubbly and heated through.
5. Sprinkle with cheese. Let stand 5 minutes for cheese to melt.

Tip:
You can prepare through Step 3 and then freeze until needed.

Exchange List Values
• Starch 0.5   • Vegetable 1.0
• Carbohydrate 0.5   • Lean Meat 2.0

Basic Nutritional Values
• Calories 190   • Sodium 440 mg
  (Calories from Fat 65) • Potassium 345 gm
• Total Fat 7 gm   • Total Carb 19 gm
  (Saturated Fat 2.2 gm, • Dietary Fiber 2 gm
  Trans Fat 0.0 gm,   • Sugars 3 gm
  Polyunsat Fat 1.8 gm, • Protein 15 gm
  Monounsat Fat 1.8 gm) • Phosphorus 190 gm
• Cholesterol 35 mg

Simmering Chicken Dinner

Trish Dick, Ladysmith, WI

Makes 6 servings,
about 8 oz. per serving

Prep. Time: 10 minutes
Cooking Time: 40 minutes

2½ cups lower-sodium, fat-free chicken broth
½ cup apple juice
1 bay leaf
½ tsp. garlic powder
½ tsp. paprika
¼ tsp. salt
1½ lbs. boneless, skinless chicken breasts, or thighs, cut into chunks

1 cup uncooked brown rice
3 cups fresh, or frozen, vegetables, including starchy and nonstarchy vegetables
½ tsp. paprika, optional
parsley as garnish, optional

1. Heat chicken broth, apple juice, bay leaf, garlic powder, paprika, and salt in large skillet until boiling, stirring occasionally.
2. Add chicken. Cover. Reduce heat and simmer 10 minutes on low.
3. Turn chicken.
4. Add 1 cup rice around chicken.
5. Top with the vegetables.
6. Cover. Simmer 25 minutes, or until rice is cooked, vegetables are as soft as you like, and chicken is done.
7. Remove bay leaf.
8. Sprinkle with paprika and parsley before serving if you wish.

Tip:
If you like a bit of zip, add curry powder in place of paprika.

Exchange List Values
• Starch 2.0   • Lean Meat 3.0
• Vegetable 1.0

Basic Nutritional Values
• Calories 320   • Sodium 390 mg
  (Calories from Fat 65) • Potassium 470 gm
• Total Fat 7 gm   • Total Carb 36 gm
  (Saturated Fat 1.7 gm, • Dietary Fiber 5 gm
  Trans Fat 0.0 gm,   • Sugars 5 gm
  Polyunsat Fat 1.6 gm, • Protein 27 gm
  Monounsat Fat 2.4 gm) • Phosphorus 310 gm
• Cholesterol 70 mg

Chicken Rice Casserole

Alma Yoder, Baltic, OH

*Makes 10 servings,
about 8 oz. per serving*

Prep. Time: 20 minutes
Baking Time: 45 minutes

2 cups uncooked long-grain rice
4 cups low-sodium, fat-free chicken broth
2 cups diced celery
1 Tbsp. canola oil
10¾-oz. can lower-sodium, lower-fat cream of mushroom soup
1¼ cups low-fat mayonnaise
2 Tbsp. chopped onion
2 cups cooked, cubed chicken
1 cup crushed cornflakes
1 Tbsp. no trans-fat tub margarine, melted

1. In large saucepan, cook rice in chicken broth, covered, for about 20 minutes over low heat.
2. While rice is cooking, sauté celery in oil in skillet.
3. When rice is tender, add celery, soup, mayonnaise, onion, and chicken to rice. Mix gently.
4. Spoon mixture into greased casserole dish.
5. Mix crushed cornflakes and melted margarine together in small bowl.
6. Scatter cornflake mixture on top.
7. Bake, covered, at 350° for 30 minutes.

8. Uncover. Bake 15 more minutes, or until bubbly and heated through.

Exchange List Values
- Starch 2.0
- Lean Meat 1.0
- Carbohydrate 0.5
- Fat 1.0

Basic Nutritional Values
- Calories 285
- (Calories from Fat 65)
- Total Fat 7 gm
- (Saturated Fat 1.4 gm, Trans Fat 0.0 gm, Polyunsat Fat 2.7 gm, Monounsat Fat 2.6 gm)
- Cholesterol 30 mg
- Sodium 485 mg
- Potassium 460 gm
- Total Carb 41 gm
- Dietary Fiber 1 gm
- Sugars 3 gm
- Protein 13 gm
- Phosphorus 135 gm

Wild-Rice Turkey-Sausage Bake

Carla Elliott, Phoenix, AZ

*Makes 10 servings,
a 2⅗"×4½" rectangle per serving*

Prep. Time: 1 hour
Baking Time: 1½ hours

1 lb. lean sweet Italian turkey sausage
¾ cup uncooked wild rice, cooked according to package directions
¾ cup uncooked long-grain rice, cooked according to package directions
1 medium onion, chopped
1 cup diced celery
10¾-oz. lower-sodium, lower-fat cream of mushroom soup
¼ tsp. salt
¼ tsp. pepper

14½-oz. can chicken broth
4-oz. can sliced mushrooms, drained, *optional*
20 oz. boneless, skinless chicken breast halves, about 4 breasts, cut into large bite-size pieces

1. Brown sausage in skillet, stirring frequently to break up clumps, until no longer pink.
2. Drain off drippings.
3. In large bowl, mix together sausage, both cooked rices, onion, celery, soup, salt, pepper, broth, and mushrooms if you wish.
4. Spoon into greased 9×13 baking pan.
5. Push chicken pieces down into rice mixture.
6. Cover. Bake at 350° for 1 hour.
7. Remove cover and check if mixture is soupy. If so, remove cover. If not, put cover back on. Continue baking 30 more minutes.

Exchange List Values
- Starch 1.0
- Lean Meat 3.0
- Carbohydrate 0.5

Basic Nutritional Values
- Calories 245
- (Calories from Fat 55)
- Total Fat 6 gm
- (Saturated Fat 1.6 gm, Trans Fat 0.1 gm, Polyunsat Fat 1.7 gm, Monounsat Fat 2.1 gm)
- Cholesterol 60 mg
- Sodium 575 mg
- Potassium 505 gm
- Total Carb 23 gm
- Dietary Fiber 1 gm
- Sugars 2 gm
- Protein 22 gm
- Phosphorus 210 gm

Company Casserole

Mary B. Sensenig
New Holland, PA

Makes 8 servings,
about 7 oz. per serving

Prep. Time: 40 minutes
Standing Time: 5 minutes
Baking Time: 45 minutes

¾ cup long-grain rice
1¾ cups water
1½ Tbsp. tub margarine,
　no trans-fat
15 oz. frozen broccoli,
　thawed and drained
1½ cups cubed cooked
　chicken
¾ cup cubed cooked 95%-
　lean ham
½ cup shredded 75%-less
　fat cheddar cheese
10¾-oz. can lower-sodium,
　lower-fat cream of
　mushroom soup
⅔ cup low-fat mayonnaise
1 tsp. prepared mustard
3 Tbsp. freshly grated
　Parmesan cheese

1. Combine rice, water, and
margarine in microwave-safe
container.
2. Cover tightly. Cook on
high 5 minutes.
3. Cook 10 minutes on
Power 5.
4. Let stand 5 minutes, covered, until water is absorbed.
5. In greased 2½- or 3-quart
casserole layer cooked rice,
broccoli, chicken, ham, and
cheddar cheese.
6. In mixing bowl, combine
soup, mayonnaise, and
mustard.

7. Spread sauce over
casserole.
8. Sprinkle with Parmesan
cheese.
9. Bake at 350° for 45–50
minutes, or until lightly
browned.

Good Go-Alongs:
　Lettuce Salad with Hot
Bacon Dressing

Exchange List Values
• Starch 1.0　　　　• Lean Meat 2.0
• Carbohydrate 0.5　• Fat 0.5

Basic Nutritional Values
• Calories 230　　　　• Sodium 595 mg
　(Calories from Fat 65)　• Potassium 470 gm
• Total Fat 7 gm　　　• Total Carb 24 gm
　(Saturated Fat 2.2 gm,　• Dietary Fiber 2 gm
　Trans Fat 0.0 gm,　　• Sugars 2 gm
　Polyunsat Fat 2.3 gm,　• Protein 17 gm
　Monounsat Fat 2.3 gm)　• Phosphorus 190 gm
• Cholesterol 35 mg

Chicken Strata Casserole

Mrs. Lewis L. Beachy
Sarasota, FL
Mary Vaughn Warye
West Liberty, OH

Makes 8 servings,
about ¾ cup per serving

Prep. Time: 20 minutes
Baking Time: 1 hour

2 cups cubed, cooked
　chicken
½ cup chopped celery
½ cup chopped onion
½ cup chopped green
　pepper

⅓ cup reduced-fat light
　mayonnaise
½ tsp. salt
¼ tsp. pepper
4 slices bread, cubed
1½ cups fat-free milk
2 eggs, beaten
14½-oz. can lower-sodium,
　lower-fat cream of
　mushroom soup
½ cup reduced-fat freshly
　grated yellow cheddar
　cheese

1. Combine chicken, celery,
onion, green pepper, mayonnaise, salt and pepper.
2. Put ½ bread into well-
greased casserole. Top with
chicken mixture and remaining bread.
3. Combine milk and eggs
and pour over other ingredients. Top with mushroom
soup and cheese.
4. Bake at 350° for 1 hour.

Exchange List Values
• Carbohydrate 1.0　• Fat 1.0
• Lean Meat 2.0

Basic Nutritional Values
• Calories 200　　　　• Sodium 560 mg
　(Calories from Fat 70)　• Potassium 490 gm
• Total Fat 8 gm　　　• Total Carb 14 gm
　(Saturated Fat 2.4 gm,　• Dietary Fiber 1 gm
　Trans Fat 0.0 gm,　　• Sugars 5 gm
　Polyunsat Fat 2.7 gm,　• Protein 16 gm
　Monounsat Fat 2.6 gm)　• Phosphorus 205 gm
• Cholesterol 85 mg

Make-Your-Own-Stuffing Chicken Bake

Mary Jane Musser, Manheim, PA

*Makes 6 servings,
about a 3" square per serving*

Prep. Time: 10 minutes
Cooking Time: 75 minutes

1½ lbs. boneless, skinless
  chicken breast,
  uncooked, cut into cubes
⅛ tsp. salt
⅛ tsp. paprika
3 slices ultra-thin cheddar
  cheese, about 1 oz. total
10¾-oz. can lower-sodium,
  lower-fat cream of
  chicken soup
½ cup water
8 slices bread, cubed
1 egg
¾ cup fat-free milk
¼ cup diced celery
2 Tbsp. diced onion

1. Place chicken in greased
7×11 glass casserole dish.
2. Sprinkle with salt and
paprika.
3. Lay cheese on top of
chicken.
4. Mix soup and water until
smooth in mixing bowl.
5. Spread soup over cheese.
6. Mix bread cubes, egg,
milk, celery, and onion
together in mixing bowl.
7. Pat filling mixture over
top of chicken.
8. Cover. Bake at 350° for
1 hour.
9. Uncover. Bake 15 minutes
more.

Exchange List Values
- Starch 1.0
- Carbohydrate 0.5
- Lean Meat 4.0

Basic Nutritional Values
- Calories 290
  (Calories from Fat 65)
- Total Fat 7 gm
  (Saturated Fat 2.5 gm,
  Trans Fat 0.0 gm,
  Polyunsat Fat 1.7 gm,
  Monounsat Fat 2.2 gm)
- Cholesterol 105 mg
- Sodium 575 mg
- Potassium 545 gm
- Total Carb 23 gm
- Dietary Fiber 1 gm
- Sugars 4 gm
- Protein 30 gm
- Phosphorus 300 gm

Chicken Cordon Bleu Casserole

Marcia S. Myer
Manheim, PA
Rachel King
Castile, NY

*Makes 24 servings,
about 3" square per serving*

Prep. Time: 30 minutes
Baking Time: 1 hour

1 lb. chipped extra-lean
  ham
5 oz. grated reduced-fat
  Swiss cheese
3 cups cooked, diced
  chicken
10¾-oz. can reduced-
  sodium, reduced-fat
  cream of chicken soup
½ cup fat-free milk

Filling:
  8 cups cubed bread
  2 Tbsp. tub margarine,
    no trans fat
  1½ cups diced celery
  1 small onion, chopped
  ½ cup egg substitute

1¾ cups fat-free milk
½ tsp. salt
¼ tsp. pepper

1. Prepare filling by sautéing celery and onion in butter
in saucepan until soft.
2. Place cubed bread in
large mixing bowl.
3. Pour sautéed vegetables,
egg substitute, 1¾ cups milk,
salt, and pepper over bread.
4. Grease 2 9×13 baking
pans.
5. Layer half of ham,
cheese, and filling into each
pan.
6. Layer half of chicken
into each pan, distributing
evenly over top of filling
mixture.
7. In mixing bowl, blend
soup and ½ cup milk
together.
8. Pour soup mixture over
top of chicken.
9. Bake at 350° for 60
minutes.

Tip:
  This makes a lot. It's great
for big groups.

Exchange List Values
- Carbohydrate 0.5
- Lean Meat 2.0

Basic Nutritional Values
- Calories 130
  (Calories from Fat 40)
- Total Fat 4.5 gm
  (Saturated Fat 1.5 gm,
  Trans Fat 0.0 gm,
  Polyunsat Fat 1.0 gm,
  Monounsat Fat 1.5 gm)
- Cholesterol 30 mg
- Sodium 430 mg
- Potassium 235 gm
- Total Carb 9 gm
- Dietary Fiber 0 gm
- Sugars 2 gm
- Protein 13 gm
- Phosphorus 145 gm

Easy Chicken Stuffing Bake

Leona M. Slabaugh
Apple Creek, OH

Makes 6 servings,
about 4" square per serving

Prep. Time: 20 minutes
Baking Time: 45 minutes

6-oz. pkg. lower-sodium
   stuffing mix for chicken
1½ lbs. boneless, skinless
   chicken breasts,
   uncooked, cut in 1"
   pieces
10¾-oz. lower-sodium,
   lower-fat cream of
   chicken soup
⅓ cup sour cream
16-oz. pkg. frozen mixed
   vegetables, including
   non-starchy vegetables
   such as broccoli and
   peppers, thawed and
   drained

1. Prepare stuffing mix
as directed on package. Set
aside.
2. In large mixing bowl,
mix chicken, soup, sour
cream, and vegetables.
3. Arrange in well-greased
9×13 baking pan.
4. Top with stuffing mix.
5. Bake uncovered 45
minutes, or until chicken is
tender.

Exchange List Values
• Starch 2.0   • Lean Meat 3.0
• Carbohydrate 0.5

Basic Nutritional Values
• Calories 340   • Sodium 505 mg
  (Calories from Fat 65)   • Potassium 645 gm
• Total Fat 7 gm   • Total Carb 36 gm
  (Saturated Fat 2.5 gm,   • Dietary Fiber 4 gm
  Trans Fat 0.0 gm,   • Sugars 5 gm
  Polyunsat Fat 1.3 gm,   • Protein 30 gm
  Monounsat Fat 2.2 gm)   • Phosphorus 275 gm
• Cholesterol 75 mg

Overnight Chicken Casserole

Lori Berezovsky
Salina, KS

Makes 12 servings,
3" square per serving

Prep. Time: 20 minutes
Chilling Time: 8 hours or
  overnight
Standing Time: 1 hour
Baking Time: 50 minutes

10½ oz. of a 14-oz. pkg.
   Pepperidge Farm herb
   stuffing
1⅔ cups hot water
4 cups diced chicken
½ cup chopped green
   onions
¼ cup light mayonnaise
4-oz. can sliced
   mushrooms, drained, *or*
   ¼ lb. fresh mushrooms,
   sliced, *optional*
½ cup egg substitute
2½ cups fat-free milk,
   divided
10¾-oz. can lower-sodium,
   lower-fat cream of
   mushroom soup
½ cup 75%-less fat
   shredded cheddar cheese

1. In large mixing bowl,
lightly mix together stuffing,
and hot water.
2. Grease 9×13 baking pan.
3. Put half of stuffing
mixture into baking pan.
4. In another bowl, mix
together chicken, onions,
mayonnaise, and mushrooms
if you wish.
5. Spread chicken layer
over stuffing layer.
6. Top with remaining
stuffing.
7. In mixing bowl, combine
egg substitute and 2 cups
milk.
8. Pour over casserole.
9. Cover and refrigerate 8
hours or overnight.
10. Remove casserole from
refrigerator 1 hour before
baking.
11. In mixing bowl, blend
soup and ½ cup milk until
smooth.
12. Spread soup over
casserole.
13. Bake at 325° for 30–40
minutes.
14. Sprinkle with grated
cheese.
15. Bake 10 minutes more,
until cheese is melted.

Exchange List Values
• Starch 1.0   • Lean Meat 3.0
• Carbohydrate 0.5

Basic Nutritional Values
• Calories 245   • Sodium 590 mg
  (Calories from Fat 65)   • Potassium 455 gm
• Total Fat 7 gm   • Total Carb 25 gm
  (Saturated Fat 1.8 gm,   • Dietary Fiber 2 gm
  Trans Fat 0.0 gm,   • Sugars 5 gm
  Polyunsat Fat 1.8 gm,   • Protein 21 gm
  Monounsat Fat 2.2 gm)   • Phosphorus 215 gm
• Cholesterol 45 mg

Really Great Chicken 'n' Chips

Jean Harris Robinson
Pemberton, NJ

*Makes 6 servings,
5–6 oz. per serving*

Prep. Time: 30 minutes
Baking Time: 30 minutes

2 Tbsp. olive oil
3 Tbsp. chopped green bell pepper
1 small onion, minced
¼ cup flour
1 cup lower-sodium, fat-free chicken broth
1 cup fat-free half-and-half
½ tsp. salt
½ tsp. pepper
¼ tsp. dried thyme
2 cups coarsely crushed baked potato chips
2 cups cubed cooked chicken, *divided*
¼ cup freshly grated Parmesan cheese

1. Place oil in saucepan.
2. Stir in green pepper and onion. Cook until soft.
3. Blend in flour. Slowly add chicken broth and cream.
4. Cook until mixture boils and thickens, stirring constantly.
5. Stir in salt, pepper, and thyme.
6. Grease a 2½- 3-quart casserole.
7. Arrange potato chips in bottom of casserole.
8. Spread 1 cup chicken over chips.
9. Top with half of sauce.

10. Top with remaining chicken.
11. Top with rest of sauce.
12. Sprinkle top with cheese.
13. Bake at 350° for about 30 minutes, or until casserole is browned, bubbly, and heated through.

Exchange List Values
- Starch 1.0
- Fat 1.0
- Lean Meat 2.0

Basic Nutritional Values
- Calories 235
- (Calories from Fat 90)
- Total Fat 10 gm
- (Saturated Fat 2.3 gm,
- Trans Fat 0.0 gm,
- Polyunsat Fat 1.7 gm,
- Monounsat Fat 5.0 gm)
- Cholesterol 45 mg
- Sodium 465 mg
- Potassium 345 gm
- Total Carb 17 gm
- Dietary Fiber 1 gm
- Sugars 4 gm
- Protein 17 gm
- Phosphorus 200 gm

Chicken Au Gratin

Joy Martin
Myerstown, PA

*Makes 6 servings,
about 6 oz. per serving*

Prep. Time: 10 minutes
Cooking/Baking Time: 30 minutes

2 cups cooked fresh *or* frozen green beans, *or* peas
2 cups diced cooked chicken

10¾-oz. can lower-sodium, lower-fat cream of chicken soup
¼ cup water
¼ tsp. salt
dash of pepper
2½ Tbsp. tub margarine, no trans-fat
2 cups soft bread cubes
½ cup 75%-less fat shredded cheddar cheese

1. Put beans and chicken in buttered shallow casserole dish.
2. In a mixing bowl, blend soup, water, and seasonings until smooth. Pour over chicken.
3. Melt margarine in saucepan. Remove from heat.
4. Mix cheese and bread cubes into margarine. Sprinkle on top of chicken and beans.
5. Bake at 350° for 30 minutes, or until browned, bubbly, and heated through-out.

Exchange List Values
- Starch 0.5
- Lean Meat 2.0
- Carbohydrate 0.5
- Fat 1.0

Basic Nutritional Values
- Calories 220
- (Calories from Fat 80)
- Total Fat 9 gm
- (Saturated Fat 2.4 gm,
- Trans Fat 0.0 gm,
- Polyunsat Fat 2.8 gm,
- Monounsat Fat 3.0 gm)
- Cholesterol 45 mg
- Sodium 495 mg
- Potassium 440 gm
- Total Carb 15 gm
- Dietary Fiber 2 gm
- Sugars 2 gm
- Protein 19 gm
- Phosphorus 175 gm

Don't be afraid to try new recipes, but learn some basic ones from cooks you trust.

Colleen Heatwole, Burton, MI

Chicken & Dumplings

Barbara Nolan
Pleasant Valley, NY

*Makes 8 servings,
about 9 oz. per serving*

Prep. Time: 15 minutes
Cooking Time: 30 minutes

4 carrots, cut into ½"-thick
   slices
2 medium onions, cut into
   eighths
1 clove garlic, sliced thin
3 celery ribs, cut into
   ½"-thick slices
2 Tbsp. canola oil
3 Tbsp. flour
2 14-oz. cans lower-sodium,
   fat-free chicken broth
1 lb. uncooked chicken
   cutlets, cut into 1" cubes
2 Tbsp. grated carrots
½ tsp. poultry seasoning
¼ tsp. garlic powder
⅛ tsp. black pepper
¼ cup half-and-half
fresh parsley, snipped, for
   garnish

Dumplings:
   1½ cups flour
   2 tsp. baking powder
   ½ tsp. salt
   1 cup milk
   1 egg
   2 Tbsp. vegetable oil

1. Sauté carrot pieces,
onions, garlic , and celery in
oil in medium saucepan for 3
minutes, or until vegetables
soften
2. Sprinkle with flour.

3. Stir to combine. Cook
1–2 minutes.
4. Stir in chicken broth,
chicken, grated carrots,
poultry seasoning, garlic
powder, and pepper until
smooth.
5. Bring to boil. Simmer 5
minutes, or until thickened,
stirring constantly.
6. To prepare dumplings,
mix together flour, baking
powder, and salt in mixing
bowl.
7. In a separate bowl,
combine milk, egg, and oil.
8. Add egg-milk mixture
to dry ingredients, barely
mixing.
9. Drop dumpling batter by
tablespoonfuls onto simmering chicken.
10. Cook 10 minutes
uncovered.
11. Then cover and cook an
additional 10 minutes.
12. Pour half-and-half
between dumplings into
broth.
13. Scatter fresh parsley
over top. Serve immediately.

Tip:
   Chop all veggies and
chicken beforehand and
refrigerate until you're ready
to make the dish. Doing so
makes it very fast to prepare
this dish.

Warm Memories:
   When my nephew was
in college, he used to come
to our place and enjoy this
dish. He often brought a few
hungry roommates along.
Now that he's married, this
is one of his family's favorite
dishes.

Exchange List Values
- Starch 1.5   • Lean Meat 1.0
- Vegetable 1.0 • Fat 1.5

Basic Nutritional Values
- Calories 260   • Sodium 565 mg
  (Calories from Fat 90) • Potassium 430 gm
- Total Fat 10 gm   • Total Carb 30 gm
  (Saturated Fat 1.7 gm, • Dietary Fiber 3 gm
  Trans Fat 0.0 gm,   • Sugars 6 gm
  Polyurisat Fat 2.6 gm, • Protein 12 gm
  Monounsat Fat 5.4 gm) • Phosphorus 270 gm
- Cholesterol 45 mg

Chicken Pie

Lavina Ebersol
Ronks, PA

*Makes 8 servings,
2¾"×3½" rectangle per serving*

Prep. Time: 45 minutes
Baking Time: 45 minutes

Filling:
   2 Tbsp. canola oil
   3 Tbsp. flour
   ¼ tsp. salt
   ⅛ tsp. pepper
   1 sodium-free chicken
      bouillon cube
   2 cups fat-free milk
   12-oz. pkg. frozen
      vegetables, including
      nonstarchy veggies like
      broccoli and peppers
   1 cup chopped cooked
      chicken

Biscuit topping:
   2 cups flour
   3 tsp. baking powder
   ¾ tsp. salt
   1 tsp. paprika
   ⅓ cup tub margarine, no
      trans-fat
   ⅔ cup fat-free milk

1. Heat oil in saucepan. Stir in flour, salt, pepper, and bouillon cube.

2. Remove from heat and gradually stir in milk.

3. Return to heat. Cook, stirring constantly until smooth and slightly thickened.

4. Add vegetables and chicken to sauce.

5. In good-sized mixing bowl, stir together flour, baking powder, salt, and paprika.

6. Cut in margarine with pastry cutter, or 2 forks, until mixture resembles small peas.

7. Stir in milk until mixture forms ball.

8. Roll out dough on lightly floured surface into 8×12 rectangle.

9. Fold dough lightly into quarters. Lift onto top of chicken mixture.

10. Unfold dough and center over greased 7×11 baking dish. Pinch dough around edges of baking dish. Cut slits in dough to allow steam to escape.

11. Bake at 350° for 45 minutes, or until pie is bubbly and crust is browned.

Exchange List Values
- Starch 2.5   • Fat 1.5
- Lean Meat 1.0

Basic Nutritional Values
- Calories 295   • Sodium 545 mg
  (Calories from Fat 100) • Potassium 350 gm
- Total Fat 11 gm   • Total Carb 36 gm
  (Saturated Fat 1.9 gm,   • Dietary Fiber 3 gm
  Trans Fat 0.0 gm,   • Sugars 6 gm
  Polyunsat Fat 3.8 gm,   • Protein 13 gm
  Monounsat Fat 4.5 gm)   • Phosphorus 350 gm
- Cholesterol 15 mg

Chicken Noodle Casserole

Leesa DeMartyn
Enola, PA

*Makes 6 servings,
7–8 oz. per serving*

Prep. Time: 15–20 minutes
Baking Time: 30 minutes

1 Tbsp. canola oil
¼ cup chopped onions
¼ cup chopped green bell pepper
8-oz. pkg. egg noodles, cooked and drained
2 cups cooked and cubed chicken
1 medium tomato, peeled and chopped
1 Tbsp. lemon juice
¼ tsp. salt
¼ tsp. pepper
½ cup fat-free mayonnaise
⅓ cup fat-free milk
⅓ cup shredded reduced-fat cheddar cheese
bread crumbs, *optional*

1. Melt butter in small skillet over medium heat.

2. Sauté onions and peppers about 5 minutes.

3. In large mixing bowl, combine sautéed vegetables with cooked noodles, chicken, tomato, lemon juice, salt, pepper, mayonnaise, and milk.

4. Turn into greased 2-quart casserole.

5. Top with cheese and bread crumbs if you wish.

6. Cover with foil. Bake at 400° for 20–25 minutes, until heated through.

7. Let baked dish stand 10 minutes before serving to allow sauce to thicken.

Exchange List Values
- Starch 2.0   • Fat 1.0
- Lean Meat 2.0

Basic Nutritional Values
- Calories 290   • Sodium 360 mg
  (Calories from Fat 90)   • Potassium 260 gm
- Total Fat 10 gm   • Total Carb 30 gm
  (Saturated Fat 2.4 gm,   • Dietary Fiber 2 gm
  Trans Fat 0.0 gm,   • Sugars 4 gm
  Polyunsat Fat 2.1 gm,   • Protein 20 gm
  Monounsat Fat 3.6 gm)   • Phosphorus 230 gm
- Cholesterol 75 mg

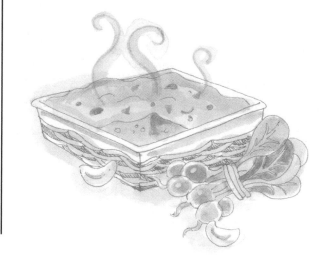

Favorite Enchilada Casserole

Janice Muller
Derwood, MD

Makes 8 servings,
3¼"×4½" rectangle per serving

Prep. Time: 20 minutes
Baking Time: 30 minutes

1 lb. 7%-fat ground turkey
2 onions, chopped
1 red, *or* green, bell
  pepper, chopped
¾ cup beef gravy
1 cup water
1 tsp. reduced-sodium beef
  bouillon granules
10½-oz. can mild
  enchilada sauce
7-oz. can pitted black
  olives, *divided*
12 corn tortillas
1 cup 75%-less fat
  shredded cheddar
  cheese, *divided*

1. In large nonstick skillet,
brown ground turkey with
onions and bell pepper, until
meat is no longer pink and
vegetables are just-tender.
Drain off any drippings.

2. In saucepan, heat gravy,
water, beef bouillon granules
and enchilada sauce together.

3. Into a well-greased
9×13 baking pan layer 6 of
the tortillas, half the turkey
mixture, half the olives,
half the sauce, and half the
cheese.

4. Repeat layers.

5. Bake at 350° for 30
minutes.

Exchange List Values
- Starch 1.0
- Vegetable 2.0
- Lean Meat 2.0
- Fat 1.0

Basic Nutritional Values
- Calories 260
  (Calories from Fat 80)
- Total Fat 9 gm
  (Saturated Fat 2.5 gm,
  Trans Fat 0.1 gm,
  Polyunsat Fat 2.2 gm,
  Monounsat Fat 3.3 gm)
- Cholesterol 50 mg
- Sodium 590 mg
- Potassium 465 gm
- Total Carb 26 gm
- Dietary Fiber 4 gm
- Sugars 3 gm
- Protein 19 gm
- Phosphorus 320 gm

Turkey Barbecue Wonder

Erma Martin
East Earl, PA

Janet Derstine
Telford, PA

Makes 8 servings,
about 3–4 oz. per serving

Prep. Time: 10 minutes
Cooking Time: 15 minutes

1 celery rib, chopped
1 medium onion, chopped
¼ cup chopped green bell
  pepper
1 Tbsp. oil
¼ cup brown sugar
¼ cup ketchup
¼ cup picante sauce
2 Tbsp. Worcestershire
  sauce
1½ tsp. chili powder
½ tsp. salt
⅓ tsp. pepper
dash of cayenne pepper
4 cups shredded, *or* cubed,
  cooked turkey

1. In a large skillet, sauté
celery, onion, and green
pepper in oil until tender.

2. Stir in brown sugar,
ketchup, picante sauce,
Worcestershire sauce, chili
powder, salt, pepper, and
cayenne pepper.

3. Bring to a boil. Reduce
heat and simmer uncovered
3–4 minutes.

4. Add turkey. Simmer
10 minutes longer, or until
heated through.

5. Serve on buns.

Exchange List Values
- Carbohydrate 0.5
- Lean Meat 3.0

Basic Nutritional Values
- Calories 175
  (Calories from Fat 45)
- Total Fat 5 gm
  (Saturated Fat 1.3 gm,
  Trans Fat 0.0 gm,
  Polyunsat Fat 1.6 gm,
  Monounsat Fat 1.9 gm)
- Cholesterol 55 mg
- Sodium 395 mg
- Potassium 360 gm
- Total Carb 10 gm
- Dietary Fiber 1 gm
- Sugars 8 gm
- Protein 21 gm
- Phosphorus 165 gm

In the fall when peppers are plentiful, chop them and freeze them in a single layer on cookie sheets. After they're frozen, store in freezer bags. We eat lots of this healthy vegetable when they are so handy for soups and casseroles.

Ann Good, Dayton, VA

Turkey and Green Bean Casserole

Melva Baumer
Mifflintown, PA

*Makes 6 servings,
about 10 oz. per serving*

Prep. Time: 35–40 minutes
Baking Time: 30–40 minutes

2 lbs. frozen French-style
  green beans
2 Tbsp. tub margarine,
  no trans-fat
3 Tbsp. flour
¼ tsp. salt
dash of pepper
½ tsp. prepared mustard
1½ cups fat-free milk
½ cup low-fat mayonnaise
1½-2 Tbsp. lemon juice
4 cups cooked turkey, cubed
½ cup freshly grated
  Parmesan cheese

1. Cook beans according to package directions. Drain.
2. Melt margarine in saucepan. Blend in flour, salt, pepper, and mustard.
3. Over low heat, add milk, stirring constantly until mixture is smooth and thickened.
4. Remove from heat. Fold in mayonnaise and lemon juice.
5. Stir in turkey.
6. Spread beans in greased shallow baking dish.
7. Spoon turkey sauce over top of beans.
8. Sprinkle with Parmesan cheese.
9. Bake at 350° for 30–40 minutes, or until bubbly and heated through.

Exchange List Values
- Carbohydrate 0.5
- Vegetable 2.0
- Lean Meat 4.0
- Fat 0.5

Basic Nutritional Values
- Calories 290
(Calories from Fat 90)
- Total Fat 10 gm
(Saturated Fat 3.0 gm,
Trans Fat 0.0 gm,
Polyunsat Fat 3.4 gm,
Monounsat Fat 2.5 gm)
- Cholesterol 75 mg
- Sodium 450 mg
- Potassium 610 gm
- Total Carb 18 gm
- Dietary Fiber 4 gm
- Sugars 6 gm
- Protein 33 gm
- Phosphorus 335 gm

Jumbulias

Lilli Unrau
Selkirk, Manitoba

*Makes 8 servings,
about ¾ cup per serving*

Prep. Time: 15 minutes
Cooking Time: 1 hour

2 Tbsp. no-trans-fat tub
  margarine
⅓ cup chopped green
  pepper
½ cup chopped onion
1 clove garlic, minced
3 cups water
1½ cups uncooked rice
2 cups cubed, cooked
  turkey
2 tsp. salt
dash pepper
2 tsp. Worcestershire sauce
4-oz. can mushroom
  pieces, drained

1. Melt margarine in large saucepan. Add green pepper, onion and garlic. Cook about 10 minutes or until tender. Add water and bring to a boil.
2. Add rice and cover saucepan. Reduce heat to simmer.
3. Cook about 25 minutes or until rice is done.
4. Add meat, salt, pepper, Worcestershire sauce and mushrooms.
5. Simmer over low heat until flavors are blended, about 15 minutes. Serve.

Exchange List Values
- Starch 2.0
- Lean Meat 2.0

Basic Nutritional Values
- Calories 230
(Calories from Fat 35)
- Total Fat 4 gm
(Saturated Fat 1.1 gm,
Trans Fat 0.0 gm,
Polyunsat Fat 1.5 gm,
Monounsat Fat 1.1 gm)
- Cholesterol 25 mg
- Sodium 395 mg
- Potassium 200 gm
- Total Carb 33 gm
- Dietary Fiber 1 gm
- Sugars 1 gm
- Protein 14 gm
- Phosphorus 135 gm

Spinach Meatloaf

Ellie Oberholtzer
Ronks, PA

Makes 6 servings, 1 slice per serving

Prep. Time: 25 minutes
Baking Time: 60 minutes
Standing Time: 10 minutes

1 lb. lean ground turkey, 93% lean
10-oz. box frozen chopped spinach, thawed and squeezed dry
¼ cup chopped fresh cilantro, *or fresh parsley*
2 oz. crumbled fat-free feta cheese
2 Tbsp. molasses
¼ cup egg substitute
3 pieces millet, *or other whole-grain, bread, toasted and crumbled*
1–2 tsp. poultry seasoning
¼ tsp. salt
¼ tsp. pepper

1. In a large bowl, mix together turkey, spinach, cilantro, cheese, molasses, egg, bread crumbs, poultry seasoning, salt, and pepper.
2. Form mixture into a loaf.
3. Place in greased loaf pan.
4. Bake at 350° for 60 minutes.
5. Allow to stand 10 minutes before slicing and serving.

Tips:
Instead of mixing the spinach into the loaf, sometimes I pat the meat mixture into a rectangular shape, about ½" thick, onto a piece of waxed paper. I spread the spinach on top, in about ½" from all the edges. I press the spinach down to make it adhere. Then, using the waxed paper to lift the meat, I roll it into a loaf, taking care to keep the spinach from falling out. Remove waxed paper. Then bake as directed above.

Exchange List Values
• Carbohydrate 1.0 • Lean Meat 3.0

Basic Nutritional Values
• Calories 195
(Calories from Fat 65)
• Total Fat 7 gm
(Saturated Fat 1.7 gm,
Trans Fat 0.1 gm,
Polyunsat Fat 2.2 gm,
Monounsat Fat 2.2 gm)
• Cholesterol 55 mg
• Sodium 405 mg
• Potassium 430 gm
• Total Carb 14 gm
• Dietary Fiber 2 gm
• Sugars 5 gm
• Protein 21 gm
• Phosphorus 225 gm

Hot Turkey Salad

Mary Herr and Elsie Lehman
Three Rivers, MI

Makes 15 servings,
a 3" square per serving

Prep. Time: 25 minutes
Baking Time: 45 minutes

4 cups cubed, cooked turkey
4 cups chopped celery
1 cup chopped almonds, blanched
¾ cup chopped green pepper
¼ cup chopped pimento
¼ cup chopped onion
1½ tsp. salt
¼ cup lemon juice
¾ cup low-fat mayonnaise
2 oz. shredded reduced-fat Swiss cheese
1 cup cracker crumbs
cooking spray

1. In a large bowl combine turkey, celery, almonds, green pepper, pimento, onion, salt, lemon juice and mayonnaise.
2. Spoon into greased 9×13 baking pan. Top with slices of cheese.
3. In small bowl combine cracker crumbs with 2 sprays of cooking spray. Sprinkle over turkey salad.
4. Bake at 350° for about 45 minutes.

Exchange List Values
• Carbohydrate 0.5 • Fat 0.5
• Lean Meat 2.0

Basic Nutritional Values
• Calories 155
(Calories from Fat 65)
• Total Fat 7 gm
(Saturated Fat 1.5 gm,
Trans Fat 0.0 gm,
Polyunsat Fat 2.1 gm,
Monounsat Fat 3.0 gm)
• Cholesterol 30 mg
• Sodium 455 mg
• Potassium 275 gm
• Total Carb 9 gm
• Dietary Fiber 2 gm
• Sugars 2 gm
• Protein 15 gm
• Phosphorus 150 gm

Deep-colored fruits and vegetables — orange, dark green, blue, red — often provide more vitamins and minerals than lighter-colored ones.

Turkey Supreme

Janet Suderman
Indianapolis, IN

Makes 6 servings,
about 1 cup per serving

Prep. Time: 15 minutes
Cooking Time: about 20 minutes

**2 cups sliced fresh
mushrooms**
1 small onion, chopped
1 cup thinly sliced celery
**10¾-oz. can lower-sodium,
lower-fat cream of
chicken soup**
1 cup fat-free milk
**2 cups cubed, cooked
turkey**
**2 cups herb-flavored
stuffing**
½ cup fat-free sour cream
¼-½ tsp. pepper
¼ cup sliced almonds

1. Combine mushrooms, onion and celery in 2-quart microwave-safe casserole dish.

2. Microwave on high, uncovered, 5–6 minutes or until vegetables are tender, stirring once.

3. Remove from microwave and add soup, milk, turkey, stuffing, sour cream and pepper. Top with sliced almonds.

4. Cover and microwave on high 10–12 minutes or until heated through. Let stand about 5 minutes before serving.

Exchange List Values
• Starch 1.0   • Lean Meat 2.0
• Carbohydrate 1.0

Basic Nutritional Values
• Calories 250
(Calories from Fat 55)
• Total Fat 6 gm
(Saturated Fat 1.5 gm,
Trans Fat 0.0 gm,
Polyunsat Fat 1.7 gm,
Monounsat Fat 2.2 gm)
• Cholesterol 40 mg
• Sodium 530 mg
• Potassium 690 gm
• Total Carb 28 gm
• Dietary Fiber 3 gm
• Sugars 6 gm
• Protein 20 gm
• Phosphorus 245 gm

Italian Sausage and White Beans

Lucille Amos
Greensboro, NC

Makes 8 servings,
about 6½ oz. per serving

Prep. Time: 15 minutes
Cooking/Baking Time: 3 hours

1 Tbsp. olive oil
1 cup chopped onion
**12-oz. pkg. 95%-fat-free
turkey kielbasa sausage**
**4½ cups cooked great
northern beans (from
approximately 2 cups
dry beans)**
14½-oz. can diced tomatoes
**1 cup red wine *or* beef
broth**
**1 tsp. Italian seasoning,
salt-free**
1 tsp. chopped garlic
½ tsp. black pepper
**⅓ cup cooked, crumbled
bacon**

1. Sauté onions in olive oil in skillet until softened. Set aside.

2. Cut sausages in ½-inch slices.

3. Put onions and sausages in casserole dish or Dutch oven.

4. Add beans, tomatoes, wine, or broth, Italian seasoning, garlic and black pepper. Mix gently.

5. Bake covered at 325° for 2 hours.

6. Remove lid. Stir. Return to oven, uncovered, for 20–40 minutes, until liquid is reduced to your preference.

7. Sprinkle top with bacon. Check seasonings. Serve.

Tip:
You can make this in a slow cooker. Combine everything except bacon in a slow cooker on high for 4–6 hours.

Exchange List Values
• Starch 1.5   • Lean Meat 2.0
• Vegetable 1.0   • Fat 0.5

Basic Nutritional Values
• Calories 265
(Calories from Fat 55)
• Total Fat 6 gm
(Saturated Fat 2.0 gm,
Trans Fat 0.0 gm,
Polyunsat Fat 0.9 gm,
Monounsat Fat 2.7 gm)
• Cholesterol 35 mg
• Sodium 580 mg
• Potassium 650 gm
• Total Carb 28 gm
• Dietary Fiber 8 gm
• Sugars 5 gm
• Protein 17 gm
• Phosphorus 280 gm

Sweet and Sour Sausage Stir-Fry

Colleen Heatwole
Burton, WI

Makes 6 servings

***Prep. Time:* 20 minutes
Cooking Time: 15 minutes**

¾ lb. 95%-reduced-fat
   turkey kielbasa, cut into
   ½"-thick slices
½–¾ cup chopped onion
1 cup shredded carrots
8-oz. can unsweetened
   pineapple chunks, *or*
   tidbits
1 Tbsp. cornstarch
½-1 tsp. ground ginger
6 Tbsp. water
⅔ tsp. lower-sodium
   soy sauce
2 cups hot cooked brown
   rice

1. In large nonstick skillet,
stir-fry sausage 3–4 minutes,
or until lightly browned.
2. Add onions and carrots.
Stir-fry until crisp-tender.
3. Drain pineapple, reserving juice. Add pineapple to
sausage-vegetable mixture.
4. In small bowl, combine
cornstarch and ginger. Stir in
water, soy sauce, and reserved
pineapple juice until smooth.
5. Add sauce to skillet.
6. Bring to boil. Cook, stirring continually 1–2 minutes,
or until sauce is thickened.
7. Serve over rice (⅓ cup
rice per serving).

Tip:
   You can double everything
in the recipe except the meat,
and it is still excellent.

Exchange List Values
• Starch 1.0   • Lean Meat 1.0
• Fruit 0.5   • Fat 0.5
• Vegetable 1.0

Basic Nutritional Values
• Calories 215   • Sodium 595 mg
  (Calories from Fat 30) • Potassium 260 gm
• Total Fat 4 gm   • Total Carb 28 gm
  (Saturated Fat 1.7 gm, • Dietary Fiber 2 gm
  Trans Fat 0.0 gm,   • Sugars 8 gm
  Polyunsat Fat 0.8 gm, • Protein 11 gm
  Monounsat Fat 1.2 gm) • Phosphorus 170 gm
• Cholesterol 40 mg

Smoked Sausage and Sauerkraut

Joan Terwilliger
Lebanon, PA

Makes 8 servings

***Prep. Time:* 20 minutes
Baking Time: 1¾-2 hours**

2 Tbsp. no-trans-fat tub
   margarine
3 apples, peeled, halved,
   thickly sliced
1 large sweet onion,
   halved, thickly sliced
1½ lbs. (about 4) Yukon
   Gold potatoes, peeled,
   cut in ½" cubes
¼ cup Splenda Brown
   Sugar Blend
1½ Tbsp. Dijon mustard
½ lb. 95%-fat-free turkey
   kielbasa, sliced ½" thick
1 cup apple cider, *or*
   Riesling
1 lb. sauerkraut, rinsed
   and drained

1. Melt butter in large
oven-proof Dutch oven over
medium-high heat.
2. Sauté apples and onions
10 minutes in butter, stirring
occasionally.
3. Add potatoes.
4. In small bowl, mix
together Splenda and
mustard. Add to onion-potato
mixture.
5. Place kielbasa slices on
top of onion-potato mixture.
6. Pour in cider or wine.
7. Place sauerkraut on top
of sausage.
8. Bake, covered, at 350°
for 1¾-2 hours, or until
potatoes are tender.

Exchange List Values
• Starch 1.0   • Lean Meat 1.0
• Fruit 0.5   • Fat 0.5
• Vegetable 1.0

Basic Nutritional Values
• Calories 200   • Sodium 600 mg
  (Calories from Fat 35) • Potassium 435 gm
• Total Fat 4 gm   • Total Carb 32 gm
  (Saturated Fat 1.3 gm, • Dietary Fiber 3 gm
  Trans Fat 0.0 gm,   • Sugars 12 gm
  Polyunsat Fat 1.2 gm, • Protein 7 gm
  Monounsat Fat 1.3 gm) • Phosphorus 105 gm
• Cholesterol 20 mg

Polish Reuben Casserole

Jean Heyerly, Shipshewana, IN

Makes 12 servings,
3" square per serving

Prep. Time: 25–30 minutes
Baking Time: 1 hour

2 10¾-oz. cans lower-
   sodium, lower-fat cream
   of mushroom soup
1⅓ cups milk
1 Tbsp. prepared mustard
½ cup chopped onion
8 oz. sauerkraut (half of a
   16-oz. can), rinsed and
   drained
2 cups shredded green
   cabbage
8-oz. pkg. uncooked
   medium-width noodles
12 oz. 95%-fat-free turkey
   kielbasa, cut in ½"-thick
   slices
1 cup reduced-fat shredded
   Swiss cheese
¾ cup whole wheat panko
   bread crumbs

1. Mix soup, milk, mustard,
and onion in a bowl. Set aside.
2. Mix sauerkraut and
cabbage. Spread mixture in
well-greased 9×13 baking dish.
3. Top with uncooked
noodles.
4. Spoon soup mixture
evenly over noodles.
5. Top with sliced kielbasa.
6. Sprinkle with shredded
cheese.
7. Sprinkle panko on top of
cheese.
8. Cover with foil and bake

at 350° for 1 hour, or until
noodles are tender.

Exchange List Values
- Starch 1.0   • Med-Fat Meat 1.0
- Carbohydrate 1.0

Basic Nutritional Values
- Calories 220   • Sodium 580 mg
  (Calories from Fat 45) • Potassium 555 gm
- Total Fat 5 gm   • Total Carb 27 gm
  (Saturated Fat 2.2 gm,   • Dietary Fiber 2 gm
  Trans Fat 0.0 gm,   • Sugars 5 gm
  Polyunsat Fat 1.0 gm,   • Protein 13 gm
  Monounsat Fat 1.4 gm)   • Phosphorus 220 gm
- Cholesterol 50 mg

Sausage Scalloped Potatoes

Karen Waggoner
Joplin, MO

Makes 6 servings,
about 7 oz. per serving

Prep. Time: 20 minutes
Cooking Time: 30–35 minutes
Standing Time: 5 minutes

12 oz. 95%-fat-free turkey
   kielbasa, cut into
   ¼"-thick slices
2 Tbsp. canola oil
2 Tbsp. flour
¼ tsp. pepper
2 cups fat-free milk
4 medium red potatoes,
   halved and thinly sliced,
   enough to make 3½–4 cups
¼ cup onions, chopped
2 Tbsp. minced fresh
   parsley, *optional*

1. Place sausage in microwave-safe dish. Microwave

uncovered on high for
3 minutes. Set aside.
2. Place oil in 2½-quart
microwave-safe dish. Microwave on high 45–60 seconds,
or until melted.
3. Whisk flour, salt, and
pepper into butter until
smooth.
4. Gradually whisk in milk.
5. Microwave on high 8–10
minutes until thickened,
stirring every 2 minutes.
6. Stir potatoes and onions
into creamy sauce.
7. Cover. Microwave on
high 4 minutes. Stir.
8. Microwave on high 4
minutes longer.
9. Stir in sausage. Cover.
10. Microwave 8–10
minutes on high, stirring
every 4 minutes. Continue
until potatoes are tender and
sausage is heated through.
Stir.
11. Let stand, covered, 5
minutes.
12. Sprinkle with parsley
and serve.

Exchange List Values
- Starch 1.5   • Lean Meat 2.0
- Carbohydrate 0.5   • Fat 0.5

Basic Nutritional Values
- Calories 270   • Sodium 600 mg
  (Calories from Fat 70) • Potassium 855 gm
- Total Fat 8 gm   • Total Carb 29 gm
  (Saturated Fat 1.9 gm,   • Dietary Fiber 2 gm
  Trans Fat 0.0 gm,   • Sugars 7 gm
  Polyunsat Fat 1.9 gm,   • Protein 15 gm
  Monounsat Fat 4.0 gm)   • Phosphorus 245 gm
- Cholesterol 40 mg

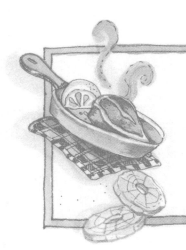

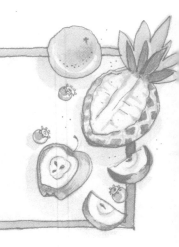

Pork Main Dishes

Gourmet Pork Chops

Elsie R. Russett, Fairbank, IA

*Makes 6 servings,
1 pork chop per serving*

*Prep. Time: 15–20 minutes
Baking Time: 60–75 minutes*

2 Tbsp. vegetable oil
2 Tbsp. flour
¼ tsp. salt
dash of pepper
6 loin pork chops, ½" thick
10½-oz. can lower-sodium,
  lower-fat cream of
  chicken soup
¾ cup water
1 tsp. ground ginger
1 tsp. dried rosemary,
  crushed
½ cup whole wheat panko
  bread crumbs

1. Place oil in good-sized skillet.
2. Combine flour, salt, and pepper in shallow but wide dish.
3. Dredge chops in mixture one at a time.
4. Place 2 or 3 chops in oil in skillet at a time, being careful not to crowd skillet. Brown chops over medium to high heat, 3–4 minutes on each side, until a browned crust forms.
5. As chops brown, place in well-greased 7×11 baking dish.
6. In bowl, combine soup, water, ginger, and rosemary.
7. Pour over chops.
8. Sprinkle with half the panko bread crumbs.
9. Cover. Bake at 350° for 50–60 minutes, or until chops are tender but not dry.
10. Uncover. Sprinkle with remaining panko bread crumbs.
11. Bake uncovered 10–15 minutes. Remove from oven and serve.

Exchange List Values
- Starch 1.0
- Fat 1.0
- Lean Meat 2.0

Basic Nutritional Values
- Calories 215
  (Calories from Fat 90)
- Total Fat 10 gm
  (Saturated Fat 2.3 gm,
  Trans Fat 0.0 gm,
  Polyunsat Fat 2.1 gm,
  Monounsat Fat 5.2 gm)
- Cholesterol 50 mg
- Sodium 315 mg
- Potassium 465 gm
- Total Carb 11 gm
- Dietary Fiber 1 gm
- Sugars 1 gm
- Protein 18 gm
- Phosphorus 130 gm

Men and children, as well as the women, should be encouraged to help with food preparations and clean-up. Church suppers provide excellent opportunities for working together and serving each other. Everyone should be included and involved.

Rachel Kauffman, Alto, MI

Pork Chops with Rice and Limas

Sandy Tinsler
Wauseon, OH

*Makes 6 servings,
about 3 oz. meat and
½ cup of the rest per serving*

*Prep. Time: 15 minutes
Baking Time: 1¼- 2½ hours*

1 cup uncooked rice
16-oz. pkg. frozen limas
1½ 10¾-oz. cans lower-sodium, lower-fat cream of mushroom soup, *divided*
6 bone-in pork chops, 2 lbs. total

1. Combine rice and limas with ½ can soup. Spoon into 8" baking dish. Top with uncooked pork chops and remaining soup.
2. Cover and bake at 325° for 1¼ hours or 275° for 2½ hours.

Exchange List Values
- Starch 3.0
- Lean Meat 3.0

Basic Nutritional Values
- Calories 390
  (Calories from Fat 70)
- Total Fat 8 gm
  (Saturated Fat 2.7 gm,
  Trans Fat 0.0 gm,
  Polyunsat Fat 1.3 gm,
  Monounsat Fat 3.1 gm)
- Cholesterol 65 mg
- Sodium 365 mg
- Potassium 1055 gm
- Total Carb 47 gm
- Dietary Fiber 6 gm
- Sugars 2 gm
- Protein 31 gm
- Phosphorus 275 gm

Pork Chops with Apple Stuffing

Arlene Yoder, Hartville, OH

*Makes 6 servings,
1 pork chop per serving*

*Prep. Time: 20 minutes
Cooking Time: 45–60 minutes*

6 bone-in pork chops, at least 1" thick, about 2 lbs. total
1 Tbsp. canola oil
¼ cup chopped celery
¼ cup chopped onion
3 apples, peeled, cored and diced
¼ cup sugar
½ cup bread crumbs, *or* cracker crumbs
¼ tsp. salt
¼ tsp. pepper
2 tsp. chopped parsley

1. Cut a pocket about 1½" deep into the side of each chop for stuffing.
2. Heat oil in skillet.
3. Stir celery and onion into oil in skillet. Cook over medium until tender, stirring frequently.
4. Stir in diced apples. Sprinkle with sugar.
5. Cover skillet. Cook apples over low heat until tender and glazed.
6. Stir in bread crumbs.
7. Stir in salt, pepper, and parsley.
8. Spreading open the pocket in each chop with your fingers, stuff with mixture.
9. Return half of stuffed chops to skillet. Brown on both sides over medium to high heat.
10. Remove browned chops to platter. Cover to keep warm.
11. Repeat Step 9 with remaining chops.
12. Return other chops to skillet.
13. Reduce heat. Add a few tablespoons of water.
14. Cover. Cook slowly over low heat until done, about 20–25 minutes.

Exchange List Values
- Carbohydrate 1.5
- Fat 0.5
- Lean Meat 3.0

Basic Nutritional Values
- Calories 270
  (Calories from Fat 80)
- Total Fat 9 gm
  (Saturated Fat 2.6 gm,
  Trans Fat 0.0 gm,
  Polyunsat Fat 1.3 gm,
  Monounsat Fat 4.3 gm)
- Cholesterol 65 mg
- Sodium 210 mg
- Potassium 370 gm
- Total Carb 24 gm
- Dietary Fiber 1 gm
- Sugars 16 gm
- Protein 24 gm
- Phosphorus 160 gm

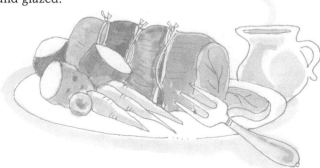

French Onion Pork Chop Skillet

Nadine Martinitz
Salina, KS

Makes 6 servings, 1 chop per serving

Prep. Time: 10 minutes
Cooking Time: 20–25 minutes

**6 boneless pork chops
(1½ lbs.), ½" thick
2 onions, thinly sliced
2 Tbsp. Worcestershire
sauce
6-oz. pkg. Stove Top
stuffing mix
1½ cups hot water**

1. Place half the chops in large nonstick skillet. Over medium to high heat, cook 10 minutes or until done, turning chops after 5 minutes.
2. Remove to platter and cover with foil to keep warm.
3. Repeat Steps 1 and 2 with remaining chops.
4. While chops are cooking, mix stuffing mix and hot water in bowl. Set aside.
5. Place onions in skillet. Cook over high heat, stirring frequently. Cook for 5 minutes, or until golden brown.
6. Stir in Worcestershire sauce.
7. Remove onions from skillet.
8. Return chops to skillet. Top with onion mixture.
9. Spoon stuffing around edge of skillet.
10. Cover and cook 5 minutes, or until cheese is melted.

Exchange List Values
- Starch 1.5
- Vegetable 1.0
- Lean Meat 3.0
- Fat 0.5

Basic Nutritional Values
- Calories 290
  (Calories from Fat 70)
- Total Fat 8 gm
  (Saturated Fat 2.6 gm,
  Trans Fat 0.0 gm,
  Polyunsat Fat 0.8 gm,
  Monounsat Fat 3.6 gm)
- Cholesterol 60 mg
- Sodium 495 mg
- Potassium 490 gm
- Total Carb 27 gm
- Dietary Fiber 2 gm
- Sugars 5 gm
- Protein 25 gm
- Phosphorus 230 gm

Pork Chop Casserole

Betty L. Moore
Plano, IL

*Makes 5 servings,
1 pork chop per serving*

Prep. Time: 15–20 minutes
Baking Time: 1 hour

**1–2 Tbsp. vegetable oil
5 bone-in pork chops,
totaling about 2 lbs.
3 Tbsp. flour
2 Tbsp. canola oil
5 cups thinly sliced potatoes,
from about 3–4 potatoes
3 cups sliced onions, from
about 2–3 onions
10¾-oz. can lower-sodium,
lower-fat cream of
mushroom soup
½ cup water**

1. Pour oil into skillet.
2. Place flour in shallow dish. Dredge chops in flour.

3. Two at a time, place chops in oil in skillet over medium-high heat. Do not crowd pan or chops will steam in their juices rather than browning.
4. Brown 2–3 minutes on each side, just until crust forms. Move browned chops to foil-covered dish and keep warm while browning rest of chops.
5. Place sliced potatoes and onions into well-greased 9×13 baking dish.
6. In a bowl, mix soup and water together until smooth.
7. Pour sauce over potatoes.
8. Place browned pork chops on top.
9. Bake, covered, at 350° for 45 minutes.
10. Remove cover from baking dish. Continue baking 15 minutes, or until lightly browned.

Exchange List Values
- Starch 1.5
- Carbohydrate 0.5
- Vegetable 1.0
- Lean Meat 4.0
- Fat 1.5

Basic Nutritional Values
- Calories 400
  (Calories from Fat 125)
- Total Fat 14 gm
  (Saturated Fat 3.4 gm,
  Trans Fat 0.0 gm,
  Polyunsat Fat 2.8 gm,
  Monounsat Fat 7.1 gm)
- Cholesterol 80 mg
- Sodium 275 mg
- Potassium 1455 gm
- Total Carb 35 gm
- Dietary Fiber 4 gm
- Sugars 6 gm
- Protein 31 gm
- Phosphorus 260 gm

Onions or garlic can increase the flavor of a dish without adding too many calories.

Pork Cutlets

Audrey Romonosky
Austin, TX

Makes 8 servings,
1 cutlet per serving

Prep. Time: 10 minutes
Cooking Time: 20–25 minutes

2 Tbsp. canola oil
½ cup egg substitute
½ cup milk
8 pork cutlets, about 4 oz.
  each, fat removed
salt and pepper
1½ cups seasoned bread
  crumbs
24½-oz. jar lower-sodium
  marinara sauce

1. Heat oil in large skillet.
2. Beat egg substitute and milk together in shallow dish.
3. Dip cutlets in egg mixture one by one.
4. Place bread crumbs in another shallow dish.
5. Dredge cutlets in bread crumbs. Discard leftover liquid and crumb mixtures.
6. Place cutlets in hot oil in skillet, one by one, being careful not to splash yourself.
7. Do not crowd skillet. Cook cutlets in 2 or 3 batches so that they brown and don't just steam in their own juices.
8. Cook each cutlet 3–3½ minutes per side, until browned.
9. Season each side of each cutlet with salt and pepper.
10. Place browned cutlets on a platter. Cover with foil while you cook the next batch.
11. Heat marinara sauce. Spoon over cooked cutlets.
12. Pass any additional sauce to ladle over individual servings.

Tips:
You can make this recipe using chicken cutlets instead.

Exchange List Values
- Starch 1.0
- Lean Meat 4.0
- Fat 1.5

Basic Nutritional Values
- Calories 335
  (Calories from Fat 145)
- Total Fat 16 gm
  (Saturated Fat 3.8 gm,
  Trans Fat 0.0 gm,
  Polyunsat Fat 3.3 gm,
  Monounsat Fat 6.9 gm)
- Cholesterol 70 mg
- Sodium 580 mg
- Potassium 660 gm
- Total Carb 19 gm
- Dietary Fiber 2 gm
- Sugars 5 gm
- Protein 27 gm
- Phosphorus 260 gm

Pork Tenderloin with Teriyaki Apricot Sauce

Jennifer Kuh
Bay Village, OH

Makes 12 servings,
about 3 oz. per serving

Prep. Time: 10 minutes
Marinating Time: 6–8 hours or
* overnight*
Grilling Time: 20–25 minutes
Standing Time: 10 minutes

3-lb. pork tenderloin
8- 12-oz. bottle light
  teriyaki sauce, *divided*
1 cup sugar-free apricot
  preserves

1. Place meat in nonmetallic pan.
2. Pour half bottle of teriyaki sauce over meat.
3. Cover. Marinade in fridge for 6–8 hours, or overnight.
4. Grill pork over medium heat, 10–12 minutes per side.
5. Meanwhile, mix preserves and 3 Tbsp. teriyaki sauce together in microwave-safe bowl.
6. Cover. Microwave until bubbly.
7. Place pork on serving platter after grilling. Pour bubbling sauce on top.
8. Allow to stand 10 minutes before cutting and serving.

Exchange List Values
- Carbohydrate 0.5
- Lean Meat 3.0

Basic Nutritional Values
- Calories 140
  (Calories from Fat 25)
- Total Fat 3 gm
  (Saturated Fat 1.0 gm,
  Trans Fat 0.0 gm,
  Polyunsat Fat 0.2 gm,
  Monounsat Fat 1.2 gm)
- Cholesterol 60 mg
- Sodium 290 mg
- Potassium 400 gm
- Total Carb 9 gm
- Dietary Fiber 0 gm
- Sugars 3 gm
- Protein 23 gm
- Phosphorus 220 gm

Ham-Potatoes-Green Bean Casserole

Sarah Miller
Harrisonburg, VA

Makes 12 servings,
3" square per serving

Prep. Time: 45 minutes
Baking Time: 30 minutes

3 Tbsp. no-trans-fat tub
   margarine
½ cup flour
3 cups fat-free milk
1¼ cups 50%-reduced fat
   grated cheddar cheese
5 medium-sized potatoes,
   cooked and sliced thin
2 lbs. fresh green beans
   with ends nipped off,
   or 2 16-oz. pkgs. frozen
   green beans, steamed
   or microwaved until
   just-tender
3 cups lower-sodium
   cooked, diced ham
1 cup panko bread crumbs

1. Melt margarine in
saucepan.
2. Stir in flour.
3. Gradually stir in milk.
Stir continually while cooking
over low heat until mixture
thickens.
4. Add cheese and stir until
it melts.
5. Arrange potatoes in well-
greased 9×13 baking dish.
6. Drain any liquid off
green beans. Spread beans
over potatoes.
7. Pour half of cheese sauce
over beans.

8. Spread ham over sauce.
9. Pour remaining sauce
over all.
10. Scatter panko crumbs
over casserole.
11. Bake at 350° for 30
minutes, or until heated
through.

Tips:
1. Instead of cooking
potatoes, you can use frozen
shredded potatoes, thawed.
2. To save more time, you
can use 2 15½-oz. cans green
beans, drained, instead of
fresh or frozen beans.

Exchange List Values
• Starch 1.5   • Lean Meat 2.0
• Vegetable 1.0

Basic Nutritional Values
• Calories 235   • Sodium 455 mg
  (Calories from Fat 55) • Potassium 565 gm
• Total Fat 6 gm   • Total Carb 31 gm
  (Saturated Fat 2.4 gm, • Dietary Fiber 4 gm
  Trans Fat 0.0 gm,   • Sugars 5 gm
  Polyunsat Fat 1.3 gm, • Protein 16 gm
  Monounsat Fat 2.1 gm) • Phosphorus 275 gm
• Cholesterol 25 mg

Scalloped Potatoes and Ham for a Crowd

Lydia Yoder
London, OH

Makes 70 servings,
about 7 oz. per serving

Prep. Time: 30 minutes
Cooking/Baking Time: 2 hours

20 lbs. potatoes, peeled
   and diced

7 lbs. lean, lower-sodium
   fully cooked ham, cut up
1 gallon milk, *divided*
1½ cups flour
1 tsp. pepper
1½ cups no-trans-fat tub
   margarine
1 lb. light reduced-fat
   Velveeta cheese

1. Place potatoes and ham
in a large roaster.
2. Take part of the milk
and make a thick paste with
the flour. Set aside.
3. Bring remaining milk
almost to boiling point. Add
flour paste, salt and pepper
and bring to a full boil. Add
butter and cheese and stir
until melted.
4. Pour cheese sauce over
ham and potatoes in roaster.
5. Bake at 450° for 30
minutes, reduce heat to 350°
and bake 30 minutes longer
or until done.

Exchange List Values
• Starch 2.0   • Fat 0.5
• Lean Meat 1.0

Basic Nutritional Values
• Calories 220   • Sodium 600 mg
  (Calories from Fat 55) • Potassium 570 gm
• Total Fat 6 gm   • Total Carb 26 gm
  (Saturated Fat 2.0 gm, • Dietary Fiber 2 gm
  Trans Fat 0.0 gm,   • Sugars 4 gm
  Polyunsat Fat 1.5 gm, • Protein 15 gm
  Monounsat Fat 2.3 gm) • Phosphorus 255 gm
• Cholesterol 30 mg

Ham Balls

Joette Droz
Kalona, IA

Makes 44 servings, 1 ball per serving

Prep. Time: 30 minutes
Baking Time: 1 hour

1¼ lbs. bulk reduced-fat
    pork sausage
2 lbs. lean, lower-sodium
    ground ham
1½ lbs. 95%-lean ground
    beef
¾ cup egg substitute
1 cup graham cracker
    crumbs
1 cup soda cracker crumbs
1½ cups fat-free milk

Glaze:
    10¾-oz. can lower-sodium,
    lower-fat tomato soup,
    undiluted
    ½-¾ cup vinegar
    ¾ cup Splenda Brown
    Sugar Blend
    ½-1 tsp. dry mustard

1. In a large bowl, combine sausage, ground ham, ground beef, egg substitute, cracker crumbs, and milk. Mix well. This is a lot of bulk, so mix either with well-washed hands, or with a hefty wooden spoon.
2. Form mixture into 44 balls, about ¼ cup each.
3. Arrange in well-greased 9×13 baking pan.
4. Bake balls at 350° for 1 hour (add glaze after 30 minutes).
5. Meanwhile, prepare glaze by mixing together soup, vinegar, brown sugar blend, and mustard in a mixing bowl.
6. Spread glaze over top after balls have baked 30 minutes.

Exchange List Values
• Carbohydrate 0.5   • Med-Fat Meat 1.0

Basic Nutritional Values
• Calories 115   • Sodium 335 mg
  (Calories from Fat 40)   • Potassium 210 gm
• Total Fat 4.5 gm   • Total Carb 8 gm
  (Saturated Fat 1.5 gm,   • Dietary Fiber 0 gm
  Trans Fat 0.1 gm,   • Sugars 3 gm
  Polyunsat Fat 0.6 gm,   • Protein 10 gm
  Monounsat Fat 1.9 gm)   • Phosphorus 100 gm
• Cholesterol 25 mg

Glazed Ham Balls

Teresa Koenig
Leola, PA
Dorothy Schrock
Arthur, IL

Makes 20 servings, 1 ball per serving

Prep. Time: 20 minutes
Baking Time: 50 minutes

8-oz. can (1 cup) crushed
    pineapple, undrained
2⅔ Tbsp. Splenda Brown
    Sugar Blend
1 Tbsp. vinegar
2–3 Tbsp. prepared
    mustard
1 lb. 50%-reduced-fat
    sausage
½ cup cooked lower-
    sodium ground ham
¾ cup bread crumbs, *or*
    crushed saltine crackers
½ cup egg substitute
½ cup ketchup, *or* milk
⅛ cup chopped onion
¼ tsp. pepper, *optional*

1. In a mixing bowl, mix together pineapple, Splenda, vinegar, and mustard. Set aside.
2. In a large mixing bowl, thoroughly combine sausage, ham, bread crumbs, egg substitute, ketchup, and onion.
3. Shape into 20 1½" balls. Place in well-greased shallow baking dish.
4. Spoon pineapple mixture over ham balls.
5. Cover. Bake at 350° for 25 minutes.
6. Uncover. Continue baking 25 more minutes.

Tip:
    You can freeze the balls, and then reheat them in the microwave. They're an easy meal after a long work day.

Exchange List Values
• Carbohydrate 0.5   • Fat 0.5
• Lean Meat 1.0

Basic Nutritional Values
• Calories 100   • Sodium 335 mg
  (Calories from Fat 35)   • Potassium 145 gm
• Total Fat 4 gm   • Total Carb 8 gm
  (Saturated Fat 1.4 gm,   • Dietary Fiber 0 gm
  Trans Fat 0.0 gm,   • Sugars 4 gm
  Polyunsat Fat 0.6 gm,   • Protein 7 gm
  Monounsat Fat 2.0 gm)   • Phosphorus 65 gm
• Cholesterol 15 mg

Fried Rice with Bacon

Millie Glick
Edmonton, Alberta

*Makes 12 servings,
about ⅔ cup per serving*

Prep. Time: 20 minutes
**Cooking Time: 1 hour and 20
  minutes**

2 cups uncooked brown rice
2 slices bacon
1 large onion, diced
8-oz. jar sliced water
  chestnuts, drained
2 Tbsp. lower-sodium light
  soy sauce

1. Cook the rice according
to directions. Do not add salt.
2. Cut bacon into small
pieces and fry in an electric
skillet. When nearly done,
add onion and sauté. Add
mushrooms and water
chestnuts and stir together
with bacon and onion.
3. Add cooked rice to
skillet and mix thoroughly.
Add soy sauce and continue
to stir until all ingredients
have blended.

Exchange List Values
• Starch 1.5   • Fat 0.5
• Vegetable 1.0

Basic Nutritional Values
• Calories 175   • Sodium 200 mg
  (Calories from Fat 40)   • Potassium 130 gm
• Total Fat 4.5 gm   • Total Carb 29 gm
  (Saturated Fat 1.5 gm,   • Dietary Fiber 3 gm
  Trans Fat 0.0 gm,   • Sugars 2 gm
  Polyunsat Fat 0.8 gm,   • Protein 5 gm
  Monounsat Fat 1.9 gm)   • Phosphorus 120 gm
• Cholesterol 5 mg

Chinese Dumplings

Jean Yan
Regina, Saskatchewan

*Makes 25 dumplings,
1 dumpling per serving*

Prep. Time: 35 minutes
Standing Time: 1 hour
Cooking Time: 7 minutes

½ lb. 96% lean ground pork
½ lb. 90% lean ground beef
2 small onions, finely
  chopped
1 Tbsp. finely chopped
  ginger root
3 cloves garlic, minced
½ tsp. salt
1 Tbsp. light reduced-
  sodium soy sauce
1 large egg
½ tsp. sugar
½ Tbsp. sesame oil
2 green onions, finely
  chopped
3 cups flour
1¼ cups water, room
  temperature

1. Combine ground pork,
beef, onions, ginger root,
garlic, salt, soy sauce, egg,
sugar, oil and green onions.
Set aside.
2. Put flour in a deep bowl.
Make a well and gradually
add water, working it into the
flour to make a soft dough.
3. Knead until smooth,
about 10 minutes. Cover with
a wet towel and set aside for
1 hour.
4. Divide dough into two
pieces. With palm of hand,
roll dough into long, narrow
roll, about 1½" in diameter.
5. Cut into ½" lengths. Roll
each piece into a 3" round.
6. Place 1 Tbsp. meat
mixture in center of each
round of dough. Pinch
edges together, sealing the
dumpling.
7. Boil in deep water in a
large pot for 7 minutes. Serve.

Exchange List Values
• Starch 1.0

Basic Nutritional Values
• Calories 90   • Sodium 85 mg
  (Calories from Fat 20)   • Potassium 80 gm
• Total Fat 2 gm   • Total Carb 12 gm
  (Saturated Fat 0.5 gm,   • Dietary Fiber 0 gm
  Trans Fat 0.0 gm,   • Sugars 0 gm
  Polyunsat Fat 0.3 gm,   • Protein 6 gm
  Monounsat Fat 0.7 gm)   • Phosphorus 55 gm
• Cholesterol 20 mg

*I love potlucks, but I find my children do
not care for the adventure of tasting new foods.
Managing two or three kids through a line can be
a headache for parents. I have found that taking
along large trays helps because one tray will hold
two or three plates plus utensils and cups.*
Melodie Davis, Harrisonburg, VA

Bubble and Squeak

Mrs. Anna Gingerich
Apple Creek, OH

Makes 8 servings

Prep. Time: 15–20 minutes
Cooking Time: 45 minutes

12 oz. reduced-fat bulk
 sausage
1 onion, diced
4 medium potatoes, sliced
 thin
½ head cabbage, sliced thin
⅓ cup vinegar, *optional*
cheese of your choice,
 sliced or grated, *optional*

1. Sauté onions and sausage together in a deep iron skillet until no pink remains in meat. Stir frequently to break up clumps of meat.

2. Stir in potatoes. Continue cooking over low heat until potatoes begin to become tender. Stir often to prevent sticking and burning, but let potatoes brown.

3. Stir in cut cabbage. Continue cooking until cabbage wilts and potatoes are tender.

4. Stir in vinegar if you wish. Cook a few minutes to blend flavors.

5. Cover contents of skillet with cheese if you wish. Let stand a few minutes until cheese melts.

Good Go-Alongs:
 Applesauce, coleslaw or salad

Exchange List Values
- Starch 1.0
- Vegetable 1.0
- Med-Fat Meat 1.0

Basic Nutritional Values
- Calories 185
 (Calories from Fat 55)
- Total Fat 6 gm
 (Saturated Fat 2.3 gm,
 Trans Fat 0.1 gm,
 Polyunsat Fat 0.9 gm,
 Monounsat Fat 3.0 gm)
- Cholesterol 20 mg
- Sodium 225 mg
- Potassium 540 gm
- Total Carb 22 gm
- Dietary Fiber 3 gm
- Sugars 4 gm
- Protein 9 gm
- Phosphorus 150 gm

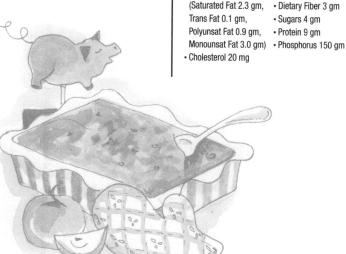

Sausage Sweet Potato Bake

Mary Hochstedler, Kokomo, IN
Cindy Gingerich, Jackson, MS

Makes 6 servings,
about ⅔ cup per serving

Prep. Time: 30 minutes
Cooking/Baking Time: 1 hour
and 10 minutes

10 oz. light pork sausage,
 50% less fat
2 medium raw sweet
 potatoes
3 medium apples
2 Tbsp. brown sugar
1 Tbsp. flour
¼ tsp. ground cinnamon
¼ tsp. salt
½ cup water

1. Brown sausage and drain excess fat.

2. Peel and slice potatoes and apples. Layer sausage, sweet potatoes and apples into 2-quart casserole dish.

3. Combine all other ingredients and pour over layers.

4. Cover and bake at 375° for 50–60 minutes or until done.

Exchange List Values
- Carbohydrate 1.5
- Med-Fat Meat 1.0

Basic Nutritional Values
- Calories 185
 (Calories from Fat 65)
- Total Fat 7 gm
 (Saturated Fat 2.5 gm,
 Trans Fat 0.1 gm,
 Polyunsat Fat 1.0 gm,
 Monounsat Fat 3.4 gm)
- Cholesterol 25 mg
- Sodium 340 mg
- Potassium 280 gm
- Total Carb 22 gm
- Dietary Fiber 2 gm
- Sugars 13 gm
- Protein 8 gm
- Phosphorus 85 gm

Hearty Farm Special

Emily Fox
Bethel, PA

Makes 6 servings

Prep. Time: 30 minutes
Baking Time: 70 minutes

9 oz. 50%-reduced-fat bulk
　sausage
2 cups chopped celery
1 medium onion, chopped
8-oz. can no-salt-added
　tomato sauce
½ cup water
2 Tbsp. prepared mustard
16-oz. can pork & beans
4 medium potatoes, peeled
　or unpeeled, sliced quite
　thin

1. In large nonstick sausage
cook sausage until no longer
pink. Stir frequently to break
up clumps of meat. Drain off
drippings.
　2. Add celery and onion.
Sauté until crisp-tender.
　3. Stir in tomato sauce,
water, mustard, and pork and
beans, and mustard. Cover.
Bring to boil.
　4. Stir in potato slices.
　5. Spoon into greased
3-quart casserole.
　6. Cover. Bake at 350°
for 60–70 minutes, or until
potatoes are tender.

Exchange List Values
- Starch 2.5
- Lean Meat 1.0
- Fat 1.0

Basic Nutritional Values
- Calories 295
　(Calories from Fat 80)
- Total Fat 9 gm
　(Saturated Fat 3.0 gm,
　Trans Fat 0.1 gm,
　Polyunsat Fat 1.2 gm,
　Monounsat Fat 3.7 gm)
- Cholesterol 30 mg
- Sodium 600 mg
- Potassium 885 gm
- Total Carb 39 gm
- Dietary Fiber 8 gm
- Sugars 9 gm
- Protein 14 gm
- Phosphorus 145 gm

Wild Rice Supper

Mamie Christopherson
Rio Rancho, NM

Makes 8 servings

Soaking Time: 8 hours, or
***　overnight***
Prep. Time: 20–30 minutes
Baking Time: 25 minutes

3 cups water
1 cup wild rice
½ lb. 50%-reduced-fat bulk
　sausage
1 finely chopped onion
½ lb. fresh mushrooms,
　sliced, *or* 8-oz. can sliced
　mushrooms, drained
¼ cup flour
¼ cup fat-free half-and-half
2½ cups fat-free lower-
　sodium chicken broth
dash of Tabasco sauce
½ tsp. dried oregano
½ tsp. dried thyme
½ tsp. dried marjoram

1. In good-sized bowl,
soak rice in water 8 hours, or
overnight.
　2. Pour rice and soaking
water into saucepan. Cover.
　3. Over medium heat, bring
to boil. Simmer, covered,
12–15 minutes, or until
tender.
　4. Meanwhile, sauté
sausage in large nonstick
skillet until no longer pink.
Stir often to break up clumps.
　5. Remove meat and keep
warm.
　6. Sauté onions and mushrooms in sausage drippings.
　7. Add sausage and rice to
skillet.
　8. In saucepan, combine
flour, cream, and chicken
broth. Cook over medium
heat, stirring continually until
mixture begins to boil and
thicken.
　9. Add Tabasco sauce,
oregano, thyme, and marjoram to saucepan.
　10. Add to sausage-rice
mixture and combine well.
　11. Spoon into well-greased
3-quart casserole dish.
　12. Cover. Bake at 375° for
25 minutes, or until bubbly
and heated through.

Exchange List Values
- Starch 1.0
- Med-Fat Meat 1.0

Basic Nutritional Values
- Calories 160
　(Calories from Fat 45)
- Total Fat 5 gm
　(Saturated Fat 1.9 gm,
　Trans Fat 0.1 gm,
　Polyunsat Fat 0.9 gm,
　Monounsat Fat 2.5 gm)
- Cholesterol 20 mg
- Sodium 335 mg
- Potassium 320 gm
- Total Carb 18 gm
- Dietary Fiber 2 gm
- Sugars 2 gm
- Protein 9 gm
- Phosphorus 140 gm

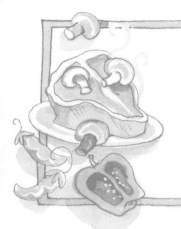
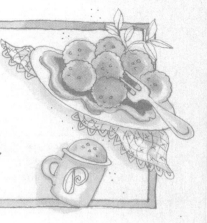

Beef
Main Dishes

Southern-Style Steak

Jeanette Oberholtzer
Lititz, PA

Makes 8 servings

Prep. Time: 20 minutes
Baking Time: 1 hour

2 lbs. lean round steak,
   ½" thick
2 Tbsp. canola oil
¼ cup flour
½ tsp. salt
¼ tsp. pepper
3 Tbsp. oil
¾ cup ketchup
¾ cup water
1 onion, thinly sliced
1 unpeeled orange, thinly
   sliced
1 unpeeled lemon, thinly
   sliced
6 whole cloves

1. Cut steak into 8 serving-size pieces.
2. Place oil in skillet.
3. Mix flour, salt, and pepper in a shallow bowl. Dredge steak pieces in mixture, pressing onto all sides of meat.
4. Place several pieces in skillet, over high heat, being careful not to crowd skillet so they brown rather than steam in each other's juices.
5. Remove pieces when browned on top and bottom and place in single layer in roaster.
6. Continue browning remaining pieces of meat and placing in roaster.
7. Combine ketchup and water in a small bowl. Pour over meat.
8. Arrange onion, orange, and lemon slices over meat. Dot with cloves.
9. Cover and bake at 350° for 1 hour, or just until tender.

Variation:
1. Add 1 tsp. dry mustard to flour, salt, and pepper in Step 3.
2. Instead of topping steak with orange and lemon slices and with whole cloves, top instead with a mixture of:

**14½-oz. can diced
   tomatoes with liquid
1 carrot, diced
1 tsp. brown sugar
2 tsp. Worcestershire
   sauce**

Jean Butzer
Batavia, NY

Exchange List Values
- Carbohydrate 1.0   • Fat 1.0
- Lean Meat 3.0

Basic Nutritional Values
- Calories 235
  (Calories from Fat 80)
- Total Fat 9 gm
  (Saturated Fat 2.2 gm,
  Trans Fat 0.2 gm,
  Polyunsat Fat 1.2 gm,
  Monounsat Fat 4.6 gm)
- Cholesterol 75 mg
- Sodium 430 mg
- Potassium 350 gm
- Total Carb 12 gm
- Dietary Fiber 1 gm
- Sugars 7 gm
- Protein 26 gm
- Phosphorus 175 gm

Tender Flank Steak

Kayla Snyder
North East, PA

Makes 6 servings

Prep. Time: 15 minutes
Marinating Time: 6–8 hours, or
overnight
Grilling Time: 20 minutes

1 cup light soy sauce
¼ cup lemon juice
¼ cup honey
6 garlic cloves, minced, *or*
**   fewer cloves if you prefer**
1½ lbs. beef flank steak

1. In a large re-sealable plastic bag, combine soy sauce, lemon juice, honey, and garlic.
2. Add steak. Seal bag and turn to coat. Place in shallow dish with sides to catch any leaks.
3. Refrigerate 6–8 hours, or overnight to marinate in sauce.
4. When ready to grill, drain meat and discard marinade.
5. Grill over medium heat 8–10 minutes, on each side or until meat reaches desired doneness (for medium-rare, a meat thermometer should read 145°; medium 160°; well-done 170°).
6. Allow to stand off heat 10 minutes before slicing.
7. Slice steak into thin slices across the grain.

Exchange List Values
• Lean Meat 3.0
• Fat 0.5

Basic Nutritional Values
• Calories 170 • Sodium 410 mg
  (Calories from Fat 55) • Potassium 305 gm
• Total Fat 6 gm • Total Carb 4 gm
  (Saturated Fat 2.5 gm, • Dietary Fiber 0 gm
  Trans Fat 0.0 gm, • Sugars 3 gm
  Polyunsat Fat 0.2 gm, • Protein 23 gm
  Monounsat Fat 2.3 gm) • Phosphorus 185 gm
• Cholesterol 40 mg

Baked Rice Moussaka

Rhoda Atzeff
Harrisburg, PA

Makes 12 servings, ½ cup per serving

Prep. Time: 30 minutes
Baking/Cooking Time: 1 hour
**   20 minutes**

1½ lbs. round steak, ground
1 Tbsp. canola oil
¼ cup chopped green
**   pepper**
½ cup chopped onion
1 clove garlic, minced
½ cup uncooked rice
1 cup stewed tomatoes
1 tsp. salt
½ tsp. pepper
½ tsp. paprika
½ tsp. dried mint
2 cups hot water
3 eggs
juice of ½ lemon

1. In a saucepan brown meat with canola oil. Add green pepper, onion, garlic, rice, tomatoes and seasonings. Sauté for 5 minutes.
2. Add water and mix well. Pour into baking dish.
3. Beat eggs well and stir in lemon juice. Pour over meat mixture.
4. Bake at 350° for 1 hour.

Exchange List Values
• Starch 0.5 • Lean Meat 2.0

Basic Nutritional Values
• Calories 145 • Sodium 275 mg
  (Calories from Fat 45) • Potassium 190 gm
• Total Fat 5 gm • Total Carb 9 gm
  (Saturated Fat 1.5 gm, • Dietary Fiber 1 gm
  Trans Fat 0.1 gm, • Sugars 1 gm
  Polyunsat Fat 0.7 gm, • Protein 15 gm
  Monounsat Fat 2.4 gm) • Phosphorus 120 gm
• Cholesterol 85 mg

Barbecued Roast

Meredith Miller
Dover, DE

Makes 10 servings, serving size
3 oz. cooked meat with a little gravy

Prep. Time: 10 minutes
Baking Time: 6 hours

3 lb. lean beef roast
1 medium onion, diced
10¾-oz. can reduced-
**   sodium, 98%-fat-free**
**   cream of mushroom soup**
½ cup water
¼ cup brown sugar
¼ cup apple cider vinegar
1 tsp. salt
1 tsp. dry mustard
1 tsp. Worcestershire sauce

1. Place roast in roaster. Cover and bake at 350° for 2 hours.
2. Meanwhile, combine onion, soup, water, brown sugar, vinegar, salt, mustard, and Worcestershire sauce

in large bowl. Whisk until smooth.

3. Remove roast from oven. Pour sauce over roast.

4. Cover. Bake at 250° for 4 hours longer. (That's not a mistake!)

5. Cut into serving pieces. Mix gravy through meat and serve.

Exchange List Values

• Carbohydrate 0.5 • Lean Meat 4.0

Basic Nutritional Values

• Calories 225
 (Calories from Fat 65)
• Total Fat 7 gm
 (Saturated Fat 2.5 gm,
 Trans Fat 0.0 gm,
 Polyunsat Fat 0.5 gm,
 Monounsat Fat 2.9 gm)
• Cholesterol 90 mg

• Sodium 385 mg
• Potassium 475 gm
• Total Carb 8 gm
• Dietary Fiber 1 gm
• Sugars 5 gm
• Protein 30 gm
• Phosphorus 205 gm

Beef Burgundy

Rosemarie Fitzgerald
Gibsonia, PA

Makes 6 servings, about 6 oz. each

Prep. Time: 20 minutes
Cooking Time: 2¾-3 hours

2 lbs. lean stewing beef cubes, trimmed of visible fat
1 cup chopped green onion
2 cloves garlic
2 cups burgundy
½ tsp. marjoram
½ lb. fresh mushrooms, sliced, *or* canned and drained
6-oz. can tomato paste
½ tsp. sugar

1. Brown beef in non-stick Dutch oven with chopped green onions and garlic.

2. Pour in burgundy. Cover and simmer 2 hours, or until tender but not dry.

3. Stir in marjoram and sliced mushrooms.

4. Cover and simmer ½ hour longer.

5. Add tomato paste and sugar.

6. Simmer uncovered until slightly thickened.

7. This is good served over noodles or potatoes (mashed, browned, steamed, or baked).

Exchange List Values

• Vegetable 1.0 • Lean Meat 4.0

Basic Nutritional Values

• Calories 220
 (Calories from Fat 55)
• Total Fat 6 gm
 (Saturated Fat 2.6 gm,
 Trans Fat 0.3 gm,
 Polyunsat Fat 0.5 gm,
 Monounsat Fat 3.1 gm)
• Cholesterol 80 mg

• Sodium 300 mg
• Potassium 835 mg
• Total Carb 8 gm
• Dietary Fiber 2 gm
• Sugars 5 gm
• Protein 32 gm
• Phosphorus 315 gm

Waldorf Astoria Stew

Barbara Longenecker
New Holland, PA

Makes 6 servings, about 1½ cups per serving

Prep. Time: 10 minutes
Baking Time: 4½-5 hours

2 lbs. boneless pot roast, visible fat removed, cubed
1 medium onion, chopped
1 cup celery, diced
2 carrots, diced
4 medium potatoes, diced
10¾-oz. can lower-sodium, lower-fat tomato soup
⅓ cup water
3 Tbsp. minute tapioca
½ tsp. salt
pepper to taste

1. Layer cubed meat, onion, celery, carrots and potatoes into small roaster. Add tomato soup and water. Sprinkle tapioca and seasonings over top.

2. Cover and bake at 250° for 4½-5 hours. Do not lift lid while baking. Serve.

Exchange List Values

• Starch 2.0 • Lean Meat 4.0
• Vegetable 1.0

Basic Nutritional Values

• Calories 350
 (Calories from Fat 65)
• Total Fat 7 gm
 (Saturated Fat 2.7 gm,
 Trans Fat 0.3 gm,
 Polyunsat Fat 0.8 gm,
 Monounsat Fat 3.2 gm)
• Cholesterol 100 mg

• Sodium 510 mg
• Potassium 1645 gm
• Total Carb 36 gm
• Dietary Fiber 4 gm
• Sugars 8 gm
• Protein 37 gm
• Phosphorus 445 gm

Oven Beef Stew

Blanche Nyce
Hatfield, PA

Makes 8 servings

Prep. Time: 25 minutes
Baking Time: 3½ hours

1½ lbs. lean beef cubes,
    trimmed of visible fat
6 carrots
6 ribs celery
6 small potatoes
6 small onions, peeled
10¾-oz. can golden
    mushroom soup
½ cup water
salt and pepper, to taste

1. Cut vegetables into large chunks.
2. Mix ingredients together. Pour into a baking dish.
3. Cover and bake at 300–325° for approximately 3 hours. Longer is better!

Good Go-Alongs:

Tossed salad, coleslaw, gelatin salad. Also peas or corn served on side or on top of stew

Exchange List Values
• Starch 1.5   • Lean Meat 2.0
• Vegetable 2.0

Basic Nutritional Values
• Calories 265
  (Calories from Fat 45)
• Total Fat 5 gm
  (Saturated Fat 1.8 gm,
  Trans Fat 0.2 gm,
  Polyunsat Fat 1.0 gm,
  Monounsat Fat 1.9 gm)
• Cholesterol 50 mg
• Sodium 395 mg
• Potassium 960 gm
• Total Carb 35 gm
• Dietary Fiber 5 gm
• Sugars 8 gm
• Protein 20 gm
• Phosphorus 285 gm

Aunt Iris's Barbecue Brisket

Carolyn Spohn
Shawnee, KS

*Makes 10 servings,
2 oz. meat with a little sauce*

Prep. Time: 20–30 minutes
Marinating Time: 8 hours, or overnight
Baking Time: 3–4 hours
Standing Time: 30 minutes

2 lb. lean beef brisket
¼ tsp. garlic powder
¼ tsp. onion powder
¼ tsp. celery salt
2 oz. liquid smoke
2 tsp. Worcestershire sauce

Barbecue sauce:
  ⅓ cup honey
  ¼ cup light soy sauce
  ⅔ cup ketchup
  ½ tsp. Tabasco
  1 tsp. dry mustard
  1 tsp. paprika
  1 cup apple cider vinegar
  1 cup orange juice
  1 tsp. salt

1. Sprinkle both sides of brisket with garlic powder, onion powder, and celery salt. Sprinkle liquid smoke on both sides.
2. Place in large bowl or roaster. Refrigerate overnight, tightly covered.
3. In morning, drain meat. Return meat to pan.
4. Sprinkle with Worcestershire sauce.
5. Bake covered at 225° for 3–4 hours, or until meat thermometer registers 175°.
6. Turn off oven, but keep meat in oven for 30 more minutes.
7. Slice and serve with barbecue sauce.
8. While brisket is roasting, prepare barbecue sauce by combining all ingredients in saucepan.
9. Cook uncovered, stirring occasionally, until sauce comes to a boil.
10. Continue simmering for 30 minutes, or until sauce thickens and reduces down.
11. Serve alongside, or spooned over, sliced brisket.

Exchange List Values
• Carbohydrate 1.0   • Lean Meat 3.0

Basic Nutritional Values
• Calories 190
  (Calories from Fat 55)
• Total Fat 6 gm
  (Saturated Fat 1.9 gm,
  Trans Fat 0.0 gm,
  Polyunsat Fat 0.2 gm,
  Monounsat Fat 2.5 gm)
• Cholesterol 50 mg
• Sodium 475 mg
• Potassium 315 gm
• Total Carb 17 gm
• Dietary Fiber 0 gm
• Sugars 15 gm
• Protein 17 gm
• Phosphorus 150 gm

Use less meat and double the vegetables in a stir-fry, pasta dish, or stew.

Hearty Pot Roast

Colleen Heatwole
Burton, MI

Makes 12 servings,
about 1 cup per serving

Prep. Time: 30 minutes
Baking Time: 2–2½ hours

½ cup flour
6-oz. can tomato paste
¼ cup water
1 tsp. instant beef
 bouillon, *or* 1 beef
 bouillon cube
¼ tsp. pepper
4 lb. beef roast, ideally
 rump roast
4 medium red potatoes,
 cut in thirds
3 medium carrots,
 quartered
2 ribs celery, chopped
2 medium onions, sliced

1. Place roast in 9×13 baking pan or roaster.
2. Arrange vegetables around roast.
3. Combine flour, tomato paste, water, bouillon, and pepper in small bowl.
4. Pour over meat and vegetables.
5. Cover. Bake at 325° for 2–2½ hours, or until meat thermometer registers 170°.
6. Allow meat to stand for 10 minutes.
7. Then slice and place on platter surrounded by vegetables.
8. Pour gravy over top. Place additional gravy in bowl and serve along with platter.

Variation:
 You can make this in a large oven cooking bag. Combine flour, tomato paste, water, bouillon, and pepper in a bowl. Pour into cooking bag.
 Place in 9×13 baking pan. Add roast to bag in pan.
 Add vegetables around roast in bag.
 Close bag with its tie. Make six ½" slits on top of bag.
 Bake according to instructions in Step 5 and following.

Exchange List Values

- Starch 1.0
- Vegetable 1.0
- Lean Meat 4.0

Basic Nutritional Values

- Calories 305
 (Calories from Fat 70)
- Total Fat 8 gm
 (Saturated Fat 2.7 gm,
 Trans Fat 0.0 gm,
 Polyunsat Fat 0.4 gm,
 Monounsat Fat 3.2 gm)
- Cholesterol 100 mg
- Sodium 255 mg
- Potassium 840 gm
- Total Carb 22 gm
- Dietary Fiber 3 gm
- Sugars 5 gm
- Protein 36 gm
- Phosphorus 280 gm

Chimichangas

Lorene Good
Armington, IL

Makes 12 servings

Prep. Time: 25 minutes
Cooking Time: 20 minutes

¾ lb. 93%-lean ground beef
2 Tbsp. diced onion
2 Tbsp. chopped green
 pepper
8-oz. can tomato sauce
2 Tbsp. chopped garlic
salt and pepper
16-oz. can pinto beans
12 whole wheat flour
 tortillas, 6" diameter

1. Brown ground beef. Drain off grease. Add onion and green pepper. Add tomato sauce, garlic, salt and pepper. Simmer.
2. Drain and mash pinto beans. Add to beef mixture. Continue cooking on low heat.
3. Microwave prepared tortillas, one at a time, between 2 paper towels for 20 seconds each.
4. Fill each tortilla with about ⅓–½ cup sauce. Roll up and serve warm, or chill and serve later.

Exchange List Values

- Starch 1.5
- Lean Meat 1.0
- Fat 0.5

Basic Nutritional Values

- Calories 175
 (Calories from Fat 40)
- Total Fat 4.5 gm
 (Saturated Fat 1.4 gm,
 Trans Fat 0.1 gm,
 Polyunsat Fat 0.6 gm,
 Monounsat Fat 2.0 gm)
- Cholesterol 15 mg
- Sodium 350 mg
- Potassium 305 gm
- Total Carb 23 gm
- Dietary Fiber 3 gm
- Sugars 2 gm
- Protein 10 gm
- Phosphorus 125 gm

Quesadilla Casserole

Lorraine Stutzman Amstutz
Akron, PA

Makes 8 servings

Prep. Time: 20 minutes
Baking Time: 15 minutes

1 lb. 95%-lean ground beef
½ cup chopped onion
8-oz. can tomato sauce
8-oz. can no-salt-added
  tomato sauce
15-oz. can black beans,
  drained
15-oz. can whole-kernel
  corn, undrained
4½-oz. can chopped green
  chilies
2 tsp. chili powder
1 tsp. ground cumin
1 tsp. minced garlic
½ tsp. dried oregano
½ tsp. crushed red pepper
8 corn tortillas, *divided*
1 cup 75%-less-fat
  shredded sharp cheddar
  cheese, *divided*

1. Brown beef and onion in skillet. Drain off any drippings.
2. Add tomato sauce, beans, corn, and chilies.
3. Stir in chili powder, cumin, garlic, oregano, and red pepper.
4. Bring to boil; simmer 5 minutes.
5. Spread half of beef mixture in greased 9×13 pan.
6. Top with 4 corn tortillas, overlapping as needed.
7. Top with half remaining beef mixture and half of cheese.

8. Top with remaining tortillas, beef mixture, and cheese.
9. Bake at 350° for 15 minutes.

Variation:

I served this with chopped lettuce, fresh tomatoes, and avocado, as well as sour cream and salsa as toppings, for each person to add as they wished.

Exchange List Values
- Starch 1.5
- Vegetable 1.0
- Lean Meat 2.0

Basic Nutritional Values
- Calories 260
  (Calories from Fat 45)
- Total Fat 5 gm
  (Saturated Fat 2.3 gm,
  Trans Fat 0.1 gm,
  Polyunsat Fat 0.7 gm,
  Monounsat Fat 1.8 gm)
- Cholesterol 40 mg
- Sodium 485 mg
- Potassium 675 gm
- Total Carb 33 gm
- Dietary Fiber 7 gm
- Sugars 5 gm
- Protein 22 gm
- Phosphorus 335 gm

Whole Enchilada Pie

Cova Rexroad
Baltimore, MD

Makes 10 servings

Prep. Time: 20–25 minutes
Baking Time: 30–40 minutes

1 lb. 95%-lean ground beef
1 medium onion, chopped
2 cloves garlic, minced fine
½ cup picante sauce
1¼ cup fat-free refried
  beans
10- *or* 12-oz. can enchilada
  sauce
1 cup sliced black olives
9 torn corn tortillas,
  divided
1½ cups freshly grated
  light (75% less fat)
  cheddar cheese
garnishes: chopped fresh
  tomatoes, green peppers,
  chopped lettuce, sliced
  green onions, *optional*

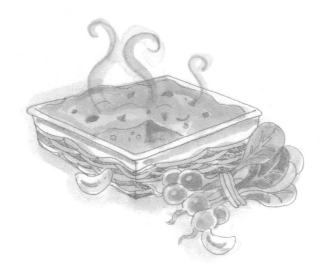

1. Brown ground beef and onion with garlic in large nonstick skillet until beef is no longer pink and onion is soft. Stir frequently to break up chunks of meat.

2. Lower heat and stir in picante sauce, beans, enchilada sauce, olives, and salt. Cook until bubbly. Remove from heat.

3. Line bottom of well-greased glass 9×13 pan with ⅓ of torn tortillas.

4. Layer half of beef mixture on top.

5. Top with layer of half the remaining tortillas.

6. Top with remaining meat mixture.

7. Top with remaining tortillas and cheese.

8. Bake 30–40 minutes at 350°, or until bubbly and heated through.

Tips:

1. Serve hot with serving bowls of garnishes.

2. Sometimes I add one 8-oz. can whole white beans, drained, to Step 2. They add good texture and nutrition.

Exchange List Values
- Starch 1.0
- Lean Meat 2.0
- Vegetable 1.0
- Fat 0.5

Basic Nutritional Values
- Calories 210
- Sodium 595 mg
(Calories from Fat 65)
- Potassium 455 gm
- Total Fat 7 gm
- Total Carb 19 gm
(Saturated Fat 2.3 gm,
- Dietary Fiber 4 gm
Trans Fat 0.1 gm,
- Sugars 2 gm
Polyunsat Fat 0.8 gm,
- Protein 18 gm
Monounsat Fat 2.7 gm)
- Phosphorus 280 gm
- Cholesterol 35 mg

Easy Taco Casserole

Orpha Herr, Andover, NY
Lori Lehman, Ephrata, PA
Gretchen Maust, Keezletown, VA

*Makes 8 servings,
2"×4" rectangle per serving*

Prep. Time: 20 minutes
Baking Time: 20–25 minutes

10 oz. 95%-lean ground beef
15-oz. can red beans, rinsed and drained
1 cup salsa, your choice of heat
½ cup fat-free mayonnaise
2 tsp. chili powder
2 cups crushed baked low-fat tortilla chips, *divided*
¾ cup shredded reduced-fat Colby cheese, *divided*
3 medium tomatoes, chopped
3 cups shredded lettuce

1. Brown beef in non-stick skillet, stirring often with wooden spoon to break up clumps. Keep stirring and cooking until pink disappears. Drain off any drippings.

2. Combine beef, beans, salsa, mayonnaise, and chili powder in skillet. Mix well.

3. In greased 8×8 baking dish, layer in half of meat mixture, topped by half of chips.

4. Repeat layers of meat mixture, followed by remaining chips.

5. Bake uncovered at 350° for 20–25 minutes or until heated through.

6. Five minutes before end of baking time, top with remaining cheese.

7. Just before serving, top with tomato and lettuce.

Variation:

Reduce ground beef to 1 cup. Add 15-oz. can black pinto beans, drained, or 2 cups cooked rice, to Step 2.
Juanita Weaver,
Johnsonville, IL

Exchange List Values
- Starch 1.5
- Lean Meat 1.0
- Vegetable 1.0
- Fat 0.5

Basic Nutritional Values
- Calories 200
- Sodium 550 mg
(Calories from Fat 45)
- Potassium 545 gm
- Total Fat 5 gm
- Total Carb 25 gm
(Saturated Fat 2.4 gm,
- Dietary Fiber 5 gm
Trans Fat 0.0 gm,
- Sugars 4 gm
Polyunsat Fat 0.5 gm,
- Protein 15 gm
Monounsat Fat 1.4 gm)
- Phosphorus 225 gm
- Cholesterol 30 mg

Each year we have a congregational Easter breakfast. We offer casseroles, rolls, juice and hard-boiled eggs which have been decorated by the children. The eggs provide decorations on the tables and are passed around near the end of the meal.
Arlene M. Mark, Elkhart, IN

Impossible Taco Pie

Esther J. Mast,
Lancaster, PA

Makes 8 servings, 1 slice per serving

Prep. Time: 15–20 minutes
Baking Time: 43–45 minutes

1 lb. 95%-lean ground beef
½ cup chopped onion
7 tsp. salt-free taco seasoning
    mix (see page 271)
1 cup egg substitute
2 cups fat-free milk
1⅓ cups reduced-fat
    baking mix
2 fresh tomatoes, sliced
4 oz. shredded reduced-fat
    cheddar cheese
3 cups chopped lettuce
2 cups fresh, chopped
    tomatoes
½ cup fat-free sour cream

1. Brown beef and onion together in non-stick skillet. Drain off drippings.
2. Stir in taco seasoning.
3. Spread mixture in greased 10" pie plate.
4. In mixing bowl, beat eggs. Add milk and baking mix and beat until smooth.
5. Pour into plate over top of meat.
6. Bake at 400° for 35 minutes.
7. Arrange 2 sliced tomatoes on top. Sprinkle cheese on top.
8. Bake 8–10 minutes more until cheese melts.
9. Serve with lettuce, chopped tomatoes, and sour cream for those at your table to add as they wish.

Variation:
If you wish, add 15-oz. can kidney beans, drained, to Step 2.

Fran Sauder
Mount Joy, PA

Exchange List Values
- Starch 1.0
- Lean Meat 2.0
- Fat-Free Milk 0.5
- Fat 0.5
- Vegetable 1.0

Basic Nutritional Values
- Calories 270
  (Calories from Fat 70)
- Total Fat 8 gm
  (Saturated Fat 3.4 gm,
  Trans Fat 0.1 gm,
  Polyunsat Fat 0.7 gm,
  Monounsat Fat 2.9 gm)
- Cholesterol 45 mg
- Sodium 505 mg
- Potassium 630 gm
- Total Carb 27 gm
- Dietary Fiber 2 gm
- Sugars 8 gm
- Protein 23 gm
- Phosphorus 425 gm

Burritos

Betty L. Moore
Plano, IL

Makes 10 servings,
1 burrito per serving

Prep. Time: 15–20 minutes
Baking Time: 30–40 minutes

12 oz. 95%-lean ground beef
1 small green pepper, diced
1 small onion, diced
4-oz. small can sliced
    mushrooms, drained
2 tsp. low-sodium taco
    seasoning (see page 271)
1 cup refried beans
10¾-oz. can lower-fat,
    lower-sodium cream of
    mushroom soup
1 pint fat-free sour cream
10 flour tortillas
8 oz. reduced-fat shredded
    sharp cheddar cheese

1. In non-stick skillet, brown ground beef, pepper, and onion. Stir frequently to break up clumps. Drain, if needed.
2. Add mushrooms, taco seasoning, and refried beans. Mix well.
3. Combine soup and sour cream in a bowl.
4. Spoon half of soup-sour cream blend in greased 9×13 baking pan.
5. Divide meat mixture evenly between tortillas. Roll up. Place rolled burritos in baking pan.
6. Cover with remaining sauce.
7. Sprinkle with cheese.
8. Bake at 350° for 30–40 minutes, or until bubbly and lightly browned.

Tip from Tester:
I used large tortillas (10 to a package), but they didn't quite fit in my 9×13 baking pan. So I cut off about 1½" from each one, and then laid 8 in a row from top to bottom. I laid the remaining 2 perpendicular to the 8. Then they all fit.

Exchange List Values
- Starch 1.5
- Lean Meat 1.0
- Fat-Free Milk 0.5
- Fat 1.0

Basic Nutritional Values
- Calories 255
  (Calories from Fat 55)
- Total Fat 6 gm
  (Saturated Fat 2.4 gm,
  Trans Fat 0.0 gm,
  Polyunsat Fat 0.9 gm,
  Monounsat Fat 2.3 gm)
- Cholesterol 30 mg
- Sodium 605 mg
- Potassium 565 gm
- Total Carb 33 gm
- Dietary Fiber 3 gm
- Sugars 4 gm
- Protein 17 gm
- Phosphorus 250 gm

Tamale Pie

Joyce Bond
Stonyford, CA

Makes 8 servings

Prep. Time: 25 minutes
Baking Time: 1 hour
Standing Time: 5–10 minutes

2 tsp. olive oil
1 medium onion, chopped
1 lb. 90%-lean ground beef
1 clove garlic, minced
¼ tsp. salt
½ tsp. pepper
3 Tbsp. chili powder
8-oz. can tomato sauce
8-oz. can no-salt-added
  tomato sauce
½ cup water
15-oz. can creamed corn
6-oz. can medium whole
  pitted olives, drained
1 cup fat-free evaporated
  milk
½ cup egg substitute
½ cup yellow cornmeal

1. Place olive oil and onion in 8-quart Dutch oven over medium heat. Cook, stirring frequently, until tender.
2. Add hamburger to onion in Dutch oven. Stir, breaking up clumps of meat, and cook until no longer pink. Drain off any drippings.
3. Off the stove, stir in garlic, salt, pepper, and chili powder.
4. Stir in tomato sauce and water.
5. Add creamed corn, olives, milk, eggs, and cornmeal. Mix together well.
6. Place Dutch oven, uncovered, in oven set at 375°. Bake 1 hour until set.
7. Let stand 5–10 minutes before serving.

Exchange List Values
- Starch 1.0
- Vegetable 2.0
- Lean Meat 2.0
- Fat 1.0

Basic Nutritional Values
- Calories 245
  (Calories from Fat 80)
- Total Fat 9 gm
  (Saturated Fat 2.5 gm,
  Trans Fat 0.3 gm,
  Polyunsat Fat 1.0 gm,
  Monounsat Fat 4.4 gm)
- Cholesterol 35 mg
- Sodium 580 mg
- Potassium 645 gm
- Total Carb 25 gm
- Dietary Fiber 4 gm
- Sugars 10 gm
- Protein 17 gm
- Phosphorus 235 gm

Tex-Mex Casserole

Ruth E. Miller
Wooster, OH

Makes 8 servings

Prep. Time: 35 minutes
Baking Time: 35 minutes

12 oz. 95%-lean ground beef
1 red bell pepper, chopped
1 onion, chopped
1 envelope dry taco
  seasoning
½ cup water
4 cups frozen, cubed hash
  brown potatoes, *or* your
  own cooked and cubed
  potatoes
10-oz. pkg. frozen corn
¾ cup reduced-fat
  shredded Mexican
  cheese, *divided*
garnishes: salsa, sour cream,
  shredded lettuce, nacho
  cheese chips, *optional*

1. In a non-stick skillet, brown meat with peppers and onions. Stir frequently to break up clumps, until meat is no longer pink.
2. Stir in taco seasoning and water.
3. Add potatoes, corn, and 2 cups cheese. Mix together well.
4. Pour into greased 9×13 baking dish.
5. Bake at 350° for 20 minutes, covered.
6. Sprinkle with remaining cheese.
7. Stir. Sprinkle with remaining cheese.
8. Bake 15 minutes uncovered.
9. Serve with bowls of garnishes for individuals to add as they wish to their servings.

Exchange List Values
- Starch 1.0
- Vegetable 1.0
- Lean Meat 1.0
- Fat 0.5

Basic Nutritional Values
- Calories 185
  (Calories from Fat 45)
- Total Fat 5 gm
  (Saturated Fat 2.5 gm,
  Trans Fat 0.1 gm,
  Polyunsat Fat 0.5 gm,
  Monounsat Fat 1.6 gm)
- Cholesterol 30 mg
- Sodium 400 mg
- Potassium 470 gm
- Total Carb 23 gm
- Dietary Fiber 3 gm
- Sugars 3 gm
- Protein 14 gm
- Phosphorus 210 gm

Taco Meat Loaf

Tammy Smith
Dorchester, WI

Makes 8 servings, 1 slice per serving

Prep. Time: 20 minutes
Baking Time: 1–1¼ hours
Standing Time: 10 minutes

¾ cup egg substitute
½ cup crushed tomatoes
¾ cup coarsely crushed
   tortilla chips
1 medium onion finely
   chopped
2 cloves garlic, minced
3 tsp. taco seasoning
2 tsp. chili powder
1 lb. 90%-lean ground beef
1 lb. 96%-lean ground pork
½ tsp. salt
¾ tsp. black pepper

1. In a large bowl, combine all ingredients well.
2. Shape into loaf.
3. Place in a well-greased shallow baking dish.
4. Bake at 350° for 1–1¼ hours, or until meat thermometer registers 160° in center of loaf.
5. Allow to stand 10 minutes before slicing.

Exchange List Values
- Carbohydrate 0.5   • Lean Meat 4.0

Basic Nutritional Values
- Calories 220   • Sodium 400 mg
  (Calories from Fat 80) • Potassium 495 gm
- Total Fat 9 gm   • Total Carb 7 gm
  (Saturated Fat 3.3 gm, • Dietary Fiber 1 gm
  Trans Fat 0.4 gm,   • Sugars 2 gm
  Polyunsat Fat 0.8 gm, • Protein 26 gm
  Monounsat Fat 4.1 gm) • Phosphorus 240 gm
- Cholesterol 70 mg

Grandma's Best Meat Loaf

Nanci Keatley
Salem, OR

Makes 10 servings,
1 slice per serving

Prep. Time: 15–25 minutes
Baking Time: 1 hour and 5 minutes

2 lbs. 90%-lean ground beef
2 Tbsp. fresh Italian
   parsley, chopped
1 tsp. dried oregano
1 small onion, chopped fine
4 cloves garlic, minced
¼ cup, plus 2 Tbsp.,
   Romano cheese, *optional*
½ cup dried bread crumbs
½ cup ketchup
½ cup egg substitute
1 tsp. black pepper
1 tsp. kosher salt

1. In a large mixing bowl, mix together ground beef, parsley, oregano, onion, garlic, optional cheese, bread crumbs, ketchup, egg substitute, pepper, and salt.
2. Roll mixture into a large ball.
3. Place in well-greased 9×13 baking dish or roaster, flattening slightly.
4. Bake at 375° for 1 hour. Keep in oven 5 more minutes with oven off and door closed.
5. Remove meatloaf from oven. Let stand 10 minutes before slicing to allow meat loaf to gather its juices and firm up.

Tip:
   This is great for meat loaf sandwiches the next day – if you have any left!

Exchange List Values
- Carbohydrate 0.5   • Fat 0.5
- Lean Meat 3.0

Basic Nutritional Values
- Calories 185   • Sodium 445 mg
  (Calories from Fat 70) • Potassium 365 gm
- Total Fat 8 gm   • Total Carb 9 gm
  (Saturated Fat 3.0 gm, • Dietary Fiber 1 gm
  Trans Fat 0.5 gm,   • Sugars 4 gm
  Polyunsat Fat 0.4 gm, • Protein 20 gm
  Monounsat Fat 3.2 gm) • Phosphorus 175 gm
- Cholesterol 55 mg

We have a fellowship meal every Sunday. This allows busy people time to visit and no one feels obliged to invite visitors to their home for Sunday dinner.
Also, in the town of Lafayette, the soup kitchen that serves free meals is closed on Sundays, so we open our fellowship meal to the local homeless population.
Marjorie Rush, West Lafayette, IN

Succulent Meat Loaf

Lizzie Ann Yoder
Hartville, OH

*Makes 6 servings,
1 slice per serving*

**Prep. Time: 20 minutes
Baking Time: 1–1½ hours**

1 lb. 90%-lean ground beef
⅔ cup dry oatmeal
½ cup fat-free milk
¼ cup egg substitute
⅓ cup chopped onions
1 Tbsp. prepared mustard
1 Tbsp. Worcestershire sauce
½ tsp. black pepper
¼ cup ketchup

1. In a large bowl, mix together beef, dry oatmeal, milk, egg substitute, onions, mustard, Worcestershire sauce, pepper, and ketchup. Blend well.

2. Shape into a loaf and place in well-greased loaf pan.

3. Bake at 350° for 1–1½ hours. Check with meat thermometer in center of loaf after 1 hour of baking to see if loaf is finished. If temperature registers 160°, it's done baking. Continue baking if it hasn't reached that temperature.

4. Allow to stand 10 minutes before slicing.

Exchange List Values
• Carbohydrate 1.0
• Lean Meat 2.0
• Fat 0.5

Basic Nutritional Values
• Calories 180 (Calories from Fat 65)
• Total Fat 7 gm (Saturated Fat 2.6 gm, Trans Fat 0.4 gm, Polyunsat Fat 0.5 gm, Monounsat Fat 2.9 gm)
• Cholesterol 45 mg
• Sodium 240 mg
• Potassium 380 gm
• Total Carb 11 gm
• Dietary Fiber 1 gm
• Sugars 4 gm
• Protein 18 gm
• Phosphorus 200 gm

Applesauce Meat Loaf

Dale Peterson
Rapid City, SD

Makes 8 servings

**Prep. Time: 15 minutes
Baking Time: 40–60 minutes**

2 lbs. 95%-lean ground beef
¾ cup dry oatmeal
¼ cup egg substitute
½ cup unsweetened applesauce
¼ cup chopped onion
1 tsp. salt
dash of pepper
1½ Tbsp. chili powder

1. Combine hamburger, dry oatmeal, egg substitute, applesauce, onions, salt, pepper, and chili powder in a good-sized mixing bowl.

2. Shape into a loaf. Place in 5×9 greased loaf pan.

3. Bake at 350° for 40–60 minutes, or until meat thermometer registers 160° in center of loaf.

4. Allow to stand 10 minutes before slicing to allow meat to gather its juices and firm up.

Variations:

1. You can use bread crumbs instead of oatmeal in this recipe.

2. You can make meatballs with this mixture.

Exchange List Values
• Carbohydrate 0.5 • Lean Meat 4.0

Basic Nutritional Values
• Calories 200 (Calories from Fat 55)
• Total Fat 6 gm (Saturated Fat 2.7 gm, Trans Fat 0.4 gm, Polyunsat Fat 0.6 gm, Monounsat Fat 2.6 gm)
• Cholesterol 70 mg
• Sodium 395 mg
• Potassium 480 gm
• Total Carb 8 gm
• Dietary Fiber 2 gm
• Sugars 2 gm
• Protein 26 gm
• Phosphorus 265 gm

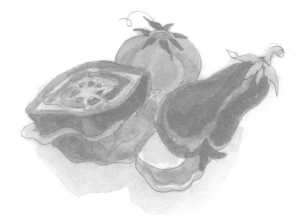

Beef and Potato Loaf

Deb Martin
Gap, PA

Makes 5 servings, 1 slice per serving

Prep. Time: 15 minutes
Baking Time: 1 hour

4 cups raw, thinly sliced
　potatoes, peeled or
　unpeeled
½ cup reduced-fat grated
　cheddar cheese
⅛ tsp. salt
¼ tsp. pepper
1 lb. 95%-lean ground beef
¾ cup fat-free evaporated
　milk, *or* tomato juice
½ cup dry oatmeal
½ cup chopped onion
dash of pepper
¾ tsp. seasoning salt
¼-½ cup ketchup

1. Arrange potatoes evenly
over bottom of greased 9×13
baking pan.
2. Layer cheese across
potatoes.
3. Sprinkle with ½ tsp. salt
and ¼ tsp. pepper.
4. In a mixing bowl, mix
together ground beef, evaporated milk or tomato juice,
dry oatmeal, onion, ketchup,
pepper, and seasoning salt.
5. When well blended,
crumble meat mixture evenly
over potatoes and cheese.
6. Drizzle with ketchup.
7. Bake at 350° for 1 hour,
or until potatoes are tender.
Check after 45 minutes of
baking. If dish is getting

too dark, cover with foil for
remainder of baking time.

Exchange List Values
- Starch 2.5　　　• Lean Meat 3.0

Basic Nutritional Values
- Calories 320
　(Calories from Fat 65)
- Total Fat 7 gm
　(Saturated Fat 3.3 gm,
　Trans Fat 0.3 gm,
　Polyunsat Fat 0.6 gm,
　Monounsat Fat 2.6 gm)
- Cholesterol 65 mg
- Sodium 600 mg
- Potassium 1055 gm
- Total Carb 36 gm
- Dietary Fiber 4 gm
- Sugars 9 gm
- Protein 28 gm
- Phosphorus 415 gm

Easy Meatballs

Cindy Krestynick
Glen Lyon, PA

Makes 8 servings,
1 meatball per serving

Prep. Time: 15 minutes
Cooking Time: 7–15 minutes

1 lb. 95%-lean ground beef
3 slices white bread, torn
　or cubed
1 small onion, chopped
4 sprigs fresh parsley,
　finely chopped
1½ Tbsp. freshly grated
　Parmesan cheese
¼ cup egg substitute
1 tsp. salt
¼ tsp. pepper
¾ cup water

1. Combine beef, bread
pieces, onions, parsley,
cheese, egg, salt, pepper, and
water in a large mixing bowl
until well mixed.
2. Form into 8 meatballs.
3. Brown in non-stick
skillet until golden brown on
each side.

Tip:
　Serve with spaghetti sauce
in hoagie rolls or over cooked
spaghetti.

Exchange List Values
- Starch 0.5　　　• Lean Meat 2.0

Basic Nutritional Values
- Calories 110
　(Calories from Fat 30)
- Total Fat 4 gm
　(Saturated Fat 1.5 gm,
　Trans Fat 0.1 gm,
　Polyunsat Fat 0.3 gm,
　Monounsat Fat 1.3 gm)
- Cholesterol 35 mg
- Sodium 415 mg
- Potassium 220 gm
- Total Carb 6 gm
- Dietary Fiber 0 gm
- Sugars 1 gm
- Protein 13 gm
- Phosphorus 120 gm

Keep a notebook of when you have guests over for a meal. List how many people attended, the weather, menus, how much you made, and how much was left over. This is handy to look at when you are planning for new guests.

Jane Geigley, Lancaster, PA

Savory Meatball Casserole

Miriam Showalter
Salem, OR

*Makes 10 servings, about 6 oz.
and includes 3 meatballs*

**Prep. Time: 30 minutes
Cooking/Baking Time: 1 hour**

1½ lbs. 93%-fat-free ground
  beef
½ cup dry bread crumbs
2⅓ cups fat-free
  evaporated milk, *divided*
2 Tbsp. chopped onion
1 tsp. chili powder
⅛ tsp. pepper
6 oz. noodles
10¾-oz. can lower-sodium,
  lower-fat cream of
  mushroom soup
1 cup evaporated milk
¼ cup water
paprika

1. Combine ground beef,
bread crumbs, ⅓ cup milk,
onion, chili powder and pepper. Shape into 30 meatballs
about the size of a tablespoon.
2. Brown meatballs under
broiler, turn once and drain.
3. Cook noodles until just
cooked. Drain.
4. In large bowl combine
mushroom soup and 1 cup
milk and mix well. Add water.
5. Fold in noodles and
meatballs.
6. Spoon into greased
1½-quart casserole dish.
Cover and bake at 375° for
20–25 minutes. Sprinkle with
paprika.

Exchange List Values
- Starch 1.0   • Lean Meat 2.0
- Carbohydrate 0.5   • Fat 0.5

Basic Nutritional Values
- Calories 225   • Sodium 230 mg
  (Calories from Fat 55) • Potassium 545 gm
- Total Fat 6 gm   • Total Carb 22 gm
  (Saturated Fat 2.3 gm, • Dietary Fiber 1 gm
  Trans Fat 0.2 gm,   • Sugars 5 gm
  Polyunsat Fat 0.8 gm, • Protein 19 gm
  Monounsat Fat 2.4 gm) • Phosphorus 235 gm
- Cholesterol 55 mg

Oven Porcupines

Clara Byler
Hartville, OH

*Makes 5 servings,
2 meatballs per serving*

**Prep. Time: 45–60 minutes
Baking Time: 50–60 minutes**

1 lb. 95%-lean ground beef
½ cup uncooked long-grain
  rice
1½ cups water, *divided*
½ cup chopped onion
½ tsp. celery, *or* seasoning,
  salt, according to your
  taste preference
⅛ tsp. garlic powder
⅛-1 tsp. pepper, according
  to your taste preference
15-oz. can low-sodium
  tomato sauce
1 Tbsp. Worcestershire
  sauce

1. In bowl, mix beef,
rice, ½ cup water, onion,
celery salt, garlic powder, and
pepper.
2. When well mixed, shape
mixture into 10 balls.

3. Cook in nonstick skillet
until brown on all sides.
Drain.
4. Place meatballs in
greased 8×8 baking dish.
5. In a mixing bowl, blend
together 1 cup water, tomato
sauce, and Worcestershire
sauce. Pour over meatballs.
6. Cover and bake at 350°
for 45–50 minutes.
7. Remove cover and
continue baking 10 more
minutes.

Exchange List Values
- Starch 1.0   • Lean Meat 3.0
- Vegetable 1.0

Basic Nutritional Values
- Calories 225   • Sodium 170 mg
  (Calories from Fat 45) • Potassium 635 gm
- Total Fat 5 gm   • Total Carb 24 gm
  (Saturated Fat 2.2 gm, • Dietary Fiber 3 gm
  Trans Fat 0.1 gm,   • Sugars 5 gm
  Polyunsat Fat 0.3 gm, • Protein 21 gm
  Monounsat Fat 2.0 gm) • Phosphorus 210 gm
- Cholesterol 55 mg

Ground Beef and Wild Rice Casserole

Lillian F. Gardner
Crystal, MN

Makes 10 servings,
a 2⅖"×4½" rectangle per serving

Prep. Time: 20 minutes
Baking/Cooking Time: 1½ hours

⅔ cup wild rice, uncooked
½ cup chopped celery
1 large onion, chopped
1⅓ lbs. 90%-fat-free
   ground beef
10¾-oz. can lower-sodium
   lower-fat cream of
   mushroom soup
10¾-oz. can lower-sodium
   lower-fat cream of
   chicken soup
8-oz. jar mushroom pieces,
   drained
4-oz. can sliced water
   chestnuts, drained
2 tsp. soy sauce
2 tsp. Worcestershire sauce
¼ cup sliced almonds

1. Prepare the rice according to package directions. Set aside.
2. Sauté celery, onion and ground beef in skillet. Drain excess fat. Add all ingredients except almonds and mix thoroughly.
3. Pour into greased 9×13 baking dish.
4. Bake at 350° for 30 minutes. Cover with sliced almonds. Bake an additional 30 minutes.

Exchange List Values
• Carbohydrate 1.0   • Fat 0.5
• Lean Meat 2.0

Basic Nutritional Values
• Calories 195   • Sodium 370 mg
  (Calories from Fat 65)   • Potassium 660 gm
• Total Fat 7 gm   • Total Carb 16 gm
  (Saturated Fat 2.3 gm,   • Dietary Fiber 3 gm
  Trans Fat 0.3 gm,   • Sugars 3 gm
  Polyunsat Fat 1.1 gm,   • Protein 16 gm
  Monounsat Fat 3.0 gm)   • Phosphorus 180 gm
• Cholesterol 40 mg

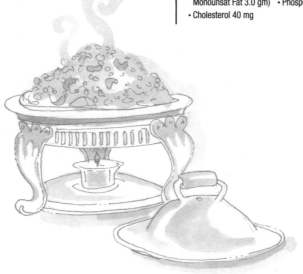

Shaggy Tigers

Shelley Burns
Elverson, PA

Makes 5 servings, 1 burger per serving

Prep. Time: 20 minutes
Baking Time: 25 minutes

1 lb. 95%-lean ground beef
¼ cup egg substitute
½ cup grated raw potatoes
½ cup grated raw carrots
¾ tsp. salt
¼ tsp. pepper
¼ cup chopped onion
¼ cup fat-free milk

1. In a good-sized mixing bowl, mix beef, egg substitute, potatoes, carrots, salt, pepper, onion, and milk or tomato juice.
2. When well blended, shape into 4 or 5 thick, oval burgers.
3. Place in greased baking dish.
4. Bake at 425° for 25 minutes, or until thermometer inserted in center of burgers registers 160°.

Tip:
   Serve with ketchup, barbecue sauce, and/or mustard.

Exchange List Values
• Starch 0.5   • Lean Meat 3.0

Basic Nutritional Values
• Calories 155   • Sodium 445 mg
  (Calories from Fat 40)   • Potassium 485 gm
• Total Fat 4.5 gm   • Total Carb 6 gm
  (Saturated Fat 2.1 gm,   • Dietary Fiber 1 gm
  Trans Fat 0.3 gm,   • Sugars 2 gm
  Polyunsat Fat 0.3 gm,   • Protein 22 gm
  Monounsat Fat 2.0 gm)   • Phosphorus 210 gm
• Cholesterol 55 mg

Beef Jambalaya

Herman Cortex Jr.
Des Allemands, LA

Makes 6 servings,
about 7 oz. per serving

Prep. Time: 15 minutes
Cooking Time: 1 hour

1 lb. 90%-lean ground beef
1 Tbsp. steak sauce
¼ cup egg substitute
8-oz. can no-salt-added
   tomato sauce
¼ cup barbecue sauce,
   lowest sodium available
¼ cup mustard
1 Tbsp. cayenne pepper
1 tsp. garlic salt
1 cup water
pepper to taste
1 cup uncooked rice

1. Combine ground beef,
steak sauce and egg. Brown
in skillet. Add all remaining
ingredients except rice. Bring
to a boil.

2. Add rice and bring to a boil
again. Reduce heat to simmer.

3. Cover and simmer for 20
minutes. Remove lid and simmer several minutes longer.

Exchange List Values

• Starch 1.5   • Lean Meat 2.0
• Carbohydrate 0.5   • Fat 0.5

Basic Nutritional Values

• Calories 275   • Sodium 425 mg
  (Calories from Fat 65) • Potassium 450 gm
• Total Fat 7 gm   • Total Carb 34 gm
  (Saturated Fat 2.5 gm, • Dietary Fiber 2 gm
  Trans Fat 0.4 gm,   • Sugars 6 gm
  Polyunsat Fat 0.4 gm, • Protein 18 gm
  Monounsat Fat 2.7 gm) • Phosphorus 180 gm
• Cholesterol 45 mg

Texas Cottage Pie

Kathy Hertzler
Lancaster, PA

Makes 8 servings,
2½"×3½" rectangle per serving

Prep. Time: 25–30 minutes
Baking Time: 30–35 minutes

1 Tbsp. oil
1½ medium onions, diced
1 lb. 95%-lean ground beef
¼ tsp. salt
½ tsp. ground cumin
½ tsp. paprika
1 tsp. chili powder
¼ tsp black pepper
¼ tsp. ground cinnamon
1 tsp. chopped garlic
15-oz. can black beans,
   drained and rinsed
2 cups frozen corn
14½-oz. can diced tomatoes
   with green chilies
3 cups leftover mashed
   potatoes
½ cup fat-free milk
½ cup reduced-fat
   shredded pepper jack
   cheese, *divided*

1. In large skillet, sauté
diced onion and ground beef in
1 Tbsp. oil until beef is almost
cooked through. Stir frequently
to break up clumps of meat.
Drain off any drippings.

2. Add salt, spices, seasonings, and garlic to skillet.

3. Cook 2 minutes more on
medium heat.

4. Add black beans, corn,
and tomatoes with chilies.
Stir well.

5. Cover. Cook on low heat
15 minutes.

6. Meanwhile, warm
mashed potatoes mixed with
½ cup milk in microwave on
low power, or in saucepan
on stove top (covered and
over very low heat for 5–10
minutes, stirring frequently to
prevent sticking).

7. Stir ¼ cup cheese into
warmed mashed potatoes.

8. Transfer meat mixture to
greased 7×10 baking dish.

9. Top with mashed
potatoes, spreading in an even
layer to edges of baking dish.

10. Sprinkle with the
remaining ¼ cup cheese.

11. Bake at 350° for 30–35
minutes.

Warm Memories:
   The first time I made
this, I got about 1 cup – my
husband, and our 2 sons
(13 and 16 years), got the rest.
It disappeared in 15 minutes.

Good Go-Alongs:
   I serve this with a tossed
green salad and cornbread.

Exchange List Values

• Starch 2.0   • Lean Meat 2.0
• Vegetable 1.0   • Fat 0.5

Basic Nutritional Values

• Calories 290   • Sodium 555 mg
  (Calories from Fat 80) • Potassium 735 gm
• Total Fat 9 gm   • Total Carb 34 gm
  (Saturated Fat 3.5 gm, • Dietary Fiber 6 gm
  Trans Fat 0.1 gm,   • Sugars 7 gm
  Polyunsat Fat 1.4 gm, • Protein 20 gm
  Monounsat Fat 3.6 gm) • Phosphorus 270 gm
• Cholesterol 40 mg

Zucchini Beef Lasagna

Dorothy VanDeest
Memphis, TN

Makes 8 servings,
3"×4" rectangle per serving

Prep. Time: 40 minutes
Cooking/Baking Time: 1 hour
Standing Time: 10 minutes

¾ lb. 95%-lean ground beef
¼ cup chopped onion
15-oz. can tomato sauce,
  or chopped tomatoes
½ tsp. dried oregano
¼ tsp. ground pepper
¼ tsp. salt
½ tsp. dried basil
1¼ lbs. zucchini, about
  4 medium zucchini,
  peeled or unpeeled,
  divided
1 cup creamed 1% cottage
  cheese
¼ cup egg substitute
3 Tbsp. flour, *divided*
¾ cup part-skim shredded
  mozzarella cheese,
  divided

1. In large skillet, brown beef and onion over medium heat. Drain off drippings.
2. Add tomato sauce, or chopped tomatoes, and seasonings to meat in skillet.
3. Bring to boil. Simmer 5 minutes.
4. Meanwhile, slice zucchini lengthwise into ¼" slices.
5. In a small bowl, combine cottage cheese and egg substitute.

6. In a greased 8×12 baking pan, place half the zucchini. Sprinkle with half the flour.
7. Top with cottage-cheese mixture and half the meat mixture.
8. Repeat layer of zucchini and flour.
9. Sprinkle with half the mozzarella cheese and remaining meat mixture.
10. Bake at 375° for about 40 minutes, or until heated through.
11. Remove from oven. Sprinkle with remaining mozzarella cheese.
12. Let stand 10 minutes before cutting and serving to allow cheeses to firm up.

Tip from Tester:
  Substitute equivalent amount of sliced eggplant (peeled or unpeeled) for zucchini.

Exchange List Values
- Vegetable 2.0   • Lean Meat 2.0

Basic Nutritional Values
- Calories 145
  (Calories from Fat 40)
- Total Fat 4.5 gm
  (Saturated Fat 2.3 gm,
  Trans Fat 0.1 gm,
  Polyunsat Fat 0.3 gm,
  Monounsat Fat 1.5 gm)
- Cholesterol 35 mg
- Sodium 575 mg
- Potassium 545 gm
- Total Carb 9 gm
- Dietary Fiber 2 gm
- Sugars 5 gm
- Protein 17 gm
- Phosphorus 210 gm

Six-Layer Casserole

Mrs. Frank Neufeld
Didsbury, Alberta

Makes 8 servings

Prep. Time: 15 minutes
Cooking/Baking Time: 2 hours
  or more

1 lb. 90%-lean ground beef
2 medium potatoes, sliced
2 medium onions,
  chopped
2 cups chopped carrots
1 cup cooked rice
1 quart canned tomatoes
  with juice

1. Brown ground beef and drain off fat.
2. Layer ingredients in greased casserole dish in following order: potatoes, onions, ground beef, carrots, rice, tomatoes and their juice.
3. Bake at 300° for at least 2 hours.

Variation:
  Sprinkle 1 Tbsp. brown sugar over dish before baking.
Hettie Conrad
Colorado Springs, CO

Tip:
  At our church we have each family bring this same dish. We then pour all dishes together into our electric roasters. This saves oven space and keeps meal warm until time for serving.
Virginia Graber
Freeman, SD

Beef and Cabbage Casserole

Lizzie Ann Yoder
Hartville, OH

*Makes 8 servings,
2"×4" rectangle per serving*

Prep. Time: 30–45 minutes
Baking Time: 1–1¼ hours

1 lb. 90%-lean ground beef
⅓ cup diced onions
¼ tsp. garlic powder
3 cups shredded cabbage
1 cup sliced carrots
½ cup low-sodium beef broth
¼ tsp. pepper
½ tsp. caraway seeds

1. Cook beef, onions, and garlic powder in non-stick skillet until meat is no longer pink. Stir to break up clumps. Drain off any drippings.

2. Stir cabbage, carrots, broth, pepper, and caraway seeds into skillet. Blend well.

3. Place in greased 8×8 baking dish.

4. Cover. Bake at 350° for 60–75 minutes, until vegetables are as tender as you like them.

Good Go-Alongs:

Slice of your favorite fresh bread or a small dinner roll, baked apples, glass of milk.

German Casserole

Lizzie Ann Yoder
Hartville, OH

*Makes 6 servings,
2⅔"×4" rectangle per serving*

Prep. Time: 40–45 minutes
Baking Time: 1½ hours

1 lb. 90%-lean ground beef
¾ cup chopped onion
15-oz. can sauerkraut, undrained
½ cup water
½ cup long-grain rice, uncooked
¼ cup finely diced green bell pepper
¼ cup low-sodium beef broth
8-oz. can low-sodium tomato sauce
¼ tsp. black pepper

1. Cook ground beef in non-stick skillet until no longer pink. Stir frequently to break up clumps. Drain off any drippings.

2. In a mixing bowl, combine sauerkraut and its juices, water, uncooked rice, green pepper, and meat and onion.

3. Stir in broth.

4. Spoon into greased 8×8 baking dish.

5. Pour tomato sauce over top. Sprinkle with black pepper.

6. Bake covered at 350° for 1 hour.

7. Cover baking dish. Continue baking 30 more minutes, or until rice is tender.

Shepherd's Pie

Judi Manos, West Islip, NY

Makes 6 servings

Prep. Time: 15 minutes
Cooking/Baking Time: 50 minutes

1¼ lb. red potatoes,
   unpeeled and cut in
   chunks
3 garlic cloves
1 lb. 95%-lean ground beef
2 Tbsp. flour
4 cups fresh vegetables of
   your choice (for example,
   carrots, corn, green
   beans, peas)
¾ cup beef broth, canned,
   or boxed, *or* your own
   homemade
2 Tbsp. ketchup
¾ cup fat-free sour cream
½ cup shredded reduced-
   fat sharp cheddar
   cheese, *divided*

1. In saucepan, cook potatoes and garlic in 1½" boiling water for 20 minutes, or until potatoes are tender.

2. Meanwhile, brown beef in large nonstick skillet.

3. Stir in flour. Cook 1 minute.

4. Stir in vegetables, broth, and ketchup. Cover. Cook 10 minutes, stirring frequently.

5. Drain cooked potatoes and garlic. Return to their pan.

6. Stir in sour cream. Mash until potatoes are smooth and mixture is well blended.

7. Stir ¼ cup cheddar cheese into mashed potatoes.

8. Spoon meat mixture into well-greased 8×8 baking dish.

9. Cover with mashed potatoes.

10. Bake at 375° for 18 minutes.

11. Top with remaining cheddar cheese. Bake 2 minutes more, or until cheese is melted.

Variation:

If you don't have access to fresh vegetables, use leftovers from your fridge or frozen ones.

Exchange List Values

- Starch 2.0
- Fat-Free Milk 0.5
- Vegetable 1.0
- Lean Meat 2.0

Basic Nutritional Values

- Calories 310
  (Calories from Fat 65)
- Total Fat 7 gm
  (Saturated Fat 3.1 gm,
  Trans Fat 0.1 gm,
  Polyunsat Fat 0.5 gm,
  Monounsat Fat 2.1 gm)
- Cholesterol 55 mg
- Sodium 360 mg
- Potassium 890 gm
- Total Carb 41 gm
- Dietary Fiber 5 gm
- Sugars 7 gm
- Protein 24 gm
- Phosphorus 370 gm

Homespun Meat Pie

Suzanne Yoder
Gap, PA

*Makes 8 servings, 1 slice and
2 Tbsp. gravy per serving*

Prep. Time: 20 minutes
Baking Time: 25–30 minutes

12 oz. 95%-lean ground beef
4-oz. can sliced mushrooms,
   drained
1 egg
⅓ cup chopped onion
¼ cup dry bread crumbs
½ tsp. salt

dash of pepper
4 cups cubed cooked
   potatoes
6 Tbsp. fat-free milk
½ cup shredded reduced-
   fat cheddar cheese
1 Tbsp. chopped parsley
¼ tsp. salt
1 cup fat-free brown gravy

1. In a mixing bowl, combine meat, mushrooms, egg, onion, bread crumbs, ½ tsp. salt and pepper. Mix lightly.

2. Press mixture onto bottom and up sides of 9" pie plate.

3. Bake at 400° for 15 minutes.

4. Meanwhile, mash potatoes and milk together.

5. Stir cheese, parsley and ¼ tsp. salt into mashed potatoes.

6. Remove meat shell from oven. Drain off any fat.

7. Reduce oven heat to 350°.

8. Fill meat shell with potato mixture.

9. Return to oven. Continue baking 10–15 minutes, or until heated through.

10. Serve with brown gravy.

Tips:

1. I keep a box of instant mashed potatoes on hand if I'm in a time squeeze, and then within 45 minutes or so, I can have this meat and potato meal ready. It's not my practice to use pre-made foods – but every now and then, they have their place.

2. I usually prepare green beans to go with this. The meat shell shrinks somewhat, so I spoon the cooked beans around the outside edge of the pie. It creates a nice presentation.

Exchange List Values
- Starch 1.5
- Lean Meat 2.0

Basic Nutritional Values
- Calories 190
  (Calories from Fat 45)
- Total Fat 5 gm
  (Saturated Fat 2.3 gm,
  Trans Fat 0.1 gm,
  Polyunsat Fat 0.4 gm,
  Monounsat Fat 1.7 gm)
- Cholesterol 55 mg
- Sodium 550 mg
- Potassium 470 gm
- Total Carb 22 gm
- Dietary Fiber 2 gm
- Sugars 3 gm
- Protein 14 gm
- Phosphorus 195 gm

Dried Beef Casserole

Mabel Eshleman
Lancaster, PA
Virginia Graybill
Hershey, PA

*Makes 6 servings,
2½"×3" rectangle per serving*

Prep. Time: 20–25 minutes
*Chilling Time: 4–6 hours, or
overnight*
Baking Time: 1 hour

10¾-oz. can lower-sodium,
  lower-fat cream of
  mushroom soup
2 cups fat-free milk
¾ cup grated reduced-fat
  cheddar cheese
1 cup uncooked elbow
  macaroni
3 Tbsp. finely chopped
  onion
¼ lb. dried beef, cut in
  bite-size pieces
2 hard-cooked eggs, sliced

1. In good-sized mixing bowl
stir soup and milk together
until of creamy consistency.

2. Stir in cheese, macaroni,
onion, and beef.
3. Fold in sliced eggs.
4. Put in well-greased 9×5
loaf pan.
5. Cover. Refrigerate at
least 4–6 hours, or overnight.
6. Bake, uncovered, at 350°
for 1 hour.

Exchange List Values
- Starch 1.0
- Fat-Free Milk 0.5
- Lean Meat 1.0
- Fat 0.5

Basic Nutritional Values
- Calories 210
  (Calories from Fat 55)
- Total Fat 6 gm
  (Saturated Fat 2.5 gm,
  Trans Fat 0.0 gm,
  Polyunsat Fat 1.0 gm,
  Monounsat Fat 1.7 gm)
- Cholesterol 80 mg
- Sodium 590 mg
- Potassium 620 gm
- Total Carb 23 gm
- Dietary Fiber 1 gm
- Sugars 6 gm
- Protein 16 gm
- Phosphorus 260 gm

Kodiak Casserole

Bev Beiler
Gap, PA

Makes 10 servings

Prep. Time: 15–25 minutes
Baking Time: 60 minutes

1 lb. 90%-lean ground beef
2 cups diced onions
½ tsp. minced garlic
3 medium bell peppers,
  chopped
1 cup low-sodium barbecue
  sauce of your choice
10¾-oz. can lower-sodium,
  lower-fat cream of
  tomato soup, undiluted
½ cup salsa of your choice
15-oz. can black beans,
  drained

4-oz. can mushroom stems
  and pieces, undrained
1 Tbsp. Worcestershire
  sauce
½ cup reduced-fat
  shredded cheddar cheese

1. In a Dutch oven, brown
beef with onions and garlic.
Stir frequently to break up
meat, cooking until no pink
remains. Drain off any
drippings.
2. Stir peppers, barbecue
sauce, soup, salsa, beans,
mushrooms, and Worcester-
shire sauce into Dutch oven.
Mix well.
3. Cover and bake at 350°
for 45 minutes.
4. Remove cover. Sprinkle
with cheese. Continue baking
15 minutes, or until bubbly
and heated through.

Exchange List Values
- Starch 0.5
- Carbohydrate 1.0
- Vegetable 1.0
- Lean Meat 1.0
- Fat 1.0

Basic Nutritional Values
- Calories 210
  (Calories from Fat 55)
- Total Fat 6 gm
  (Saturated Fat 2.4 gm,
  Trans Fat 0.2 gm,
  Polyunsat Fat 0.5 gm,
  Monounsat Fat 1.9 gm)
- Cholesterol 30 mg
- Sodium 525 mg
- Potassium 625 gm
- Total Carb 27 gm
- Dietary Fiber 4 gm
- Sugars 15 gm
- Protein 14 gm
- Phosphorus 185 gm

Upside-Down Pizza

Julia Rohrer
Aaronsburg, PA
Janet L. Roggie
Lowville, NY

*Makes 10 servings,
2½"×4½" rectangle*

Prep. Time: 20–30 minutes
Baking Time: 25–30 minutes

14 oz. 95%-lean ground beef
1 chopped onion
1 medium red, *or* green,
    bell pepper, chopped
1 tsp. dried basil
1 tsp. dried oregano
2 cups pizza, *or* spaghetti,
    sauce
¼ lb. fresh mushrooms,
    chopped, *or* 4-oz. can
    chopped mushrooms,
    drained
1 cup grated part-skim
    mozzarella cheese
sprinkling of dried
    oregano
sprinkling of grated
    Parmesan cheese

Batter:
    ¾ cup egg substitute
    1½ cups fat-free milk
    1½ Tbsp. oil
    ½ tsp. salt
    1 tsp. baking soda
    1¾ cups flour

1. Brown meat with onion
and pepper in large nonstick
skillet.
2. Stir in seasonings, sauce,
and mushrooms. Simmer 5–8
minutes.

3. Place in well-greased
9×13 baking pan.
4. Cover with grated cheese.
5. Prepare batter by
beating egg substitute, milk,
and oil together in good-sized
mixing bowl.
6. Add salt, baking soda,
and flour. Stir just until
mixed.
7. Pour over cheese-meat
mixture. Do not stir.
8. Sprinkle with oregano
and Parmesan cheese.
9. Bake at 400° for 25
minutes or until toothpick
inserted in center of dough
comes out clean.

Exchange List Values
- Starch 1.5
- Lean Meat 2.0
- Fat 0.5

Basic Nutritional Values
- Calories 235
  (Calories from Fat 65)
- Total Fat 7 gm
  (Saturated Fat 2.5 gm,
  Trans Fat 0.1 gm,
  Polyunsat Fat 1.2 gm,
  Monounsat Fat 2.9 gm)
- Cholesterol 30 mg
- Sodium 580 mg
- Potassium 510 gm
- Total Carb 26 gm
- Dietary Fiber 2 gm
- Sugars 6 gm
- Protein 17 gm
- Phosphorus 230 gm

Pizza Cups

Alice Miller
Stuarts Draft, VA

*Makes 8 servings,
1 pizza cup per serving*

Prep. Time: 20–25 minutes
Baking Time: 10–12 minutes

8 oz. 95%-lean ground beef
6-oz. can no-salt-added
    tomato paste
1 Tbsp. instant minced
    onion
½ tsp. dried oregano
½ tsp. dried basil
¼ tsp. salt

Biscuits:
    2 cups flour
    3 tsp. baking powder
    ½ tsp. salt
    ¼ cup canola oil
    ¾ cup fat-free milk

2⅔ Tbsp. shredded
    part-skim mozzarella
    cheese, *divided*

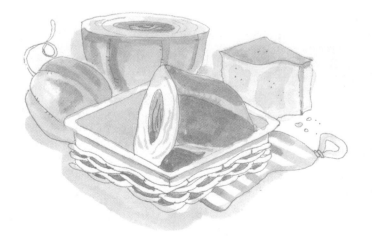

1. Cook ground beef in large skillet, stirring frequently to break up clumps, until no pink remains. Drain off drippings.

2. Stir in tomato paste, onion, and seasonings.

3. Cook over medium heat an additional 5 minutes, stirring frequently.

4. Prepare biscuits by sifting flour, baking powder, and salt together in large bowl.

5. Add milk and oil together. Add to flour mixture and stir with fork until a ball forms.

6. Roll ball onto lightly floured counter. Knead lightly, about 20 turns.

7. Divide ball into 8 pieces.

8. Place a ball in each of 8 muffin cups, pressing to cover bottom and sides as evenly as you can.

9. Spoon meat mixture into cups, distributing evenly.

10. Sprinkle each cup with 1 tsp. cheese.

11. Bake at 400° for 10–12 minutes.

Exchange List Values
- Starch 1.5
- Lean Meat 1.0
- Vegetable 1.0
- Fat 1.5

Basic Nutritional Values
- Calories 250
  (Calories from Fat 80)
- Total Fat 9 gm
  (Saturated Fat 1.5 gm,
  Trans Fat 0.1 gm,
  Polyunsat Fat 2.2 gm,
  Monounsat Fat 5.2 gm)
- Cholesterol 20 mg
- Sodium 415 mg
- Potassium 390 gm
- Total Carb 30 gm
- Dietary Fiber 2 gm
- Sugars 5 gm
- Protein 11 gm
- Phosphorus 310 gm

Hearty Ground Meat and Veggies Pilaf

Linda Yoder
Fresno, OH

*Makes 6 servings,
about 6 oz. per serving*

Prep. Time: 15 minutes
Cooking Time: 20 minutes

½ lb. 90%-lean ground
  beef, *or* venison
2 tsp. olive oil
1 cup sliced onions
1 clove garlic, minced
2 cups water
1 cup long-grain rice,
  uncooked
¼ lb. fresh mushrooms,
  sliced, *or* 4-oz. can sliced
  or cut-up mushrooms,
  drained
1 beef bouillon cube
¾ tsp. salt
1 pint fresh green beans, *or*
  1 lb. frozen green beans,
  thawed
½ tsp. dried basil
½ tsp. dried sage
½ tsp. dried oregano
½ tsp. dried marjoram
½ tsp. dried rosemary
½ tsp. dried thyme
¼ tsp. black pepper

1. In large nonstick skillet brown ground beef in oil. Stir frequently to break up clumps, until no longer pink. Drain off any drippings.

2. Stir in onions and garlic, sautéing until tender.

3. Add water, cover, and bring to boil.

4. Stir in rice, mushrooms, bouillon, salt, green beans, basil, sage, oregano, marjoram, rosemary, thyme and pepper.

5. Bring mixture again to boil, stirring once or twice.

6. Reduce heat, cover, and simmer 20 minutes, or until rice and green beans are tender.

Tip:

If you prefer your green beans to have some crunch, you can add them to the skillet 10 minutes before the end of the cooking time.

Exchange List Values
- Starch 1.5
- Lean Meat 1.0
- Vegetable 1.0
- Fat 0.5

Basic Nutritional Values
- Calories 205
  (Calories from Fat 40)
- Total Fat 4.5 gm
  (Saturated Fat 1.5 gm,
  Trans Fat 0.2 gm,
  Polyunsat Fat 0.4 gm,
  Monounsat Fat 2.2 gm)
- Cholesterol 25 mg
- Sodium 395 mg
- Potassium 285 gm
- Total Carb 30 gm
- Dietary Fiber 2 gm
- Sugars 2 gm
- Protein 11 gm
- Phosphorus 135 gm

Curried Beef Rice

Erma J. Sider
Fort Erie, Ontario

*Makes 10 servings,
about ⅔ cup per serving*

**Prep. Time: 25 minutes
Cooking/Baking Time: 50
minutes**

2 cups uncooked brown
   rice
1 lb. 90% lean ground beef
1 medium onion, chopped
1 Tbsp. canola oil
2–3 tsp. curry powder,
   depending on your taste
   preference
1 tsp. ground coriander
1 tsp. ground cumin
½ tsp. ground cinnamon
¼ tsp. black pepper
1 tsp. salt
2 Tbsp. lemon juice, *or*
   vinegar
1 cup tomato juice

1. Prepare rice according
to directions, omitting salt or
any fat.
2. Brown ground beef and
drain off grease.
3. Sauté onion in cooking
oil until golden brown.
4. Mix together all spices
and lemon juice or vinegar.
Add mixture to onions. Stir
fry lightly.
5. Add drained ground
beef. Add tomato juice and
simmer for 15 minutes. If
necessary, add water.
6. Pour mixture into baking
dish; add rice and toss lightly.
7. Bake at 325° for 20
minutes.

Exchange List Values
- Starch 2.5   • Fat 0.5
- Lean Meat 1.0

Basic Nutritional Values
- Calories 245   • Sodium 330 mg
  (Calories from Fat 55)   • Potassium 265 gm
- Total Fat 6 gm   • Total Carb 35 gm
  (Saturated Fat 1.7 gm, • Dietary Fiber 1 gm
  Trans Fat 0.2 gm,   • Sugars 2 gm
  Polyunsat Fat 0.6 gm, • Protein 12 gm
  Monounsat Fat 2.6 gm) • Phosphorus 140 gm
- Cholesterol 25 mg

Chili Rice Bake

Lucy St. Pierre
Peru, NY

*Makes 8 servings,
3¼"×4½" rectangle per serving*

**Prep. Time: 25 minutes
Baking Time: 50–60 minutes**

1 lb. 90%-lean ground beef
1 small onion, diced
2 celery ribs, diced
14½-oz. can diced tomatoes
   with juice
1 cup water
15-oz. can chili with beans
1 cup long-grain rice,
   uncooked

1. Sauté beef, onions, and
celery in nonstick medium
skillet until meat is no longer

pink. Stir frequently to break
up clumps of me at. Drain off
any fat.
2. In well-greased 9×13
casserole dish, mix together
tomatoes, water, chili, and
uncooked rice.
3. Stir in beef mixture.
4. Cover. Bake at 350° for 1
hour, or until rice is tender.

Variations from Tester:
1. For more kick, add 1–2
tsp. chili powder to Step 2.
2. Top fully baked cas-
serole with ½ cup grated
cheddar cheese. Allow to
stand 10 minutes before
serving, until cheese melts.
Barb Carper
Lancaster, PA

Exchange List Values
- Starch 1.5   • Lean Meat 2.0
- Vegetable 1.0   • Fat 0.5

Basic Nutritional Values
- Calories 250   • Sodium 355 mg
  (Calories from Fat 65)   • Potassium 490 gm
- Total Fat 7 gm   • Total Carb 29 gm
  (Saturated Fat 2.7 gm, • Dietary Fiber 3 gm
  Trans Fat 0.3 gm,   • Sugars 3 gm
  Polyunsat Fat 0.4 gm, • Protein 17 gm
  Monounsat Fat 2.8 gm) • Phosphorus 180 gm
- Cholesterol 40 mg

It's helpful to have potluck dishes labeled with their ingredients for people who need to know exactly what they're eating. Add the nutritional information per serving, if you know it.

Pita Burgers

Willard and Alice Roth
Elkhart, IN

Makes 12 servings

Prep. Time: 15 minutes
Cooking Time: 4–6 hours

2 lbs. 93%-fat-free ground
  beef
1 cup dry rolled oats
1 egg
1 medium onion, finely
  chopped
15-oz. can no-salt-added
  tomato sauce
2 Tbsp. brown sugar
2 Tbsp. cider vinegar
1 Tbsp. Worcestershire
  sauce
1 Tbsp. reduced-sodium
  soy sauce
12 pita breads

1. Combine ground chuck,
dry oats, egg and onion.
Shape mixture into 12
burgers.
2. Combine tomato sauce,
brown sugar, vinegar, Worcestershire sauce and soy sauce.
Coat each burger with sauce.
3. Place burgers with any
remaining sauce in slow
cooker. Cover and cook on
low 6 hours (or high 4 hours).
4. Invite diners to lift a
burger with tongs from slow
cooker and put into pita
pocket.

Exchange List Values
- Starch 2.5
- Vegetable 1.0
- Lean Meat 2.0
- Fat 0.5

Basic Nutritional Values
- Calories 335
  (Calories from Fat 65)
- Total Fat 7 gm
  (Saturated Fat 2.4 gm,
  Trans Fat 0.3 gm,
  Polyunsat Fat 0.8 gm,
  Monounsat Fat 2.5 gm)
- Cholesterol 60 mg
- Sodium 445 mg
- Potassium 480 gm
- Total Carb 45 gm
- Dietary Fiber 3 gm
- Sugars 5 gm
- Protein 22 gm
- Phosphorus 240 gm

Homemade Hamburgers

Janet Derstine
Telford, PA

Makes 6 servings,
1 burger per serving

Prep. Time: 30–35 minutes
Baking Time: 60 minutes

1 cup dry bread crumbs
½ cup fat-free milk
1 lb. 90%-lean ground beef
¼ cup chopped onion
¼ tsp. pepper

Sauce:
  3 Tbsp. brown sugar
  1 Tbsp. vinegar
  ¼ cup ketchup
  1 Tbsp. Worcestershire
    sauce
  ¼ cup barbecue sauce
  ½ cup water

1. In good-sized
mixing bowl,
moisten bread
crumbs with milk.
2. Add ground
beef, onion, and
pepper. Mix well.
Set aside.

3. In a mixing bowl, make
sauce by mixing together
thoroughly brown sugar,
vinegar, ketchup, Worcestershire sauce, barbecue sauce,
and water.
4. Shape hamburger
mixture into 6 patties.
5. Place in single layer in
baking dish.
6. Pour barbecue sauce
over patties.
7. Cover and bake at 375°
for 30 minutes.
8. Remove cover and bake
another 30 minutes, basting
occasionally with sauce.

Tips:
  You can double or triple
this recipe and freeze the
patties for a later meal. I
make the sauce then, when I
bake them.

Exchange List Values
- Starch 1.0
- Carbohydrate 1.0
- Lean Meat 2.0
- Fat 0.5

Basic Nutritional Values
- Calories 255
  (Calories from Fat 65)
- Total Fat 7 gm
  (Saturated Fat 2.7 gm,
  Trans Fat 0.4 gm,
  Polyunsat Fat 0.6 gm,
  Monounsat Fat 2.8 gm)
- Cholesterol 45 mg
- Sodium 445 mg
- Potassium 395 gm
- Total Carb 28 gm
- Dietary Fiber 1 gm
- Sugars 14 gm
- Protein 18 gm
- Phosphorus 190 gm

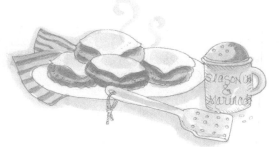

So-Good Sloppy Joes

Judy Diller
Bluffton, OH

Makes 18 servings,
1 sandwich per serving

Prep. Time: 15–20 minutes
Cooking or Baking Time: 1–2 hours

3 lbs. 90%-lean ground beef
1 medium onion, chopped
1 green bell pepper, chopped fine
10¾-oz. can lower-sodium, lower-fat tomato soup
¾ cup + 2 Tbsp. ketchup
2 Tbsp. prepared mustard
2 Tbsp. vinegar
1 Tbsp. brown sugar
2 Tbsp. Worcestershire sauce
18 whole wheat hamburger buns

1. Brown ground beef in large skillet or saucepan. Stir frequently to break up clumps and to brown thoroughly. Drain off drippings.
2. Stir onion, pepper, soup, ketchup, mustard, vinegar, brown sugar, and Worcestershire sauce into beef.
3. Simmer slowly on stovetop for 2 hours, or spoon into a Dutch oven or baking dish and bake at 325° for 1 hour.
4. Divide evenly among the rolls. Serve.

Exchange List Values
• Starch 2.0   • Fat 0.5
• Lean Meat 2.0

Basic Nutritional Values
• Calories 265   • Sodium 475 mg
  (Calories from Fat 80) • Potassium 525 gm
• Total Fat 9 gm   • Total Carb 30 gm
  (Saturated Fat 2.9 gm, • Dietary Fiber 4 gm
  Trans Fat 0.4 gm,   • Sugars 9 gm
  Polyunsat Fat 1.3 gm, • Protein 19 gm
  Monounsat Fat 3.2 gm) • Phosphorus 240 gm
• Cholesterol 45 mg

Barbecue Sloppy Joes

Winifred Paul
Scottdale, PA

Makes 5 sandwiches, 1 per serving

Prep. Time: 10 minutes
Cooking Time: 15 minutes

¾ lb. 90%-lean ground beef
1 Tbsp. oil
1 tsp. lemon juice
1 Tbsp. vinegar
3 Tbsp. water
6 Tbsp. ketchup
1 tsp. brown sugar
1 tsp. onion chopped fine
⅓ cup chopped celery
1 tsp. dry mustard
5 whole wheat hamburger buns

1. Brown beef in oil in skillet. Stir frequently to break up clumps and to make sure meat browns completely. Drain off drippings.
2. Make sauce by combining lemon juice, vinegar, water, ketchup, brown sugar, onion, celery, and dry mustard in saucepan.
3. Heat thoroughly, but do not cook enough to soften vegetables.
4. When beginning to simmer, combine with meat. Serve on buns.

Exchange List Values
• Starch 2.0   • Fat 1.0
• Lean Meat 2.0

Basic Nutritional Values
• Calories 270   • Sodium 455 mg
  (Calories from Fat 100) • Potassium 410 gm
• Total Fat 11 gm   • Total Carb 28 gm
  (Saturated Fat 2.8 gm, • Dietary Fiber 3 gm
  Trans Fat 0.4 gm,   • Sugars 9 gm
  Polyunsat Fat 1.9 gm, • Protein 17 gm
  Monounsat Fat 4.6 gm) • Phosphorus 220 gm
• Cholesterol 40 mg

Skilled cooks need to be sensitive about people who may not have the same training and understanding of how to prepare a meal as they do. All contributions to the meal should be appreciated and praised, even those which come directly from a grocery store or even fast-food restaurant.

Rachel Kauffman, Alto, MI

Delicious Sub Casserole

Janice Nolt
Ephrata, PA

Makes 8 servings

Prep. Time: 25 minutes
Baking Time: 30 minutes

**12 slices multi-grain bread,
12 oz. total, crusts
retained and bread cubed
½ cup fat-free Ranch salad
dressing
½ cup fat-free mayonnaise
1 cup sliced green bell
peppers
½ cup thinly sliced onions
¾ cup + 1 Tbsp. pizza
sauce of your choice
1 lb. 95%-lean ground beef
½ cup grated part-skim
mozzarella cheese**

1. Brown ground beef in non-stick skillet. Stir frequently to break up clumps, cooking until no pink remains. Drain off any drippings.
2. Stir pizza sauce into beef.
3. Layer bread cubes into greased 9×13 baking pan.
4. Mix salad dressing and mayonnaise together in mixing bowl.
5. Spoon over bread.
6. Layer the green pepper and onion slices over the mayo mixture.
7. Spoon beef-pizza sauce mixture over top the green peppers and onions.
8. Sprinkle with grated cheese.

9. Bake at 350° for 30 minutes, or until bubbly and heated through.

Exchange List Values
- Starch 1.5
- Carbohydrate 0.5
- Lean Meat 2.0

Basic Nutritional Values
- Calories 235 (Calories from Fat 55)
- Total Fat 6 gm (Saturated Fat 2.5 gm, Trans Fat 0.1 gm, Polyunsat Fat 0.9 gm, Monounsat Fat 1.9 gm)
- Cholesterol 40 mg
- Sodium 595 mg
- Potassium 430 gm
- Total Carb 29 gm
- Dietary Fiber 4 gm
- Sugars 5 gm
- Protein 17 gm
- Phosphorus 275 gm

Meat Pasties (Turnovers)

Jeanette Zacharias
Morden, Manitoba

Makes 12 servings

Prep. Time: 30 minutes
Cooking/Baking Time: 1 hour

Dough:
**2 cups all-purpose flour
½ cup no-trans-fat
shortening
½ tsp. salt
7 Tbsp. fat-free milk, *or*
more**

Filling:
**¾ lb. 90%-lean ground
beef
2 Tbsp. chopped onion
1 Tbsp. chopped bell
pepper
1 Tbsp. chopped celery
1 tsp. dried oregano
1 tsp. dried basil**

**2 Tbsp. barbecue
sauce, lowest sodium
available**

1. Combine all ingredients for dough and mix well. Add as much milk as needed to make a soft dough.
2. Divide dough into four parts. Roll each part out thin and cut into three 6" circles for a total of 12.
3. Combine all filling ingredients. Heat until meat has browned.
4. Place 1 Tbsp. meat on each circle. Moisten edges of dough with water and fold in half to make a turnover. Seal edges will with fork. Prick top to allow steam to escape. Place on ungreased cookie sheet.
5. Bake at 375° for 40 minutes. Serve hot or cold.

Exchange List Values
- Starch 1.0
- Lean Meat 1.0

Basic Nutritional Values
- Calories 135 (Calories from Fat 25)
- Total Fat 3 gm (Saturated Fat 1.1 gm, Trans Fat 0.1 gm, Polyunsat Fat 0.4 gm, Monounsat Fat 1.2 gm)
- Cholesterol 15 mg
- Sodium 140 mg
- Potassium 145 gm
- Total Carb 18 gm
- Dietary Fiber 1 gm
- Sugars 2 gm
- Protein 8 gm
- Phosphorus 80 gm

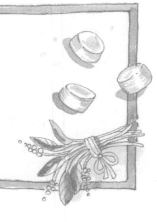

Seafood Main Dishes

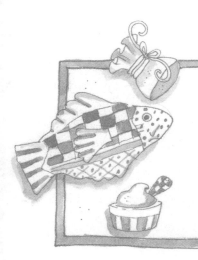

Holiday Salmon Bake

Rhoda Atzeff
Lancaster, PA

Makes 8 servings,
3¼"×4½" rectangle per serving

Prep. Time: 15–20 minutes
Baking Time: 35–40 minutes

⅔ cup shredded 75%-less-
   fat cheddar cheese,
   divided
⅔ cup shredded reduced-
   fat Swiss cheese, *divided*
3 cups cubed day old
   sourdough bread, *or*
   bagels
10-oz. bag frozen chopped
   broccoli, thawed and
   drained
8-oz. bag frozen cut
   asparagus, thawed and
   drained
4½-oz. can sliced
   mushrooms, drained
½ cup sliced green onions,
   or red onions

1 cup egg substitute
2 eggs, beaten
1 cup fat-free milk
1 tsp. garlic salt
1 tsp. pepper
½ lb. salmon fillet, *or*
   7.1-oz. pouch boneless,
   skinless pink salmon

1. In large bowl, combine
⅓ cup cheddar cheese, ⅓ cup
Swiss cheese, bread, broccoli,
asparagus, mushrooms, and
onions.

2. In another bowl, whisk
together egg substitute, milk,
garlic salt, and pepper.

3. Add egg mixture to
vegetable mixture. Blend
well.

4. If using fresh salmon,
remove skin. Flake salmon
and fold into mixture.

5. Spoon into well-greased
9×13 baking dish.

6. Bake uncovered at 375°
for 35–40 minutes, or until
firm.

7. During last 7 minutes
of baking time, sprinkle on
remaining cheeses.

8. Bake uncovered until

cheeses melt. Serve immediately.

Tips:
   You can make this up to
24 hours before baking and
serving. Prepare through Step
5, cover, and then refrigerate.

Exchange List Values
- Starch 1.0
- Vegetable 1.0
- Lean Meat 3.0

Basic Nutritional Values
- Calories 245
  (Calories from Fat 65)
- Total Fat 7 gm
  (Saturated Fat 2.4 gm,
  Trans Fat 0.0 gm,
  Polyunsat Fat 1.2 gm,
  Monounsat Fat 2.3 gm)
- Cholesterol 75 mg
- Sodium 585 mg
- Potassium 395 gm
- Total Carb 22 gm
- Dietary Fiber 3 gm
- Sugars 4 gm
- Protein 24 gm
- Phosphorus 300 gm

Nutty Salmon

Mary Seielstad
Sparks, NV

Makes 6 servings
Prep. Time: 5–10 minutes
Baking Time: 20 minutes

2 Tbsp. Dijon mustard
2 Tbsp. olive oil
½ cup ground pecans
6 4-oz. salmon fillets

1. In a mixing bowl, mix together mustard, oil, and pecans.
2. Spread on salmon fillets.
3. Place on an oiled or baking pan.
4. Bake at 375° for 15–18 minutes, or until fish flakes easily.

Tips:
You can cook this recipe on the grill. Watch closely to see that the topping doesn't burn and that you don't over-cook the fish.

Exchange List Values
• Lean Meat 4.0   • Fat 2.0

Basic Nutritional Values
• Calories 300   • Sodium 180 mg
  (Calories from Fat 190) • Potassium 385 gm
• Total Fat 21 gm   • Total Carb 2 gm
  (Saturated Fat 2.9 gm, • Dietary Fiber 1 gm
  Trans Fat 0.0 gm,   • Sugars 1 gm
  Polyunsat Fat 4.3 gm, • Protein 26 gm
  Monounsat Fat 11.7 gm) • Phosphorus 280 gm
• Cholesterol 80 mg

Salmon Loaf

Clara Yoder Byler
Hartville, OH

Makes 6 servings, 1 slice per serving
Prep. Time: 15 minutes
Cooking Time: 1 hour
Standing Time: 10 minutes

14¾-oz. can sockeye salmon canned without salt, drained and flaked
¼ cup fat-free milk
10¾-oz. can lower-sodium, lower-fat cream of celery soup
¼ cup egg substitute
1 cup dry bread crumbs
½ cup chopped onion
1 Tbsp. lemon juice

1. Combine salmon, milk, soup, egg substitute, bread crumbs, onion, and lemon juice in a bowl.
2. Shape into loaf. Place in greased 8½×4½ loaf pan.
3. Bake at 350° for 1 hour.
4. Allow to stand 10 minutes before slicing.

Exchange List Values
• Starch 1.0   • Lean Meat 2.0
• Carbohydrate 0.5

Basic Nutritional Values
• Calories 210   • Sodium 370 mg
  (Calories from Fat 55) • Potassium 565 gm
• Total Fat 6 gm   • Total Carb 20 gm
  (Saturated Fat 1.4 gm, • Dietary Fiber 1 gm
  Trans Fat 0.0 gm,   • Sugars 3 gm
  Polyunsat Fat 2.2 gm, • Protein 17 gm
  Monounsat Fat 2.1 gm) • Phosphorus 265 gm
• Cholesterol 30 mg

Crab and Zucchini Casserole

Virginia Bender, Dover, DE

*Makes 6 servings,
about 1 cup per serving*
Prep. Time: 20 minutes
Baking Time: 35–40 minutes

2 medium zucchini, sliced
½ cup chopped onion
2 cloves garlic, crushed
2 Tbsp. canola oil
⅛ tsp. pepper
1 tsp. dried basil
1 lb. crab meat
1 cup freshly grated reduced-fat Swiss cheese
1 cup soft bread crumbs
3 medium tomatoes

1. Cook zucchini, onion and garlic in oil about 5 minutes or until tender.
2. Remove from skillet and add seasonings, crab meat, cheese and bread crumbs.
3. Chop tomatoes, removing seeds. Add tomatoes and toss lightly.
4. Place in glass casserole dish. Bake at 375° for 30–35 minutes or until heated through.

Exchange List Values
• Carbohydrate 0.5   • Lean Meat 3.0
• Vegetable 1.0   • Fat 0.5

Basic Nutritional Values
• Calories 210   • Sodium 300 mg
  (Calories from Fat 80) • Potassium 655 gm
• Total Fat 9 gm   • Total Carb 12 gm
  (Saturated Fat 2.2 gm, • Dietary Fiber 2 gm
  Trans Fat 0.0 gm,   • Sugars 4 gm
  Polyunsat Fat 1.8 gm, • Protein 21 gm
  Monounsat Fat 4.0 gm) • Phosphorus 300 gm
• Cholesterol 55 mg

Flounder Zucchini Bundles

Betty L. Moore
Plano, IL

Makes 4 servings, 1 bundle per serving

Prep. Time: 15 minutes
Cooking/Baking Time: 20 minutes

4 6-oz. flounder fillets
¼ tsp. lemon pepper, *divided*
1 medium lemon, thinly sliced, *divided*
1 medium zucchini, cut into ¼"-thick slices, *divided*
12 cherry tomatoes, sliced, *divided*
¼ tsp. dill weed, *divided*
¼ tsp. dried basil, *divided*

1. Place 1 fillet on double thickness of 15"×18" piece of heavy duty foil.
2. Sprinkle with ¼ of lemon pepper.
3. Top with ¼ of lemon slices, zucchini, and tomatoes.
4. Sprinkle with ¼ of dill and basil.

5. Fold foil around fish and seal tightly. Place on baking sheet.
6. Repeat with other fillets.
7. Bake at 425° for 15–20 minutes, or until fish flakes easily.

Exchange List Values
• Lean Meat 4.0

Basic Nutritional Values
• Calories 170
 (Calories from Fat 20)
• Total Fat 2 gm
 (Saturated Fat 0.5 gm,
 Trans Fat 0.0 gm,
 Polyunsat Fat 0.9 gm,
 Monounsat Fat 0.4 gm)
• Cholesterol 90 mg
• Sodium 170 mg
• Potassium 690 gm
• Total Carb 4 gm
• Dietary Fiber 1 gm
• Sugars 2 gm
• Protein 33 gm
• Phosphorus 410 gm

Easy Dill Sauce for Fish Fillets

Mary Seielstad
Sparks, NV

Makes 1¼ cups sauce,
10 servings, 2 Tbsp. per serving

Prep. Time: 10 minutes
Baking Time: 18–20 minutes

7 Tbsp. tub margarine, no trans-fat

¼ tsp. dried thyme
1 large bay leaf
1 Tbsp. minced onion
¾ tsp. dill weed
¼ tsp. salt
⅛ tsp. pepper
1 tsp. sugar
1 cup fat-free sour cream

1. Melt margarine in small saucepan.
2. Remove from heat. Add thyme, bay leaf, onion, dill weed, salt, pepper, sugar, and sour cream.
3. Mix well.
4. Lay fish fillets on greased baking pan.
5. Spread sauce over top of fish fillets to cover.
6. Bake until sauce is bubbly, about 18–20 minutes at 375°.
7. Offer remaining sauce when serving fish.

Tip:
 We like this on white fillets, as well as on salmon.

Exchange List Values
• Carbohydrate 0.5 • Fat 1.0

Basic Nutritional Values
• Calories 75
 (Calories from Fat 55)
• Total Fat 6 gm
 (Saturated Fat 1.4 gm,
 Trans Fat 0.0 gm,
 Polyunsat Fat 2.5 gm,
 Monounsat Fat 1.9 gm)
• Cholesterol 0 mg
• Sodium 145 mg
• Potassium 40 gm
• Total Carb 5 gm
• Dietary Fiber 0 gm
• Sugars 1 gm
• Protein 1 gm
• Phosphorus 25 gm

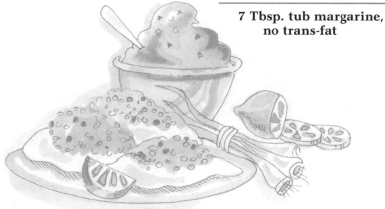

Red Snapper Creole

Dorothy L. Ealy
Los Angeles, CA

*Makes 6 servings,
about 3 oz. fish and
about ¾ cup sauce*

Prep. Time: 20 minutes
Baking Time: 40 minutes

6 4-oz. red snapper fillets
salt and pepper to taste
1 Tbsp. butter
1–2 Tbsp. flour
6 slices bacon
2 large onions, chopped
1 clove garlic, minced
1 Tbsp. canola oil
2 16-oz. cans tomatoes
1 cup water
1 Tbsp. chopped parsley
½ tsp. thyme
2 bay leaves
lemon wedges

1. Wash fish thoroughly. Rub with salt and pepper. Lay into baking pan, dot with butter and sprinkle with flour.
2. Bake at 350° for 15 minutes.
3. Fry and drain bacon. Set aside.
4. Brown onions and garlic in canola oil. Add tomatoes, water and seasonings. Cook until sauce is thickened.
5. Pour sauce over fish and bake 15 minutes longer. Remove bay leaves.
6. Garnish with bacon slices and lemon wedges. Serve.

Exchange List Values
• Vegetable 3.0   • Fat 0.5
• Lean Meat 3.0

Basic Nutritional Values
• Calories 240   • Sodium 425 mg
  (Calories from Fat 70) • Potassium 900 gm
• Total Fat 8 gm   • Total Carb 14 gm
  (Saturated Fat 1.7 gm, • Dietary Fiber 3 gm
  Trans Fat 0.0 gm,   • Sugars 7 gm
  Polyunsat Fat 2.1 gm,   • Protein 28 gm
  Monounsat Fat 3.4 gm)   • Phosphorus 265 gm
• Cholesterol 50 mg

Shrimp Creole

Ethel Camardelle
Des Allemands, LA

*Makes 8 servings,
about 1 cup per serving*

Prep. Time: 20 minutes
Cooking Time: 1½ hours

1¾ lbs. raw shrimp, peeled
pepper to taste
2 Tbsp. canola oil
1 cup chopped onions
1 cup chopped celery
½ cup chopped bell peppers
8-oz. can no-salt-added tomato paste
8-oz. can no-salt-added tomato sauce
1 Tbsp. Louisiana hot sauce
2½ cups water
3 cloves garlic, minced
1 cup chopped green onions
parsley

1. Peel shrimp. Pepper to taste and set aside.
2. In a heavy saucepan heat oil. Sauté onions, celery and peppers until wilted.
3. Add tomato paste and cook 5 minutes over low heat, stirring constantly.
4. Add tomato sauce, hot sauce and water. Cook for 1 hour, stirring occasionally.
5. Stir in shrimp and garlic. Cook another 15 minutes.
6. Sprinkle with green onions and parsley. Cook 2–3 more minutes.
7. Serve with rice.

Exchange List Values
• Vegetable 3.0   • Fat 0.5
• Lean Meat 1.0

Basic Nutritional Values
• Calories 150   • Sodium 600 mg
  (Calories from Fat 40) • Potassium 600 gm
• Total Fat 4.5 gm   • Total Carb 13 gm
  (Saturated Fat 0.6 gm, • Dietary Fiber 3 gm
  Trans Fat 0.0 gm,   • Sugars 6 gm
  Polyunsat Fat 1.4 gm,   • Protein 15 gm
  Monounsat Fat 2.5 gm)   • Phosphorus 220 gm
• Cholesterol 120 mg

Be sure to check around to see if any of the attendees have dietary restrictions. Some people have allergies or prefer not to eat certain foods, so it's nice to make sure there's some food on the table that they can eat.

Scalloped Scallops

Flossie Sultzaberger
Mechanicsburg, PA

*Makes 6 servings,
about 2 oz. per serving*

**Prep. Time: 15 minutes
Baking Time: 25 minutes**

2 Tbsp. tub margarine, no
   trans-fat
2 Tbsp. canola oil
½ cup snack-cracker,
   preferably wheat thins,
   crumbs
¼ cup soft bread crumbs
1 lb. scallops (if large, cut
   in half)
dash of salt
dash of pepper
cooking spray

1. Melt margarine and oil together in saucepan.
2. Stir in cracker crumbs and bread crumbs.
3. Spray a 1½- 2 –quart casserole lightly with cooking spray.
4. Place half the scallops in bottom of baking dish.
5. Sprinkle with salt and pepper.
6. Cover with half buttered crumbs.
7. Repeat layers.
8. Bake at 400° for 25 minutes.

Tip:
   Add a few shrimp to the scallops for a very special dish.

Exchange List Values
- Starch 0.5
- Fat 1.5
- Lean Meat 1.0

Basic Nutritional Values
- Calories 155
  (Calories from Fat 80)
- Total Fat 9 gm
  (Saturated Fat 1.2 gm,
  Trans Fat 0.1 gm,
  Polyunsat Fat 3.2 gm,
  Monounsat Fat 4.2 gm)
- Cholesterol 20 mg
- Sodium 450 mg
- Potassium 170 gm
- Total Carb 8 gm
- Dietary Fiber 0 gm
- Sugars 1 gm
- Protein 11 gm
- Phosphorus 225 gm

Spanish Paella

Melodie Davis
Harrisonburg, VA

*Makes 10 servings,
about 11 oz. per serving*

**Prep. Time: 20 minutes
Cooking Time: 50 minutes**

1¼ lbs. boneless skinless
   chicken thighs, cut in 5
   pieces
1¼ lbs. boneless skinless
   chicken breasts, cut in 5
   pieces
¼ cup olive oil
¼ lb. lean boneless pork
   chop, cubed
¼ lb. bulk lean Italian
   turkey sweet sausage
8 slices onion
4 medium tomatoes, diced
1 green pepper, chopped
2 cups uncooked rice
3 cups lower-sodium, fat-
   free chicken broth
2 Tbsp. paprika
½ tsp. pepper
¼ tsp. red pepper
⅛ tsp. saffron
pinch of minced garlic
1¾ cups shrimp, shelled
   and deveined
10-oz. pkg. green peas
4 oz. sliced pimento, drained

1. Wash chicken pieces and dry. In Dutch oven or heavy kettle, brown chicken in oil. Remove chicken and drain excess fat.
2. Brown pork and sausage. Remove and drain excess fat.
3. Sauté onions, tomatoes and green pepper, stirring until onion is tender. Stir in rice, chicken broth and seasonings. Add chicken.
4. Cover tightly and simmer for 20 minutes.
5. Gently fold in shrimp, pork, sausage and peas. Cover and simmer another 15 minutes.
6. Add pimento, heat through and serve.

Exchange List Values
- Starch 2.0
- Lean Meat 4.0
- Vegetable 1.0
- Fat 1.5

Basic Nutritional Values
- Calories 435
  (Calories from Fat 125)
- Total Fat 14 gm
  (Saturated Fat 3.1 gm,
  Trans Fat 0.0 gm,
  Polyunsat Fat 2.5 gm,
  Monounsat Fat 6.9 gm)
- Cholesterol 135 mg
- Sodium 575 mg
- Potassium 610 gm
- Total Carb 39 gm
- Dietary Fiber 4 gm
- Sugars 4 gm
- Protein 37 gm
- Phosphorus 365 gm

Seafood Noodles

Helen Rose Pauls
Sardis, British Columbia

Makes 8 servings, about ⅔ cup

Prep. Time: 20 minutes
Cooking/Baking Time: 40 minutes

10-oz. pkg. broad noodles
2 7-oz. cans tuna, *or* shrimp, *or* salmon
½ cup fat-free milk
celery salt to taste
pepper to taste
2 Tbsp. no-salt-added dry onion soup mix (see page 271)

1. Cook noodles according to directions, omitting salt, and drain.
2. Drain seafood of liquid.
3. Combine all ingredients and spoon into 2-quart baking dish.
4. Bake at 350° for 30 minutes.

Exchange List Values
- Starch 1.5
- Lean Meat 1.0

Basic Nutritional Values
- Calories 175
  (Calories from Fat 20)
- Total Fat 2.5 gm
  (Saturated Fat 0.5 gm,
  Trans Fat 0.0 gm,
  Polyunsat Fat 0.7 gm,
  Monounsat Fat 0.6 gm)
- Cholesterol 45 mg
- Sodium 155 mg
- Potassium 285 gm
- Total Carb 25 gm
- Dietary Fiber 1 gm
- Sugars 2 gm
- Protein 13 gm
- Phosphorus 160 gm

Seafood Quiche

Anne Jones
Ballston Lake, NY

Makes 8 servings,
1 slice per serving

Prep. Time: 10–15 minutes
Baking Time: 30–40 minutes
Standing Time: 10 minutes

8" pie crust, made from Basic Pie Crust by Graham Kerr (see page 203)
1 Tbsp. chopped onion
7-oz. pkg. crab and shrimp
1 cup egg substitute
½ cup fat-free milk
½ tsp. salt
¼ tsp. pepper
2 oz. shredded reduced-fat Swiss cheese
dash of nutmeg, *optional*

1. Sprinkle chopped onion in crust.
2. Spread crab and shrimp over top.
3. In mixing bowl, beat eggs substitute, milk, salt, and pepper together.
4. Add shredded cheese.
5. Pour over crab meat mixture in pie crust.
6. Sprinkle with nutmeg if you wish.
7. Bake at 375° for 30–40 minutes, or until knife inserted in center of quiche comes out clean.
8. Allow to stand 10 minutes before cutting into wedges.

Exchange List Values
- Starch 0.5
- Lean Meat 2.0

Basic Nutritional Values
- Calories 105
  (Calories from Fat 30)
- Total Fat 4 gm
  (Saturated Fat 1.1 gm,
  Trans Fat 0.2 gm,
  Polyunsat Fat 0.6 gm,
  Monounsat Fat 1.2 gm)
- Cholesterol 50 mg
- Sodium 395 mg
- Potassium 145 gm
- Total Carb 7 gm
- Dietary Fiber 0 gm
- Sugars 1 gm
- Protein 11 gm
- Phosphorus 135 gm

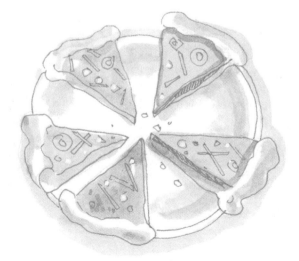

Tuna Bake with Cheese Swirls

Mary Ann Lefever
Lancaster, PA

Makes 8 servings,
3¼"×4½" rectangle per serving

Prep. Time: 30 minutes
Baking Time: 25 minutes

½ cup diced green bell
  peppers
½ cup chopped onions
2 Tbsp. canola oil
6 Tbsp. flour
2 cups fat-free milk
6½- *or* 7-oz. can *or* pouch
  tuna

Cheese Swirls:
  1½ cups reduced-fat
    buttermilk biscuit mix
  ¾ cup grated 50%-less
    fat cheddar cheese
  ½ cup fat-free milk
  2 chopped pimentos
    (from jar)

1. In saucepan, sauté green
pepper and onions in butter
until soft but not brown.
2. Blend in flour and cook
over low heat a few minutes
to get rid of raw flour taste.
3. Gradually stir in milk.
Cook over low heat, stirring
continually until smooth.

4. Add tuna.
5. Spoon into greased 9×13
baking pan. Set aside.
6. To make cheese swirls,
prepare biscuits with milk
according to package directions.
7. On lightly floured board,
roll out to 8×13 rectangle.
8. Sprinkle with cheese and
chopped pimento. Press into
dough to help adhere.
9. Roll up jelly-roll fashion.
10. Cut roll into 8 slices.
11. Flatten slightly and
place on top of tuna mixture.
12. Bake at 450° for 25
minutes, or until tuna mix
is bubbly and biscuits are
browned.

Exchange List Values
- Starch 1.5   • Lean Meat 2.0

Basic Nutritional Values
- Calories 215   • Sodium 440 mg
  (Calories from Fat 65)   • Potassium 270 gm
- Total Fat 7 gm   • Total Carb 26 gm
  (Saturated Fat 1.7 gm,   • Dietary Fiber 1 gm
  Trans Fat 0.0 gm,   • Sugars 7 gm
  Polyunsat Fat 1.5 gm,   • Protein 13 gm
  Monounsat Fat 3.6 gm)   • Phosphorus 310 gm
- Cholesterol 15 mg

Tuna Tempties

Lois Ostrander
Lebanon, PA

Makes 6 servings,
1 sandwich per serving

Prep. Time: 15 minutes
Baking Time: 15 minutes

3½ oz. 75%-less-fat
  cheddar cheese, cubed
6-oz. can low-sodium tuna,
  flaked
2 Tbsp. chopped green bell
  pepper
2 Tbsp. minced onion
2 Tbsp. sweet pickle
¼ cup fat-free mayonnaise
dash of pepper
6 whole-grain hot dog buns

1. Combine cheese, tuna,
green pepper, minced onion,
sweet pickle, mayonnaise,
salt, and pepper in mixing
bowl.
2. Split buns and fill with
tuna mixture.
3. Wrap each bun in foil.
4. Bake in oven at 350°
for 15 minutes until filling is
heated and cheese melts.

Exchange List Values
- Starch 2.0   • Lean Meat 1.0

Basic Nutritional Values
- Calories 200   • Sodium 470 mg
  (Calories from Fat 35)   • Potassium 235 gm
- Total Fat 4 gm   • Total Carb 26 gm
  (Saturated Fat 1.4 gm,   • Dietary Fiber 4 gm
  Trans Fat 0.0 gm,   • Sugars 6 gm
  Polyunsat Fat 1.0 gm,   • Protein 17 gm
  Monounsat Fat 0.9 gm)   • Phosphorus 235 gm
- Cholesterol 20 mg

Let your kids help in the kitchen. They love to
crack eggs, add ingredients, and mix. Yes, the mess
will be bigger, but the time together is well spent.
                              Beth Maurer, West Liberty, OH

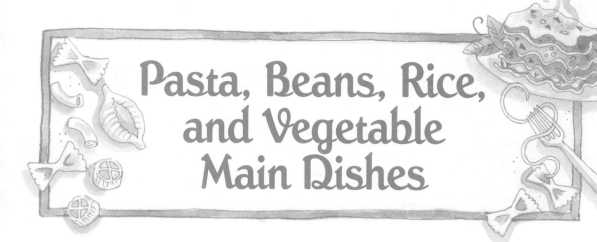

Pasta, Beans, Rice, and Vegetable Main Dishes

Creamy Crunchy Mac & Cheese

Kathy Hertzler
Lancaster, PA

Makes 10 servings, a 2⅗"×4½" rectangle per serving

Prep. Time: 25 minutes
Cooking/Baking Time: 30 minutes

1 lb. uncooked macaroni
2 cups fat-free milk
1½ Tbsp. canola oil
3 Tbsp. flour
3½ cups shredded 75%-less-fat cheddar cheese, *divided*
½ tsp. seasoned salt
½ tsp. ground black pepper
1 tsp. dry mustard
1 tsp. garlic powder, *or* 2 cloves garlic, minced
1 tsp. onion powder, *or* ¼ cup onions, chopped
¾ cup crushed cornflakes

1. Cook macaroni until al dente in unsalted water, according to package directions, about 7 minutes. Drain well.

2. While pasta is cooking, warm milk until steamy but not boiling.

3. In another, medium-sized saucepan, warm oil. Add flour, and whisk until smooth.

4. Add warm milk to oil/flour mixture. Whisk until smooth.

5. Cook, stirring constantly, on low heat for 2 minutes.

6. Add 3 cups shredded cheddar. Stir well, and then remove from heat. Set aside.

7. Stir salt, pepper, mustard, minced garlic or garlic powder, and chopped onions or onion powder into creamy sauce.

8. Place cooked macaroni in large mixing bowl.

9. Stir in cheese sauce.

10. Transfer mixture to greased 9×13 baking dish.

11. Sprinkle with cornflakes, and then remaining shredded cheddar.

12. Bake at 400° for 10–12 minutes, or until hot and bubbly.

Tips:

Don't boil the sauce after the cheese has been added. It's best to add the cheese to the sauce, stir, and remove from heat. Boiled cheese sauces usually curdle a bit or separate and don't look appetizing.

Exchange List Values
• Starch 3.0   • Lean Meat 2.0

Basic Nutritional Values
• Calories 320 (Calories from Fat 65)
• Total Fat 7 gm (Saturated Fat 2.4 gm, Trans Fat 0.0 gm, Polyunsat Fat 1.0 gm, Monounsat Fat 2.2 gm)
• Cholesterol 15 mg
• Sodium 400 mg
• Potassium 185 gm
• Total Carb 43 gm
• Dietary Fiber 2 gm
• Sugars 4 gm
• Protein 21 gm
• Phosphorus 310 gm

Homemade Mac and Cheese

Sherry L. Lapp
Lancaster, PA

Karissa Newswanger
Denver, PA

Karen Burkholder
Narvon, PA

Jen Hoover
Akron, PA

*Makes 8 servings,
about 6 oz. per serving*

Prep. Time: 20 minutes
Cooking/Baking Time: 35 minutes

½ lb. (2 cups) small shell macaroni
¼ cup water
1½ Tbsp. no-trans-fat tub margarine
3 Tbsp. flour
3 cups fat-free milk
11 oz. extra-sharp 75%-reduced-fat shredded cheddar cheese
½ tsp. salt
2 tsp. Dijon mustard

1. Cook macaroni according to package direction in unsalted water until al dente. Drain.
2. Transfer to greased 3-quart baking dish.
3. Stir ¼ cup water into cooked macaroni.
4. Melt margarine in medium-sized saucepan. Sprinkle in flour and stir constantly over medium heat, about 2 minutes.
5. Increase heat a bit. Add milk ½ cup at a time.

6. When milk is fully mixed in, reduce heat and stir continually until mixture bubbles and begins to thicken.
7. Add cheese 1 cup at a time, stirring continually.
8. Add salt and mustard. Mix well.
9. Transfer to casserole dish. Blend with macaroni.
10. Bake at 375° for 25 minutes, or until bubbly and heated through.

Exchange List Values
- Starch 1.5
- Lean Meat 1.0
- Fat-Free Milk 0.5
- Fat 0.5

Basic Nutritional Values
- Calories 240
  (Calories from Fat 55)
- Total Fat 6 gm
  (Saturated Fat 2.5 gm,
  Trans Fat 0.0 gm,
  Polyunsat Fat 0.9 gm,
  Monounsat Fat 1.3 gm)
- Cholesterol 15 mg
- Sodium 505 mg
- Potassium 225 gm
- Total Carb 28 gm
- Dietary Fiber 1 gm
- Sugars 5 gm
- Protein 20 gm
- Phosphorus 320 gm

Baked Macaroni

Ann Good
Perry, NY

*Makes 12 servings,
3" square per serving*

Prep. Time: 5 minutes
Cooking/Baking Time: 3 hours

2½ Tbsp. tub margarine, no trans-fat
3 cups *uncooked* macaroni
2 quarts fat-free milk
4 cups 75%-less-fat shredded cheddar cheese
1 tsp. salt
½ tsp. pepper

1. In large bowl, mix together butter, macaroni, milk, cheese, salt, and pepper.
2. Pour into greased 9×13 casserole dish.
3. Cover. Bake at 225° for 2¾ hours.
4. Remove cover. Bake 15 minutes longer to brown dish.

Warm Memories:
This was the first recipe I got as a newly-wed from my mother-in-law. My husband loves when I make it. It has been a long-time favorite Sunday dinner side dish for his family.

Exchange List Values
- Starch 1.5
- Lean Meat 2.0
- Fat-Free Milk 0.5

Basic Nutritional Values
- Calories 250
  (Calories from Fat 55)
- Total Fat 6 gm
  (Saturated Fat 2.5 gm,
  Trans Fat 0.0 gm,
  Polyunsat Fat 0.9 gm,
  Monounsat Fat 1.3 gm)
- Cholesterol 15 mg
- Sodium 550 mg
- Potassium 360 gm
- Total Carb 29 gm
- Dietary Fiber 1 gm
- Sugars 9 gm
- Protein 21 gm
- Phosphorus 395 gm

Ham and Macaroni Casserole

Jena Hammond
Traverse City, MI

Makes 10 servings,
2⅗"×4½" rectangle per serving

Prep. Time: 20 minutes
Chilling Time: 8 hours, or
overnight
Cooking/Baking Time: 1–1½ hours

¼ cup chopped onions
1½ tsp. canola oil
1¾ cups low-sodium cubed
   ham
2 10¾-oz. cans lower-
   sodium, lower-fat
   mushroom soup
2 cups fat-free milk
2½ cups uncooked
   macaroni
1½ cups 75%-less-fat
   shredded cheddar cheese

1. Sauté onion in oil in saucepan.
2. Add ham, soup, milk, macaroni, and cheese. Stir until well blended.
3. Pour into greased 9×13 pan or 2-quart baking dish.
4. Cover. Refrigerate at least 8 hours or overnight.
5. Bake, covered, at 325° for 45–60 minutes, or until beginning to bubble around edges.
6. Remove cover. Bake an additional 15 minutes, or until lightly browned.

Exchange List Values
• Starch 1.5
• Carbohydrate 0.5
• Lean Meat 2.0

Basic Nutritional Values
• Calories 240   • Sodium 575 mg
   (Calories from Fat 45)   • Potassium 595 gm
• Total Fat 5 gm   • Total Carb 30 gm
   (Saturated Fat 1.8 gm,   • Dietary Fiber 2 gm
   Trans Fat 0.0 gm,   • Sugars 4 gm
   Polyunsat Fat 1.0 gm,   • Protein 17 gm
   Monounsat Fat 1.7 gm)   • Phosphorus 240 gm
• Cholesterol 20 mg

Rigatoni Royal

Gloria Julien
Gladstone, MI

Makes 15 servings,
2⅗"×3" rectangle per serving

Prep. Time: 50 minutes
Baking Time: 45 minutes

1¾ lbs. 95%-lean ground
   beef
1 large onion, chopped
2 cloves garlic, diced
8 cups marinara sauce,
   light in sodium
1 lb. uncooked rigatoni
   noodles, *divided*
4 oz. reduced-fat provolone
   cheese, grated
1½ cups fat-free sour
   cream
4 oz. part-skim mozzarella
   cheese, grated
Italian seasoning
Parmesan cheese, *optional*

1. Brown hamburger with onion and garlic in large stock-pot. Stir frequently to break up clumps of meat, cooking until no pink remains.
2. Drain off drippings.
3. Stir in marinara sauce. Simmer slowly for 30 minutes.

4. Meanwhile, cook noodles in unsalted water until slightly under-done. Drain.
5. Grease deep 9×13 baking dish or lasagna pan. Layer in half the noodles.
6. Top with provolone cheese.
7. Spoon sour cream over provolone, spreading as well as possible.
8. Top with half of meat sauce.
9. Add another layer of noodles, using all that remain.
10. Top with mozzarella cheese.
11. Spoon over remainder of sauce.
12. Sprinkle generously with Italian seasoning and optional Parmesan cheese.
13. Bake at 350° for 45 minutes, or until bubbly and heated throughout.

Tip:
   You can prepare this dish through Step 12 the night before you want to serve it. Bake it just before serving. If you're going to serve this at a church potluck, bake it at a low heat (300°) during church, and it will be ready to eat at noon.

Exchange List Values
• Starch 2.0   • Lean Meat 2.0
• Fat-Free Milk 0.5   • Fat 1.0

Basic Nutritional Values
• Calories 335   • Sodium 470 mg
   (Calories from Fat 100) • Potassium 660 gm
• Total Fat 11 gm   • Total Carb 38 gm
   (Saturated Fat 3.5 gm,   • Dietary Fiber 3 gm
   Trans Fat 0.1 gm,   • Sugars 8 gm
   Polyunsat Fat 2.2 gm,   • Protein 21 gm
   Monounsat Fat 3.1 gm)   • Phosphorus 280 gm
• Cholesterol 45 mg

Creamy Baked Ziti

Judi Manos
West Islip, NY

Makes 12 servings,
3" square per serving

Prep. Time: 20 minutes
Baking Time: 20 minutes

4 cups uncooked ziti pasta
24½-oz. jar lower-sodium marinara sauce
14½-oz. can diced tomatoes, undrained
2 3-oz. pkgs. fat-free cream cheese, cubed
¾ cup fat-free sour cream
8 oz. shredded part-skim mozzarella cheese, *divided*
⅓ cup freshly grated Parmesan cheese

1. Cook pasta as directed on package, but omit salt. Drain cooked pasta well.
2. While pasta drains, add marinara sauce, tomatoes, and cream cheese to cooking pot.
3. Cook on medium heat 5 minutes, or until cream cheese is melted and mixture is well blended. Stir frequently.
4. Return pasta to pan. Mix well.
5. Layer half the pasta mixture in greased 9×13 baking dish.
6. Cover with layer of sour cream.
7. Top with 1 cup mozzarella.
8. Spoon over remaining pasta mixture.
9. Top with remaining mozzarella.
10. Sprinkle with Parmesan cheese.
11. Bake 20 minutes, or until bubbly and heated through.

Tips:
1. You can use penne pasta instead of ziti.
2. You can make this dish ahead of the day you want to serve it. Prepare through Step 10. Cover and refrigerate before baking. If you put the casserole in the oven cold, Increase baking time to 30–35 minutes, or until heated through.

Exchange List Values
- Starch 2.0
- Med-Fat Meat 1.0

Basic Nutritional Values
- Calories 230 (Calories from Fat 55)
- Total Fat 6 gm (Saturated Fat 2.5 gm, Trans Fat 0.0 gm, Polyunsat Fat 1.1 gm, Monounsat Fat 1.6 gm)
- Cholesterol 15 mg
- Sodium 440 mg
- Potassium 350 gm
- Total Carb 31 gm
- Dietary Fiber 2 gm
- Sugars 6 gm
- Protein 12 gm
- Phosphorus 255 gm

Baked Ziti with Vegetables

Sandra Haverstraw
Hummelstown, PA

Makes 12 servings,
3" square per serving

Prep. Time: 15–20 minutes
Baking Time: 30 minutes
Standing Time: 10 minutes

12-oz. pkg. ziti, uncooked
10-oz. pkg. frozen broccoli
10-oz. pkg. frozen cauliflower
15-oz. container fat-free ricotta cheese
¾ tsp. dried oregano
1 cup part-skim shredded mozzarella
2 tsp. hot sauce
24½-oz. jar marinara low-sodium spaghetti sauce, *divided*
¾ cup freshly grated Parmesan cheese

1. Cook ziti in boiling water for 6 minutes.
2. Add broccoli and cauliflower to ziti and boiling water. Cook for 2 additional minutes. Drain.
3. Blend ricotta, oregano, mozzarella, and red pepper sauce in bowl.
4. Toss ziti and veggies with 1 cup spaghetti sauce.
5. Spoon half of ziti-veggie-sauce mix into bottom of

Roasting fruits and vegetables is a healthy way to enhance their natural flavors.

well-greased 9×13 baking dish.

6. Spoon ⅔ of cheese mixture over ziti.

7. Cover with remaining ziti.

8. Spoon remaining spaghetti sauce over ziti. Top with remaining ⅓ of cheese mixture.

9. Cover with foil. Bake at 450° for 25 minutes.

10. Uncover. Sprinkle with Parmesan cheese.

11. Bake 5 minutes longer.

12. Allow to stand 10 minutes before cutting and serving to allow cheeses to firm up.

Exchange List Values

• Starch 2.0   • Med-Fat Meat 1.0

Basic Nutritional Values

• Calories 225   • Sodium 320 mg
  (Calories from Fat 45) • Potassium 335 gm
• Total Fat 5 gm   • Total Carb 30 gm
  (Saturated Fat 2.0 gm, • Dietary Fiber 3 gm
  Trans Fat 0.0 gm,   • Sugars 6 gm
  Polyunsat Fat 1.1 gm, • Protein 14 gm
  Monounsat Fat 1.4 gm) • Phosphorus 215 gm
• Cholesterol 20 mg

Ziti Bake— BIG, Big Batch

Joy Reiff
Mount Joy, PA

*Makes 60 servings,
3" square per serving*

Prep. Time: 45–50 minutes
Baking Time: 1½ hours

5 lbs. uncooked ziti, *or* rigatoni
5 lbs. 90%-lean ground beef
5 lbs. fat-free ricotta cheese, *or* cottage cheese
2½ cups grated Parmesan cheese
1 cup chopped parsley
5 eggs, beaten
1 Tbsp. salt
1 tsp. pepper
6½ quarts marinara pasta sauce, lower in sodium, *divided*
1½ lbs. part-skim mozzarella cheese, shredded

1. Prepare ziti according to package directions.(Do in several batches if you don't have a large enough stockpot to do all at once.) Drain and set aside.

2. Brown ground beef in large stockpot. Stir frequently to break up clumps. Cook until pink no longer remains. Drain off drippings.

3. Stir in ricotta cheese, Parmesan cheese, parsley, eggs, and seasonings.

4. Add 5 quarts spaghetti sauce. Stir until well mixed.

5. Add ziti. Toss gently to coat well.

6. Pour mixture into 5 9×13 pans 3-quart baking pans. Or spoon into 18-quart electric roaster.

7. Pour remaining spaghetti sauce over ziti mixture. Sprinkle with cheese.

8. Bake at 350° for 1–1½ hours, if using smaller roasters or baking pans, until bubbly and hot through. If using large electric roaster, bake up to 2 hours, or until hot through.

Tip:

Stir occasionally, to prevent a thick layer of cheese from forming on top and making it hard to scoop out.

Exchange List Values

• Starch 2.5   • Med-Fat Meat 2.0

Basic Nutritional Values

• Calories 340   • Sodium 550 mg
  (Calories from Fat 90) • Potassium 535 gm
• Total Fat 10 gm   • Total Carb 39 gm
  (Saturated Fat 3.4 gm, • Dietary Fiber 3 gm
  Trans Fat 0.2 gm,   • Sugars 8 gm
  Polyunsat Fat 1.8 gm, • Protein 23 gm
  Monounsat Fat 3.1 gm) • Phosphorus 295 gm
• Cholesterol 45 mg

To reduce your sodium intake, avoid salting the water when cooking pasta or rice.

Sesame Noodles

Sheila Ann Plock
Boalsburg, PA

Makes 12 servings,
about ⅔ cup per serving

Prep. Time: 15 minutes
Chilling Time: 8 hours or
overnight
Cooking Time: 11 minutes

2 Tbsp. soy sauce
3 Tbsp. sesame oil
2 Tbsp. red wine vinegar
2 Tbsp. olive oil
1½ Tbsp. sugar
1 Tbsp. prepared chili
   sauce with garlic
12-oz. box linguine noodles
4 green onions
1 red bell pepper, cut into
   thin match-stick strips

1. One day before serving noodles, combine soy sauce, 2 Tbsp. sesame oil, vinegar, olive oil, sugar, and chili sauce in food processor or blender. Blend until well combined.
2. Cover. Chill in fridge for 8 hours or overnight to allow flavors to blend.
3. Cook noodles according to package directions in unsalted water. Rinse, drain, and cool.
4. In large bowl, toss cooked noodles with 1 Tbsp. sesame oil.
5. Stir in green onions and peppers.
6. Toss with dressing.
7. Serve chilled or at room temperature.

Exchange List Values
• Starch 1.5   • Fat 1.0

Basic Nutritional Values
• Calories 170   • Sodium 180 mg
(Calories from Fat 55) • Potassium 75 gm
• Total Fat 6 gm   • Total Carb 25 gm
(Saturated Fat 0.9 gm, • Dietary Fiber 1 gm
Trans Fat 0.0 gm,   • Sugars 3 gm
Polyunsat Fat 1.8 gm,   • Protein 4 gm
Monounsat Fat 3.0 gm)   • Phosphorus 50 gm
• Cholesterol 0 mg

Sukiyake

Cincy Jordan
Ambler, PA

Makes 8 servings, about ¼ cup
cooked spaghetti, 2 oz. meat,
½ cup rest of ingredients

Prep. Time: 20 minutes
Cooking Time: about 25 minutes

4 oz. thin spaghetti
3 eggs, beaten
2 small onions, sliced
12–16 green onions, sliced
½ lb. mushrooms, sliced
5 ribs celery, diced
1 lb. spinach leaves, torn
   in pieces
1½ lbs. boneless beef
   flank steak, fat removed
⅓ cup reduced-sodium
   soy sauce
2 Tbsp. sugar
2 Tbsp. canola oil
1½ Tbsp. sesame oil

1. Cook spaghetti according to directions, but without using salt. Rinse and drain.
2. Pour eggs into nonstick skillet and cook on low until set. Cut into ½" squares. Set aside.
3. Trim fat from steak and cut into thin slices.
4. In a 10" frying pan, combine and heat soy sauce, sugar, cooking oil and sesame oil.
5. Add meat and vegetables and cook until tender, stirring frequently. Immediately before serving, fold in egg.
6. Serve over cooked spaghetti.

Exchange List Values
• Starch 1.0   • Lean Meat 2.0
• Vegetable 2.0   • Fat 2.0

Basic Nutritional Values
• Calories 305   • Sodium 500 mg
(Calories from Fat 115) • Potassium 820 gm
• Total Fat 13 gm   • Total Carb 22 gm
(Saturated Fat 3.2 gm, • Dietary Fiber 3 gm
Trans Fat 0.0 gm,   • Sugars 6 gm
Polyunsat Fat 2.8 gm,   • Protein 25 gm
Monounsat Fat 5.7 gm)   • Phosphorus 260 gm
• Cholesterol 100 mg

Party Spaghetti

Sheila Ann Plock
Boalsburg, PA

Makes 12 servings

Prep. Time: 30–45 minutes
Baking Time: 30–40 minutes

1 lb. uncooked linguine,
   divided
2 lbs. 90%-lean ground beef
1 Tbsp. canola oil
½ lb. mushrooms, sliced
   thin
2 medium onions, chopped

¼ cup chopped parsley
2 8-oz. cans tomato sauce
6-oz. can no-salt-added
    tomato paste
1 tsp. dried oregano
1 tsp. garlic powder
¼ tsp. pepper
2 8-oz. cans tomato sauce
6-oz. can tomato paste
1 tsp. dried oregano
1 tsp. garlic powder
8-oz. pkg. fat-free cream
    cheese, softened
2 cups fat-free cottage
    cheese
½ cup fat-free sour cream
½ cup chives
2 Tbsp. no trans-fat tub
    margarine
½ cup dried bread crumbs

1. Prepare linguini according to package directions. Drain well.

2. Heat oil in large skillet. Add meat and cook until browned, stirring frequently to break up clumps.

3. Stir in mushrooms, onions, parsley, tomato sauce, tomato paste, oregano, and garlic powder.

4. Season to taste with salt and pepper.

5. Simmer, uncovered, 15 minutes.

6. Combine cream cheese, cottage cheese, sour cream, and chives in mixing bowl. Blend well.

7. Pour half of linguine into 3½-4-quart buttered casserole.

8. Cover with all of cheese mixture.

9. Spoon in rest of linguine.

10. Top with meat mixture.

11. Melt margarine in small saucepan.

12. Stir in bread crumbs.

13. Sprinkle over top of casserole.

14. Bake at 350° for 30–40 minutes, or until browned and bubbly.

Exchange List Values

- Starch 2.0   • Lean Meat 3.0
- Fat-Free Milk 0.5   • Fat 0.5
- Vegetable 1.0

Basic Nutritional Values

- Calories 395   Trans Fat 0.4 gm,
  (Calories from Fat 90)   Polyunsat Fat 1.6 gm,
- Total Fat 10 gm   Monounsat Fat 4.0 gm)
  (Saturated Fat 3.2 gm, • Cholesterol 50 mg

Mazetti

Sally Holzem
Schofield, WI

*Makes 8 servings,
about 8 oz. per serving*

Prep. Time: 30 minutes
Baking Time: 25–30 minutes

¾ lb. 90%-lean ground beef
8-oz. pkg. uncooked wide
    noodles
1 cup chopped onion
1½ cups chopped celery
1 Tbsp. canola oil
8-oz. can corn, undrained
10¾-oz. can lower-sodium,
    lower-fat tomato soup
4-oz. can mushrooms,
    undrained
½ cup fat-free milk
½ tsp. salt
½ tsp. pepper
¼ tsp. garlic powder
⅔ cup 75%-less-fat
    shredded cheddar cheese

1. Brown beef in large skillet. Stir frequently to break up clumps. When pink no longer remains, remove from heat and drain off drippings.

2. Prepare noodles in unsalted water according to package directions. Drain well.

3. Add beef to drained noodles.

4. In same skillet as you cooked beef, sauté onion and celery in oil. Add to beef-noodle mixture.

5. Stir corn, soup, mushrooms, milk, salt, pepper, and garlic powder into beef-noodle mixture.

6. Turn into greased 3-quart casserole.

7. Sprinkle with cheese.

8. Bake uncovered at 400° for 25–30 minutes, or until bubbly and heated through.

Exchange List Values

- Starch 1.5   • Lean Meat 2.0
- Carbohydrate 0.5   • Fat 1.0

Basic Nutritional Values

- Calories 280   • Sodium 550 mg
  (Calories from Fat 70) • Potassium 580 gm
- Total Fat 8 gm   • Total Carb 34 gm
  (Saturated Fat 2.5 gm, • Dietary Fiber 3 gm
  Trans Fat 0.2 gm,   • Sugars 7 gm
  Polyunsat Fat 1.3 gm,   • Protein 17 gm
  Monounsat Fat 3.2 gm)   • Phosphorus 245 gm
- Cholesterol 50 mg

Creamy Beef and Pasta Casserole

Virginia Graybill
Hershey, PA

Makes 6 servings,
4" square per serving

Prep. Time: 25 minutes
Baking Time: 30 minutes

1 lb. 90% lean ground beef
8-oz. pkg. noodles, *or* macaroni
8-oz. pkg. fat-free cream cheese, softened
10¾-oz. can lower-fat, lower-sodium cream of mushroom soup
1 cup fat-free milk
½ cup no-salt ketchup

1. Cook ground beef in non-stick skillet until no longer pink, stirring frequently to break up clumps. Drain off any drippings.
2. Cook noodles or macaroni al dente as directed on package. Drain.
3. Mix pasta and hamburger in large mixing bowl.
4. In another mixing bowl, blend together cream cheese, soup, milk, ketchup, and salt if you wish.
5. Stir sauce into pasta and hamburger.
6. Pour into greased 9×13 baking pan.
7. Bake at 350° for 30 minutes, or until bubbly and heated through.

Exchange List Values
• Starch 2.0   • Lean Meat 3.0
• Carbohydrate 0.5   • Fat 0.5

Basic Nutritional Values
• Calories 360   • Sodium 485 mg
(Calories from Fat 80)   • Potassium 855 gm
• Total Fat 9 gm   • Total Carb 40 gm
(Saturated Fat 3.1 gm,   • Dietary Fiber 2 gm
Trans Fat 0.4 gm,   • Sugars 10 gm
Polyunsat Fat 1.2 gm,   • Protein 26 gm
Monounsat Fat 3.4 gm)   • Phosphorus 470 gm
• Cholesterol 85 mg

Pizza Noodle Casserole

Arianne Hochstetler
Goshen, IN

Makes 15 servings,
a 2⅗"×3" rectangle per serving

Prep. Time: 30 minutes
Baking Time: 45 minutes

12-oz. pkg. kluski noodles
¾ lb. 90%-lean ground beef
1 small onion, chopped
24½-oz. jar marinara pasta sauce, light in sodium
1½ cups pizza sauce
4-oz. can sliced mushrooms, drained
½ cup green bell pepper, chopped, *optional*
⅓ cup green, *or* black, olives, chopped, *optional*
4 oz. shredded 75%-less-fat cheddar cheese
2 oz. shredded part-skim mozzarella cheese
2 oz. sliced reduced-fat turkey pepperoni

1. Cook noodles according to package directions, using unsalted water. Drain.
2. Brown ground beef and onion in large saucepan.

Stir frequently to break up clumps. Drain off drippings.
3. Add marinara and pizza sauces to meat.
4. Cover. Simmer over low heat for 10 minutes.
5. Stir mushrooms, and chopped peppers and olives into meat sauce if you wish.
6. Grease 9×13 baking pan. Layer in half of noodles.
7. Follow with half of meat sauce.
8. Top with half of cheeses.
9. Scatter half of pepperoni over top.
10. Repeat layers.
11. Bake in 9×13 baking pan at 350° for 45 minutes.

Tips:
1. You can use 1 pound of spaghetti instead of the kluski noodles.
2. You can make this casserole through Step 10 the day before serving. Cover and refrigerate. Bake chilled casserole up to 1¼ hours, or until bubbly and heated through.

Exchange List Values
• Starch 1.5   • Med-Fat Meat 1.0

Basic Nutritional Values
• Calories 210   • Sodium 410 mg
(Calories from Fat 65)   • Potassium 405 gm
• Total Fat 7 gm   • Total Carb 23 gm
(Saturated Fat 2.4 gm,   • Dietary Fiber 2 gm
Trans Fat 0.1 gm,   • Sugars 4 gm
Polyunsat Fat 1.6 gm,   • Protein 14 gm
Monounsat Fat 2.3 gm)   • Phosphorus 200 gm
• Cholesterol 70 mg

Spinach Cheese Manicotti

Kimberly Richard
Mars, PA

Makes 7 servings, 2 stuffed shells and about ⅔ cup sauce per serving

Prep. Time: 35 minutes
Baking Time: 45–60 minutes

15-oz. container fat-free ricotta cheese
10-oz. pkg. frozen chopped spinach, thawed and squeezed dry
½ cup minced onion
¼ cup egg substitute
2 tsp. parsley
½ tsp. black pepper
½ tsp. garlic powder
2 tsp. dried basil
1¼ cups part-skim shredded mozzarella, *divided*
½ cup freshly grated Parmesan, *divided*
24½-oz. jar marinara pasta sauce, light in sodium
1½ cups water
1 cup diced fresh tomatoes
8-oz. pkg. manicotti shells

1. In large bowl combine ricotta, spinach, onion, and egg substitute.
2. Stir in parsley, basil, garlic, and black pepper.
3. Mix in 1 cup mozzarella and ¼ cup Parmesan cheese.
4. In separate bowl, mix together sauce, water, and tomatoes.
5. Grease 9×13 baking pan. Spread 1 cup spaghetti sauce in bottom of pan.

6. Stuff uncooked manicotti with ricotta mixture. Arrange in single layer in baking pan.
7. Cover stuffed manicotti with remaining sauce.
8. Sprinkle with remaining cheeses.
9. Cover. Bake 45–60 minutes, or until noodles are soft.

Exchange List Values

- Starch 2.0
- Vegetable 1.0
- Lean Meat 2.0
- Fat 1.0

Basic Nutritional Values

- Calories 325
  (Calories from Fat 80)
- Total Fat 9 gm
  (Saturated Fat 3.4 gm,
  Trans Fat 0.0 gm,
  Polyunsat Fat 1.8 gm,
  Monounsat Fat 2.3 gm)
- Cholesterol 35 mg
- Sodium 555 mg
- Potassium 640 gm
- Total Carb 40 gm
- Dietary Fiber 5 gm
- Sugars 9 gm
- Protein 22 gm
- Phosphorus 350 gm

Lazy Lasagna

Elaine Rineer
Lancaster, PA

*Makes 10 servings,
3" square per serving*

Prep. Time: 45 minutes
Baking Time: 30–45 minutes

1 lb. 90%-lean ground beef
1-lb. pkg. malfada noodles, *divided*
1-lb. container fat-free ricotta cheese
1 cup shredded part-skim mozzarella cheese, *divided*
4 cups marinara pasta sauce, light in sodium
2 oz. reduced-fat sliced turkey pepperoni

1. Brown ground beef in skillet. Stir frequently to break up clumps. Cook until no pink remains. Drain off drippings.
2. Cook noodles according to package instructions in unsalted water. Drain well.
3. In large bowl, toss cooked noodles with all of cottage cheese and 1 cup mozzarella cheese.
4. In a greased 4-quart, or 9×13 baking pan, spoon in enough sauce to just cover bottom.
5. Stir rest of marinara sauce into browned beef.
6. Add half of beef-marinara sauce to baking dish.
7. Layer in half of noodles.
8. Top with half of remaining sauce.
9. Place sliced pepperoni over sauce.
10. Repeat layers, using all of remaining noodles and beef-marinara sauce.
11. Sprinkle with remaining mozzarella cheese.
12. Bake at 375° for 30–45 minutes, or until bubbly and heated through.

Exchange List Values

- Starch 3.0
- Lean Meat 3.0

Basic Nutritional Values

- Calories 380
  (Calories from Fat 100)
- Total Fat 11 gm
  (Saturated Fat 3.4 gm,
  Trans Fat 0.2 gm,
  Polyunsat Fat 1.9 gm,
  Monounsat Fat 3.3 gm)
- Cholesterol 55 mg
- Sodium 490 mg
- Potassium 570 gm
- Total Carb 44 gm
- Dietary Fiber 3 gm
- Sugars 7 gm
- Protein 27 gm
- Phosphorus 340 gm

Lasagna

Colleen Heatwole
Burton, MI

Makes 12 servings,
3" square per serving

Prep. Time: 45 minutes
Baking Time: 30 minutes at
375°; 2 hours at 200°

⅔ lb. 90%-lean ground
  beef
1 clove garlic, minced
1 Tbsp. dried basil
½ tsp. salt
28-oz. can no-salt-added
  stewed tomatoes
6-oz. can tomato paste
½ tsp. dried oregano
10 oz. lasagna noodles,
  divided
3 cups fat-free cottage
  cheese
½ cup freshly grated
  Parmesan cheese
4 oz. part-skim mozzarella
  cheese, grated
2 Tbsp. parsley flakes
½ cup egg substitute
½ tsp. pepper

1. Brown beef slowly in
stockpot. Stir frequently to
break up clumps. Pour off
drippings.
2. Stir in garlic, basil, salt,
tomatoes or pasta sauce,
tomato paste, and oregano.
Mix well.
3. Simmer, uncovered, 30
minutes.
4. Meanwhile, cook pasta
al dente, according to package
directions. Drain well.
5. In large bowl, combine
cottage cheese, Parmesan

cheese, mozzarella cheese,
parsley flakes, egg substitute,
and pepper.
6. Place half the noodles in
greased 9×13 baking dish.
7. Cover with half the meat
sauce.
8. Top with half the cheese
mixture.
9. Repeat layers, ending
with cheese mixture.
10. Bake at 375° for 30
minutes, or until bubbly and
heated through.

Tip:
    You can assemble this
lasagna ahead of time through
Step 9. Cover and refrigerate.
When ready to bake, allow
15 minutes longer in oven,
or bake at 200° for 2 hours
if baking during church or a
noon potluck. Cover during
baking if baking 2 hours.

Exchange List Values
- Starch 1.0   • Vegetable 1.0
- Fat-Free Milk 0.5   • Lean Meat 2.0

Basic Nutritional Values
- Calories 240   • Sodium 560 mg
  (Calories from Fat 45) • Potassium 515 gm
- Total Fat 5 gm   • Total Carb 30 gm
  (Saturated Fat 2.5 gm, • Dietary Fiber 3 gm
  Trans Fat 0.1 gm,   • Sugars 8 gm
  Polyunsat Fat 0.4 gm, • Protein 19 gm
  Monounsat Fat 1.7 gm) • Phosphorus 275 gm
- Cholesterol 25 mg

Weekday Lasagna

Karen Burkholder
Narvon, PA

Makes 9 servings,
a 3"×4⅓" rectangle per serving

Prep. Time: 25–35 minutes
Baking Time: 60–65 minutes
Standing Time: 15 minutes

1 lb. 90%-lean ground beef
1 small onion, chopped
28-oz. can no-added-salt
  crushed tomatoes
1¾ cups water
6-oz. can no-added-salt
  tomato paste
1 pkg. Italian-style
  spaghetti sauce mix
1 egg, slightly beaten
2 cups fat-free cottage
  cheese
2 Tbsp. freshly grated
  Parmesan cheese
6 uncooked lasagna
  noodles, *divided*
1 cup shredded part-skim
  mozzarella cheese

1. In a large saucepan, cook
beef and onion over medium
heat until meat is no longer
pink, stirring frequently to
break up clumps. Drain off
any drippings.
2. Stir tomatoes, water,
tomato paste, and spaghetti
sauce mix into skillet.
3. Bring mixture to a boil.
Reduce heat. Cover and simmer 15–20 minutes, stirring
occasionally.
4. In a small bowl, combine
egg, cottage cheese, and
Parmesan cheese.
5. Spread 2 cups meat

sauce in greased 9×13 baking dish.

6. Top with three uncooked noodles.

7. Layer on half of cottage cheese mixture.

8. Top with half remaining meat sauce.

9. Repeat layers.

10. Cover and bake at 350° for 50 minutes.

11. Uncover. Sprinkle with mozzarella cheese.

12. Bake uncovered 10–15 minutes longer, or until bubbly and cheese is melted.

13. Let stand 15 minutes before cutting.

Exchange List Values

- Starch 1.0
- Lean Meat 3.0
- Vegetable 2.0

Basic Nutritional Values

- Calories 280
  (Calories from Fat 70)
- Total Fat 8 gm
  (Saturated Fat 3.4 gm,
  Trans Fat 0.3 gm,
  Polyunsat Fat 0.6 gm,
  Monounsat Fat 2.7 gm)
- Cholesterol 65 mg
- Sodium 520 mg
- Potassium 720 gm
- Total Carb 28 gm
- Dietary Fiber 3 gm
- Sugars 9 gm
- Protein 23 gm
- Phosphorus 340 gm

Garden Lasagna

Deb Martin
Gap, PA

*Makes 12 servings,
3" square per serving*

Prep. Time: 30 minutes
Baking Time: 70–75 minutes

8 oz. lasagna noodles, *divided*

2 10¾-oz. cans lower-sodium, fat-free cream of chicken soup

1 cup fat-free sour cream

¾ cup lower-sodium, lower-fat chicken broth

½ cup egg substitute

3 cups cooked chopped chicken, *divided*

1 lb. bag frozen broccoli, cauliflower, and carrots, *divided*

½ cup freshly grated Parmesan cheese, *divided*

1 cup part-skim mozzarella cheese, shredded

1. Cook noodles according to package directions. Drain well.

2. Steam vegetables until lightly cooked. Drain well.

3. In large bowl, mix soup, sour cream, broth, and egg substitute.

4. Place small amount of sauce on bottom of greased 9×13 baking pan. Swirl to cover bottom.

5. Layer 3 lasagna noodles on top of sauce.

6. Add half of soup mixture.

7. Top with half of chicken.

8. Top with half of vegetables.

9. Sprinkle with half of Parmesan cheese.

10. Repeat layers, using all remaining amounts of ingredients.

11. Top with mozzarella cheese.

12. Bake, covered, at 350° for 1 hour.

13. Uncover. Bake another 10–15 minutes.

Exchange List Values

- Starch 1.0
- Lean Meat 2.0
- Carbohydrate 0.5
- Fat 0.5

Basic Nutritional Values

- Calories 235
  (Calories from Fat 55)
- Total Fat 6 gm
  (Saturated Fat 2.5 gm,
  Trans Fat 0.0 gm,
  Polyunsat Fat 1.3 gm,
  Monounsat Fat 1.8 gm)
- Cholesterol 45 mg
- Sodium 395 mg
- Potassium 460 gm
- Total Carb 24 gm
- Dietary Fiber 2 gm
- Sugars 3 gm
- Protein 19 gm
- Phosphorus 215 gm

Meatless Lasagna Roll-Ups

Judy Buller
Bluffton, OH

Makes 12 servings, 1 roll per serving

Prep. Time: 30 minutes
Baking Time: 25–30 minutes

12 uncooked whole-grain
  lasagna noodles
2 eggs, slightly beaten
2½ cups fat-free ricotta
  cheese
1½ cups shredded part-
  skim mozzarella cheese,
  divided
½ cup freshly grated
  Parmesan cheese
1 pkg. frozen, chopped
  spinach, thawed and
  squeezed dry, *or* 4 cups
  chopped fresh spinach
  that has been microwaved
  on HIGH 1–2 minutes and
  squeezed dry
¼ tsp. salt
¼ tsp. pepper
1–2 cups cooked black
  beans, rinsed and
  drained
24½-oz. jar marinara pasta
  sauce, light in sodium,
  divided

1. Cook lasagna noodles
according to box directions
in unsalted water. Drain and
rinse well. Lay flat.
2. In a good-sized mixing
bowl, mix together eggs,
ricotta cheese, 1½ cups
mozzarella cheese, Parmesan
cheese, spinach, salt, and
pepper.

3. Spread about ⅓ cup
mixture on each noodle.
4. Sprinkle each noodle
with black beans. Press down
to make beans adhere.
5. Spread 1 cup spaghetti
sauce in bottom of well
greased 9×13 baking pan.
6. Roll up noodles and
place seam side down in
baking pan.
7. Top rolls with remaining
sauce. Sprinkle with 1 cup
mozzarella cheese.
8. Bake uncovered at 350°
for 25–30 minutes, or until
heated through.

Tips:
   You can assemble this
dish ahead of time, and then
freeze or refrigerate it until
you're ready to use it. Allow
more time to bake if the
dish is cold, probably 45–50
minutes. But check while
baking so as not to have it dry
out or be over-baked.

Exchange List Values
• Starch 2.0   • Lean Meat 2.0

Basic Nutritional Values
• Calories 250
  (Calories from Fat 65)
• Total Fat 7 gm
  (Saturated Fat 2.5 gm,
  Trans Fat 0.0 gm,
  Polyunsat Fat 1.2 gm,
  Monounsat Fat 1.8 gm)
• Cholesterol 60 mg
• Sodium 420 mg
• Potassium 405 gm
• Total Carb 29 gm
• Dietary Fiber 5 gm
• Sugars 5 gm
• Protein 19 gm
• Phosphorus 285 gm

Pesto Lasagna Rolls

Joy Uhler
Richardson, TX

*Makes 12 servings, 1 roll-up per
serving*

Prep. Time: 25 minutes
Baking Time: 30–40 minutes

12 uncooked lasagna
  noodles
24½-oz. jar marinara pasta
  sauce, light in sodium
2 cloves garlic, minced
24 oz. fat-free ricotta
  cheese
10-oz. pkg. frozen chopped
  spinach, thawed and
  squeezed dry
3½-oz. jar prepared pesto
1 egg
½ cup freshly grated
  Parmesan cheese
½ tsp. salt
¼ tsp. pepper
1 cup shredded part-skim
  mozzarella cheese

1. Cook noodles according
to package directions. Drain.
2. Spread 2 cups pasta
sauce in bottom of greased
9×13 baking pan.
3. Combine garlic, ricotta,
spinach, pesto, egg, Parmesan, salt, and pepper in bowl.
4. Place cooked noodle on
clean kitchen towel or clean
cutting board. Spread ¼ cup
ricotta mixture on noodle.
5. Roll noodle up. Place
seam-side down in baking pan.
6. Repeat with remaining
noodles. Place 4 in a row the

length of the pan. Make 3 such rows.

7. Pour remaining pasta sauce over noodles.

8. Sprinkle with mozzarella.

9. Cover pan with foil. Bake 20 minutes at 350°.

10. Uncover. Bake until cheese is golden brown, about 10–15 minutes longer.

Warm Memories:

I recently served this for my granddaughter's birthday; it was her pick for a main dish. She and everyone present loved the dish, eating 2 rolls apiece.

Tip:

Divide the ricotta mixture into 12 parts (with hand or knife) before using it on the noodles.

Exchange List Values

- Starch 1.5   • Fat 0.5
- Lean Meat 2.0

Basic Nutritional Values

- Calories 235   • Sodium 515 mg
  (Calories from Fat 70) • Potassium 350 gm
- Total Fat 8 gm   • Total Carb 26 gm
  (Saturated Fat 2.3 gm, • Dietary Fiber 3 gm
  Trans Fat 0.0 gm,   • Sugars 6 gm
  Polyunsat Fat 1.4 gm, • Protein 16 gm
  Monounsat Fat 3.0 gm) • Phosphorus 240 gm
- Cholesterol 40 mg

Verenike Casserole

Jenelle Miller
Marion, SD

Makes 10 servings, a 2⅗"×4½" rectangle per serving

Prep. Time: 30 minutes
Cooking/Baking Time: 45 minutes

9 lasagna noodles
3 cups fat-free cottage cheese
3 eggs
½ tsp. pepper
1 cup fat-free sour cream
2 Tbsp. flour
1 cup fat-free half-and-half
2 cups cooked lean, low-sodium ham chunks

1. Cook noodles according to package directions until al dente. Rinse and drain.

2. In a mixing bowl, stir together cottage cheese, eggs, salt, and pepper.

3. In a greased 9×13 baking pan, layer in all noodles.

4. Follow with layer of cottage cheese mixture

5. Scatter ham chunks over all.

6. Mix flour with sour cream in saucepan until smooth.

7. Whisk in half-and-half.

8. Cook over medium heat until slightly thickened, stirring constantly.

9. Pour white sauce over noodles.

10. Bake at 300° for 45 minutes, or until bubbly and heated through.

Tip:

You can make this the night before you want to serve it, through Step 9. Cover and refrigerate. When ready to bake, allow about 10 minutes more than stated in instructions.

Warm Memories:

We eat verenike (cheese pockets) a lot in our area of South Dakota. This is an easier version, but you get the same great taste!

Exchange List Values

- Starch 1.0   • Lean Meat 1.0
- Fat-Free Milk 1.0

Basic Nutritional Values

- Calories 225   • Sodium 550 mg
  (Calories from Fat 35) • Potassium 290 gm
- Total Fat 4 gm   • Total Carb 28 gm
  (Saturated Fat 1.4 gm, • Dietary Fiber 1 gm
  Trans Fat 0.0 gm,   • Sugars 5 gm
  Polyunsat Fat 0.6 gm, • Protein 19 gm
  Monounsat Fat 1.4 gm) • Phosphorus 300 gm
- Cholesterol 80 mg

You may want to appoint someone to be responsible for taking a plate of food to shut-ins. This is a nice way to say, "You are a part of us. We have not forgotten you."
Marnetta Brilhart, Scottdale, PA

Creamy Chicken Lasagna

Joanne E. Martin
Stevens, PA

Makes 10 servings,
2⅗"×4½" rectangle per serving

Prep. Time: 30 minutes
Cooking/Baking Time: 45 minutes

8 oz. uncooked lasagna noodles, *divided*
10¾-oz. can lower-sodium, lower-fat cream of mushroom soup
10¾-oz. can lower-sodium, lower-fat cream of chicken soup
½ cup freshly grated Parmesan cheese
1 cup fat-free sour cream
3 cups diced, cooked chicken
½ cup shredded part-skim mozzarella cheese, *divided*

1. Cook noodles according to package directions in unsalted water. Drain.
2. In mixing bowl, blend together soups, Parmesan cheese, and sour cream.
3. Stir in chicken.
4. Put ¼ of chicken mixture in greased 9×13 baking pan.
5. Top with half the cooked noodles.
6. Spoon in half the chicken mixture.
7. Sprinkle with half the mozzarella cheese.
8. Repeat layers, using all remaining ingredients.

9. Bake at 350° for 40–45 minutes, or until heated through.

Exchange List Values
- Starch 1.0
- Carbohydrate 1.0
- Lean Meat 2.0

Basic Nutritional Values
- Calories 245
  (Calories from Fat 65)
- Total Fat 7 gm
  (Saturated Fat 2.4 gm,
  Trans Fat 0.0 gm,
  Polyunsat Fat 1.4 gm,
  Monounsat Fat 1.9 gm)
- Cholesterol 50 mg
- Sodium 365 mg
- Potassium 500 gm
- Total Carb 26 gm
- Dietary Fiber 1 gm
- Sugars 3 gm
- Protein 19 gm
- Phosphorus 205 gm

Our Favorite Tetrazzini

Carolyn Spohn
Shawnee, KS

Makes 8 servings,
3¼"×4½" rectangle per serving

Prep. Time: 30 minutes
Baking Time: 30–40 minutes

5 oz. spaghetti, broken
1 medium onion, chopped
1 medium green bell pepper, chopped
10¾-oz. can lower-sodium, lower-fat cream of chicken soup
⅓ cup fat-free milk
1 cup fat-free plain yogurt
3–4 cups diced cooked chicken, *or* turkey
8-oz. can sliced ripe olives, drained
8-oz. can mushroom stems/pieces, drained
4-oz. jar chopped pimento, drained

1 cup 75%-less-fat shredded cheddar cheese

1. Cook spaghetti according to package directions. Drain well.
2. Sauté onion and green pepper in non-stick skillet until soft.
3. Mix soup, milk, and yogurt together in large mixing bowl until smooth.
4. Stir into soup mixture the onion and green pepper, spaghetti, meat, olives, yogurt, mushrooms, and pimento. Fold together until well mixed.
5. Pour into greased 9×13 baking dish.
6. Bake at 350° for 30 minutes, until bubbly.
7. Sprinkle with shredded cheddar cheese. Bake 10 more minutes.

Tips:
1. You can extend the number of servings easily by using more pasta.
2. This is a great way to use leftover Thanksgiving turkey.

Exchange List Values
- Starch 1.0
- Carbohydrate 0.5
- Lean Meat 3.0
- Fat 0.5

Basic Nutritional Values
- Calories 275
  (Calories from Fat 70)
- Total Fat 8 gm
  (Saturated Fat 2.3 gm,
  Trans Fat 0.0 gm,
  Polyunsat Fat 1.5 gm,
  Monounsat Fat 2.9 gm)
- Cholesterol 55 mg
- Sodium 530 mg
- Potassium 525 gm
- Total Carb 25 gm
- Dietary Fiber 3 gm
- Sugars 5 gm
- Protein 26 gm
- Phosphorus 290 gm

Chicken and Bows

Arianne Hochstetler
Goshen, IN

*Makes 12 servings,
about 8 oz. per serving*

Prep. Time: 15–20 minutes
Cooking Time: 10–20 minutes

16-oz. pkg. bowtie pasta
2 lbs. uncooked boneless,
  skinless chicken breasts,
  cut into strips
1 cup chopped red bell
  pepper
3 Tbsp. canola oil
2 10¾-oz. cans lower-
  sodium, lower-fat cream
  of chicken soup
2 cups frozen peas
1½ cups 1% milk
1 tsp. garlic powder
¼ -½ tsp. salt
¼ tsp. pepper
⅔ cup freshly grated
  Parmesan cheese

1. Cook pasta according to
package directions. Drain.
2. In large saucepan, cook
chicken and red pepper in oil
for 5–6 minutes until juices
run clear.
3. Stir in soup, peas, milk,
garlic powder, salt, and
pepper.
4. Bring to boil. Simmer,
uncovered, 1–2 minutes.
5. Stir in Parmesan cheese.
6. Add pasta and toss to
coat.
7. Serve immediately, or
refrigerate or freeze.
8. To heat, thaw frozen
casserole in refrigerator overnight. Place in microwave-safe

dish. Cover, and microwave
8–10 minutes or until heated
through, stirring once.
Or warm thawed dish in
oven—350° for 1 hour, or
until bubbly and heated
through.

Exchange List Values
- Starch 2.0
- Carbohydrate 0.5
- Lean Meat 3.0

Basic Nutritional Values
- Calories 330
  (Calories from Fat 70)
- Total Fat 8 gm
  (Saturated Fat 1.9 gm,
  Trans Fat 0.0 gm,
  Polyunsat Fat 2.2 gm,
  Monounsat Fat 3.5 gm)
- Cholesterol 50 mg
- Sodium 355 mg
- Potassium 495 gm
- Total Carb 37 gm
- Dietary Fiber 3 gm
- Sugars 6 gm
- Protein 25 gm
- Phosphorus 260 gm

Pasta Turkey Bake

Joy Sutter
Perkasie, PA

*Makes 8 servings,
3¼"×4½" rectangle per serving*

Prep. Time: 20 minutes
Baking Time: 25 minutes

3 cups uncooked penne
  pasta
1 lb. 7%-fat ground turkey
½ cup chopped onion
½ cup chopped green bell
  pepper
15-oz. can tomato sauce
15-oz. can no-salt-added
  tomato sauce
1 Tbsp. sugar
½ tsp. salt
1 tsp. pepper
1 tsp. dried basil
1 tsp. dried oregano

½ cup 75%-less-fat
  shredded cheddar cheese
½ cup shredded mozzarella
  cheese

1. Cook penne according to
package directions. Drain. Set
aside.
2. Meanwhile, brown the
ground turkey in large skillet,
stirring frequently to break
up clumps until no pink
remains.
3. Add onion and green
pepper to skillet. Simmer 10
minutes.
4. Add tomato sauce,
sugar, salt, pepper, basil, and
oregano.
5. Mix together with penne.
6. Pour into greased 9×13
baking pan.
7. Top with shredded
cheeses.
8. Bake at 350° for 25
minutes, or until bubbly and
heated through.

Exchange List Values
- Starch 1.5
- Vegetable 2.0
- Lean Meat 2.0
- Fat 0.5

Basic Nutritional Values
- Calories 280
  (Calories from Fat 65)
- Total Fat 7 gm
  (Saturated Fat 2.5 gm,
  Trans Fat 0.1 gm,
  Polyunsat Fat 1.8 gm,
  Monounsat Fat 2.2 gm)
- Cholesterol 50 mg
- Sodium 575 mg
- Potassium 560 gm
- Total Carb 34 gm
- Dietary Fiber 4 gm
- Sugars 7 gm
- Protein 21 gm
- Phosphorus 245 gm

Baked Pasta with Turkey Sausage

Kim Rapp, Longmont, CO

Makes 12 servings,
3" square per serving

Prep. Time: 40 minutes
Baking Time: 20–30 minutes

1 lb. uncooked rigatoni
10-oz. pkg. fresh baby
   spinach
1 Tbsp. olive oil
1 medium red onion,
   chopped
4 cloves garlic, minced
¼ cup vodka, *optional*
28-oz. can whole tomatoes
   with juice, lightly
   crushed with hands
½ tsp. dried oregano
½ cup fat-free half-and-half
12-oz. lean smoked
   turkey sausage, halved
   lengthwise then cut into
   ¼"-thick slices
5 oz. part-skim mozzarella:
   3½ oz. cubed and 1½ oz.
   shredded
¼ cup Parmesan cheese,
   freshly grated

1. Cook rigatoni according
to package directions for 4
minutes.
2. Stir in baby spinach.
Continue cooking 3 minutes.
Drain pasta and spinach well.
Return to cooking pot and
keep warm,
3. Heat oil in large skillet
over medium heat. Add
onion. Cook about 3 minutes.
4. Stir in garlic. Remove
from heat.

5. Add vodka if you wish.
6. Return to fairly high
heat and cook until liquid is
almost evaporated, about 1
minute.
7. Stir in tomatoes and
oregano. Cook 10–15 minutes.
8. Add half-and-half and
warm, cooking gently about 5
minutes.
9. Add sausage and cubed
mozzarella to pot. Toss to
coat.
10. Season with several
grinds salt and pepper.
11. Spoon into greased
9×13 baking dish.
12. Top with grated
mozzarella and Parmesan
cheeses.
13. Bake at 400° until
browned, about 20–30
minutes.

Tip:
   Add ¼ cup water or broth
if mixture seems dry before
baking.

Exchange List Values
• Starch 2.0   • Med-Fat Meat 1.0
• Vegetable 1.0

Basic Nutritional Values
• Calories 265   • Sodium 595 mg
  (Calories from Fat 55) • Potassium 395 gm
• Total Fat 6 gm   • Total Carb 36 gm
  (Saturated Fat 2.5 gm, • Dietary Fiber 3 gm
  Trans Fat 0.0 gm,   • Sugars 5 gm
  Polyunsat Fat 0.8 gm, • Protein 14 gm
  Monounsat Fat 2.0 gm) • Phosphorus 215 gm
• Cholesterol 30 mg

Italian Pork Spaghetti Pie

Char Hagner
Montague, MI

Makes 8 servings,
about 6½ oz. per serving

Prep. Time: 30 minutes
Baking Time: 10–15 minutes
Standing Time: 5 minutes

8 oz. dry spaghetti
½ cup fat-free milk
1 egg
1 lb. 96%-lean ground
   pork, no added salt
½ tsp. black pepper
½ tsp. dried parsley
1½ tsp. Italian herb
   seasoning
¼ tsp. garlic powder
pinch red pepper flakes
½ tsp. anise seeds
¼ tsp. paprika
¼ tsp. dried minced onion
½ cup chopped onions
½ cup chopped green bell
   pepper
1 clove garlic, minced
½-1 Tbsp. chili powder,
   depending upon how
   much heat you like
15-oz. can tomato sauce
2 oz. reduced-fat pepper
   Jack cheese
½ cup shredded 75%-less-
   fat cheddar cheese

1. Cook spaghetti according
to package directions. Drain
well. Return to pan.
2. Combine milk and egg
in small bowl. Stir into hot
pasta.
3. Butter 3-quart baking

dish. Spoon in prepared spaghetti.

4. Mix together pork, black pepper, parsley, Italian herb seasoning, garlic powder, red pepper flakes, anise seeds, paprika, and dried onion.

5. In a large skillet, cook pork mixture with onions, green peppers, garlic, and chili powder. Stir frequently to break up clumps of meat.

6. Stir in tomato sauce. Simmer, uncovered, 5 minutes.

7. Spoon over pasta in baking dish.

8. Sprinkle with cheeses.

9. Bake uncovered at 425° for 10–15 minutes, or until bubbly around edges.

10. Let stand 5 minutes before serving.

Warm Memories:

This is a favorite because it's easier for small children to eat than spaghetti with sauce.

Exchange List Values

- Starch 1.5   • Lean Meat 2.0
- Vegetable 1.0

Basic Nutritional Values

- Calories 250   • Sodium 430 mg
  (Calories from Fat 55)   • Potassium 465 gm
- Total Fat 6 gm   • Total Carb 27 gm
  (Saturated Fat 2.4 gm,   • Dietary Fiber 2 gm
  Trans Fat 0.0 gm,   • Sugars 4 gm
  Polyunsat Fat 0.7 gm,   • Protein 22 gm
  Monounsat Fat 2.0 gm)   • Phosphorus 255 gm
- Cholesterol 60 mg

Mostaccioli

Sally Holzem
Schofield, WI

*Makes 10 servings,
2⅗"×3½" rectangle per serving*

**Prep. Time: 45 minutes
Cooking/Baking Time: 30–45
minutes**

½ **lb. fresh lean turkey Italian sweet sausage**
½ **cup chopped onion**
16-oz. **can no-added-salt tomato paste**
½ **cup water**
½ **tsp. dried oregano**
¼ **tsp. pepper**
4-oz. **can sliced mushrooms, drained**
14½-oz. **can diced tomatoes, undrained**
¾ **cup tomato juice**
8-oz. **pkg. mostaccioli noodles,** *divided*
5 oz. **shredded reduced-fat mozzarella cheese,** *divided*
1½ **cups fat-free cottage cheese**
½ **tsp. dried marjoram**
¼ **cup freshly grated Parmesan cheese**

1. Brown sausage and onions in saucepan, stirring often to break up clumps.

When pink no longer remains, drain off drippings.

2. Stir in tomato paste, water, oregano, pepper, mushrooms, tomatoes, and tomato juice.

3. Cover. Simmer 30 minutes over medium heat.

4. Meanwhile, prepare noodles according to package directions. Drain well.

5. In mixing bowl, combine cottage cheese and marjoram.

6. In greased 9×13 baking pan, layer in half of noodles.

7. Top with half of meat sauce.

8. Sprinkle with half of mozzarella.

9. Spoon cottage-cheese mixture over top and spread as well as you can.

10. Layer on remaining noodles.

11. Top with remaining meat sauce.

12. Sprinkle with remaining mozzarella cheese.

13. Sprinkle with Parmesan cheese.

14. Bake at 350° for 30–45 minutes, or until bubbly, heated through, and lightly browned.

Exchange List Values

- Starch 1.0   • Med-Fat Meat 1.0
- Vegetable 2.0

Basic Nutritional Values

- Calories 225   • Sodium 490 mg
  (Calories from Fat 55)   • Potassium 595 gm
- Total Fat 6 gm   • Total Carb 29 gm
  (Saturated Fat 2.4 gm,   • Dietary Fiber 3 gm
  Trans Fat 0.1 gm,   • Sugars 7 gm
  Polyunsat Fat 0.8 gm,   • Protein 16 gm
  Monounsat Fat 1.6 gm)   • Phosphorus 245 gm
- Cholesterol 25 mg

You can cut back on the number of calories you get each day and still eat your favorite foods — just reduce how much of them you eat. Control your portion sizes to control your weight!

Ham Noodle Casserole

Edna E. Miller
Shipshewana, IN

Makes 12 servings,
3" square per serving

Prep. Time: 45 minutes
Baking Time: 30 minutes

3 Tbsp. canola oil
4 Tbsp. flour
2 cups fat-free milk
2 cups shredded 75%-less-
  fat cheddar cheese
¼ cup ketchup
2 Tbsp. horseradish
3¼ cups lean, lower-
  sodium chopped ham
2 cups peas, *or* green beans
  (if using frozen beans,
  cook lightly first)
6 cups noodles, cooked and
  well drained
2 cups panko bread crumbs

1. Heat oil in large saucepan. Blend in flour, stir well.
2. Add milk slowly. Over low
to medium heat, stir continually
until sauce thickens.
3. Add cheese. Continue
over low heat, stirring until
cheese melts.
4. Stir in ketchup, horseradish, ham, and vegetables.
5. Stir in noodles, mixing
together well.
6. Spoon into greased 9×13
baking dish.
7. Sprinkle panko over top
of casserole.
8. Bake at 350° 30–45
minutes, or until bubbly and
heated through.

Exchange List Values
- Starch 2.5 • Fat 0.5
- Lean Meat 2.0

Basic Nutritional Values
- Calories 320 • Sodium 580 mg
  (Calories from Fat 80) • Potassium 330 gm
- Total Fat 9 gm • Total Carb 39 gm
  (Saturated Fat 2.3 gm, • Dietary Fiber 3 gm
  Trans Fat 0.0 gm, • Sugars 6 gm
  Polyunsat Fat 1.7 gm, • Protein 21 gm
  Monounsat Fat 4.0 gm) • Phosphorus 310 gm
- Cholesterol 50 mg

Pepperoni and Macaroni

Karen Ceneviva
Seymour, CT

Makes 12 servings,
about 5 oz. per serving

Prep. Time: 10 minutes
Cooking Time: 30 minutes

1 lb. uncooked macaroni
2 Tbsp. olive oil
8 oz. sliced reduced-fat
  turkey pepperoni
1–2 tsp. chopped garlic
8-oz. can tomato sauce
8-oz. can no-added-salt
  tomato sauce
½ cup water
dash thyme
1-lb. can chickpeas, *or*
  cannellini beans, drained

1. Cook macaroni accord-
ing to package directions,
using unsalted water. Drain
well.
2. Meanwhile, sauté
pepperoni with garlic in olive
oil in large stockpot.

3. Add tomato sauce and
water to meat.
4. Add thyme and beans.
5. Stir in cooked noodles
Mix all together.
6. Warm over low heat
until heated through.

Exchange List Values
- Starch 2.5 • Med-Fat Meat 1.0

Basic Nutritional Values
- Calories 260 • Sodium 550 mg
  (Calories from Fat 55) • Potassium 315 gm
- Total Fat 6 gm • Total Carb 38 gm
  (Saturated Fat 1.4 gm, • Dietary Fiber 4 gm
  Trans Fat 0.0 gm, • Sugars 3 gm
  Polyunsat Fat 1.4 gm, • Protein 14 gm
  Monounsat Fat 2.8 gm) • Phosphorus 215 gm
- Cholesterol 25 mg

Quiche

Marjorie Weaver Nafziger
Harman, WV

Makes 6 servings,
1 slice of the pie per serving

Prep. Time: 25 minutes
Cooking/Baking Time: 1 hour
Standing Time: 5–10 minutes

9" unbaked pie shell (see
  page 203)
2 cups chopped tomatoes,
  green beans, onions, *or*
  mushrooms
½ cup chopped chicken
  breast
½ tsp. basil, sage, thyme,
  or oregano
¾ tsp. salt
dash pepper
½ cup grated reduced-fat
  Swiss

½ cup egg substitute
2 Tbsp. flour
1 cup fat-free evaporated
   milk

1. Bake pie shell for 10 minutes at 375°. Set aside.
2. Lightly sauté choice of vegetables and chicken. Spoon into pie shell.
3. Sprinkle choice of seasonings over vegetable mixture. Add salt and dash of pepper. Cover with grated cheese.
4. Combine egg substitute, flour and milk. Pour over ingredients.
5. Bake at 375° for 40–45 minutes or until set. Let sit at least 5 minutes before serving.

Variation:

Instead of using regular pie shell, combine 3 Tbsp. cooking oil with 3–4 cups grated potatoes. Press mixture into 9" pie pan and bake at 425° for 15 minutes.

Exchange List Values
• Carbohydrate 1.0   • Lean Meat 2.0

Basic Nutritional Values
• Calories 160
  (Calories from Fat 45)
• Total Fat 5 gm
  (Saturated Fat 1.5 gm,
  Trans Fat 0.2 gm,
  Polyunsat Fat 0.8 gm,
  Monounsat Fat 1.8 gm)
• Cholesterol 20 mg
• Sodium 430 mg
• Potassium 365 gm
• Total Carb 16 gm
• Dietary Fiber 1 gm
• Sugars 7 gm
• Protein 13 gm
• Phosphorus 195 gm

Crustless Spinach Quiche

Elaine Vigoda
Rochester, NY

Makes 16 servings, 1 slice of an 8-slice pie per serving

Prep. Time: 10 minutes
Baking Time: 30–35 minutes
Standing Time: 10 minutes

1 cup flour
1 tsp. salt
1 tsp. baking powder
¾ cup egg substitute
1 cup fat-free milk
2 Tbsp. no trans-fat tub
   margarine, melted
½ medium onion, chopped
10-oz. pkg. frozen spinach,
   thawed and squeezed
   dry
12 oz. 75%-less-fat
   shredded cheddar cheese
¼ tsp. nutmeg

1. In a large mixing bowl, blend together flour, salt, baking powder, egg substitute, milk, and margarine.
2. Stir in onion, spinach, and cheese.
3. Pour into 2 greased pie pans. Sprinkle with nutmeg.
4. Bake at 350° until set and light golden brown, about 30–35 minutes. To test if the quiche is done, put the blade of a knife into the center of the baking dish. If the knife comes out clean, the quiche is finished. If it doesn't, continue baking for another 5 minutes. Test again. Repeat if necessary.

5. Allow quiche to stand 10 minutes before cutting and serving. The standing time will allow the filling to firm up.

Tips:
1. You'll need to defrost the package of spinach before making this recipe. If you have time (8 hours or so), you can let it thaw in a bowl in the fridge. If you decided to make this quiche on short notice, and the spinach is frozen solid, lay the spinach in a shallow, microwave-safe dish, and defrost it in the microwave until thawed. (You can remove the box either before or after thawing the spinach.) When thawed, place the spinach in a strainer and press a spoon against it to remove as much of the water as possible. Or squeeze the spinach in your hand to remove the water. Then mix the spinach in with the rest of the ingredients and proceed with Step 3.
2. You can freeze the quiche after you've baked it. When ready to serve, allow to thaw. Then bake for 10 minutes, or until heated through.

Exchange List Values
• Starch 0.5   • Lean Meat 1.0

Basic Nutritional Values
• Calories 100
  (Calories from Fat 25)
• Total Fat 3 gm
  (Saturated Fat 1.4 gm,
  Trans Fat 0.0 gm,
  Polyunsat Fat 0.5 gm,
  Monounsat Fat 0.7 gm)
• Cholesterol 10 mg
• Sodium 370 mg
• Potassium 125 gm
• Total Carb 9 gm
• Dietary Fiber 1 gm
• Sugars 1 gm
• Protein 10 gm
• Phosphorus 165 gm

Crustless Veggie Quiche

Susan Kasting
Jenks, OK

*Makes 15 servings,
about 5 oz. per serving*

Prep. Time: 30 minutes
Baking Time: 45–50 minutes
Standing Time: 10 minutes

2¼ cups egg substitute
1½ cups shredded
　75%-less-fat sharp
　cheddar cheese, *divided*
1½ cups shredded reduced-
　fat Monterey Jack
　cheese, *divided*
½ cup fat-free milk
½ cup flour
1 tsp. baking powder
16 oz. 1%-fat cottage cheese
2 cups diced potatoes
½ onion, chopped
½ cup water
4 cups sliced zucchini
1 cup chopped green bell
　pepper
½ cup chopped parsley
2 tomatoes, thinly sliced

1. In a large mixer, bowl, beat egg substitute until fluffy. Add 1 cup cheddar, 1 cup Monterey Jack cheese, milk, flour, baking powder, and cottage cheese. Stir together well.
2. Place potatoes in a medium-sized saucepan, along with onions and ½ cup water. Cover and cook gently until potatoes and onions are nearly tender.
3. Add zucchini and green pepper. Continue cooking

until just-tender. Drain off water.
4. Add vegetable mixture and parsley to egg-cheese mixture.
5. Pour into greased 3-quart baking dish.
6. Top with remaining cheese and tomato slices.
7. Bake at 400° for 15 minutes. Then reduce temperature to 350° and bake for an additional 35 minutes, or until set.
8. To test if quiche is done, insert blade of knife into center. If knife comes out clean, quiche is fully baked. If it doesn't, continue baking for another 5 minutes. Test again. Repeat if not fully cooked.
9. Allow quiche to stand 10 minutes before slicing to allow it to firm up.

Tips:
　You can serve this hot or at room temperature.
2. You can use leftover potatoes and vegetables.

Exchange List Values
- Starch 0.5
- Lean Meat 2.0
- Vegetable 1.0

Basic Nutritional Values
- Calories 150
　(Calories from Fat 35)
- Total Fat 4 gm
　(Saturated Fat 2.2 gm,
　Trans Fat 0.0 gm,
　Polyunsat Fat 0.1 gm,
　Monounsat Fat 0.9 gm)
- Cholesterol 15 mg
- Sodium 400 mg
- Potassium 365 gm
- Total Carb 13 gm
- Dietary Fiber 1 gm
- Sugars 3 gm
- Protein 16 gm
- Phosphorus 235 gm

Mexican Lasagna

Jeanne Heyerly
Shipshewana, IN

*Makes 12 servings, 3" square per
serving*

Prep. Time: 20 minutes
Baking Time: 30–45 minutes
Standing Time: 10 minutes

¾ lb. 90%-lean ground
　beef
half large onion, chopped
1 large clove garlic, minced
2½ cups low-sodium salsa,
　divided
4 (6") whole-wheat
　tortillas, halved
1½ cups fat-free cottage
　cheese
1 cup fat-free sour cream
8-oz. can chopped green
　chilies
½ cup fresh cilantro,
　chopped
2 tsp. ground cumin
4-oz. can sliced ripe olives,
　drained, *optional*
1¼ cups shredded reduced-
　fat Monterey Jack cheese

1. Brown ground beef in skillet, stirring frequently to break up clumps. Remove meat to platter. Discard drippings.
2. Cook onion and garlic in same pan for 2 minutes.
3. Spread 1 cup salsa on bottom of greased 9×13 baking dish.
4. Layer half of tortillas over salsa.
5. In bowl, stir together cottage cheese, sour cream, green chilies, cilantro, cumin,

and black olives if you wish.

6. Spread half cottage cheese mixture on tortillas.

7. Spread half beef mixture on cheese mixture.

8. Repeat layers using rest of salsa, tortillas, cottage cheese mixture, and beef mixture.

9. Top with Monterey Jack cheese.

10. Bake at 350° for 30–45 minutes, until dish is bubbly and heated through. Cover loosely with foil if getting too brown or beginning to dry out.

11. Remove from oven and let stand 10 minutes before serving.

Exchange List Values
- Carbohydrate 1.0 • Lean Meat 2.0

Basic Nutritional Values
- Calories 165
  (Calories from Fat 45)
- Total Fat 5 gm
  (Saturated Fat 2.5 gm,
  Trans Fat 0.1 gm,
  Polyunsat Fat 0.3 gm,
  Monounsat Fat 1.7 gm)
- Cholesterol 30 mg
- Sodium 495 mg
- Potassium 390 gm
- Total Carb 16 gm
- Dietary Fiber 2 gm
- Sugars 4 gm
- Protein 14 gm
- Phosphorus 215 gm

Spinach in Phyllo

Jeanette Zacharias
Morden, Manitoba

Makes 20 slices, 1 slice per serving

Prep. Time: 25 minutes
Cooling Time: 20 minutes
Cooking/Baking Time: 45 minutes

1 medium onion, finely chopped
10-oz. pkg. frozen spinach
1 cup finely chopped mushrooms
1 clove garlic, crushed
1 Tbsp. dried oregano
2 Tbsp. white wine
1 cup lowfat 1% milkfat cottage cheese
1 egg
salt and pepper to taste
12 14" × 18" sheets phyllo dough
¼ cup melted trans-fat-free tub margarine

1. Sauté onion in non-stick skillet until transparent.

2. Thaw and drain spinach. Chop into fine pieces.

3. To onions in skillet add spinach, mushrooms, garlic, oregano and wine. Cook until most of moisture has evaporated. Cool at least 20 minutes.

4. Combine cottage cheese and egg. Add cooled spinach mixture. Add salt and pepper.

5. Spread phyllo sheets out and layer one on top of the other, brushing melted margarine over each sheet.

6. On last phyllo sheet put spinach filling. Roll up, being careful to fold in ends.

7. Lay seam-side down on greased cookie sheet. Brush phyllo roll with melted margarine.

8. Bake at 350° for 30–35 minutes or until golden brown and crisp.

9. Slice in 20 slices and serve either hot or cold.

Exchange List Values
- Starch 0.5 • Fat 0.5

Basic Nutritional Values
- Calories 75
  (Calories from Fat 20)
- Total Fat 2.5 gm
  (Saturated Fat 0.5 gm,
  Trans Fat 0.0 gm,
  Polyunsat Fat 0.9 gm,
  Monounsat Fat 0.7 gm)
- Cholesterol 10 mg
- Sodium 130 mg
- Potassium 80 gm
- Total Carb 10 gm
- Dietary Fiber 1 gm
- Sugars 1 gm
- Protein 3 gm
- Phosphorus 40 gm

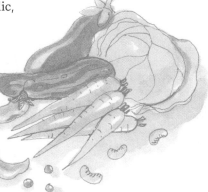

Zucchini Supper

Susan Kastings
Jenks, OK

Makes 8 servings,
3¼"×4½" rectangle per serving

Prep. Time: 15 minutes
Cooking/Baking Time: 25–30 minutes

4 cups thinly sliced
  zucchini
1 cup reduced-fat
  buttermilk baking mix
½ cup chopped green
  onions
½ cup freshly grated
  Parmesan cheese
2 Tbsp. chopped parsley,
  fresh *or* dried
½ tsp. dried oregano
½ tsp. pepper
½ tsp. garlic powder
½ tsp. seasoned salt
¼ cup canola oil
½ cup fat-free milk
1 cup egg substitute

1. In a large mixing bowl, mix together zucchini, baking mix, green onions, cheese, parsley, oregano, pepper, garlic powder, seasoned salt, oil, milk, and eggs.
2. Pour into well-greased 9×13 baking pan.
3. Bake at 350° for 25–30 minutes, or until firm.
4. Serve warm or at room temperature.

Exchange List Values
• Starch 1.0   • Fat 1.0
• Lean Meat 1.0

Basic Nutritional Values
• Calories 165   • Sodium 400 mg
 (Calories from Fat 80)   • Potassium 265 gm
• Total Fat 9 gm   • Total Carb 14 gm
 (Saturated Fat 1.4 gm,   • Dietary Fiber 1 gm
 Trans Fat 0.0 gm,   • Sugars 3 gm
 Polyunsat Fat 2.2 gm,   • Protein 7 gm
 Monounsat Fat 5.2 gm)   • Phosphorus 165 gm
• Cholesterol 5 mg

Carrot Pie

Jean Harris Robinson
Pemberton, NJ

Makes 8 servings,
⅛ of pie per serving

Prep. Time: 20 minutes
Baking Time: 40 minutes

1 cup egg substitute
½ cup freshly grated
  Parmesan cheese
¼ cup canola oil
1 cup reduced-fat
  buttermilk baking mix
1 medium onion, chopped
3 cups raw shredded
  carrots

1. In a large mixing bowl, mix egg substitute, cheese, oil, baking mix, onion, and carrots together.
2. Pour into buttered 9" pie plate.
3. Bake on the middle rack at 350° for 40 minutes, or until set in center. To test, insert blade of knife in center of pie. If it comes out clean, the pie is finished baking. If it doesn't, continue baking 5 more minutes. Test again. Continue baking in 5-minute intervals, and testing, until done.

Exchange List Values
• Starch 0.5   • Lean Meat 1.0
• Vegetable 1.0   • Fat 1.0

Basic Nutritional Values
• Calories 170   • Sodium 315 mg
 (Calories from Fat 80)   • Potassium 210 gm
• Total Fat 9 gm   • Total Carb 16 gm
 (Saturated Fat 1.4 gm,   • Dietary Fiber 2 gm
 Trans Fat 0.0 gm,   • Sugars 4 gm
 Polyunsat Fat 2.2 gm,   • Protein 6 gm
 Monounsat Fat 5.2 gm)   • Phosphorus 140 gm
• Cholesterol 5 mg

Corn and Green Chili Casserole

Marilyn Mowry
Irving, TX

Makes 6 servings,
4¼" square per serving

Prep. Time: 10 minutes
Baking Time: 45–55 minutes
Standing Time: 10 minutes

14¾-oz. can creamed corn
4-oz. can chopped green
  chilies
½ cup egg substitute
½ tsp. garlic salt
½ cup cornmeal
2 Tbsp. canola oil
4 oz. 75%-less-fat shredded
  cheddar cheese

1. In a mixing bowl, mix corn, green chilies, egg substitute, garlic salt, cornmeal, and oil together.
2. Spread half the corn mixture in a well-greased 9×13 baking pan.
3. Top with all of the cheese.

4. Top with the rest of the corn mixture.

5. Bake uncovered at 350° for 45–55 minutes, or until mixture is set. Insert knife blade in center of casserole to determine if set. If knife comes out clean, the casserole is finished baking. If not, continue baking for 5 more minutes. Test again with knife. If needed, bake another 5 minutes. Repeat test, and baking if necessary.

6. Allow to stand 10 minutes after baking to allow casserole to firm up before serving.

Exchange List Values
- Starch 1.5
- Fat 0.5
- Lean Meat 1.0

Basic Nutritional Values
- Calories 180
  (Calories from Fat 65)
- Total Fat 7 gm
  (Saturated Fat 1.4 gm,
  Trans Fat 0.0 gm,
  Polyunsat Fat 1.6 gm,
  Monounsat Fat 3.4 gm)
- Cholesterol 5 mg
- Sodium 460 mg
- Potassium 175 gm
- Total Carb 20 gm
- Dietary Fiber 1 gm
- Sugars 5 gm
- Protein 9 gm
- Phosphorus 145 gm

Corn Casserole

Beth Nafziger
Lowville, NY

*Makes 10 servings,
about 5–6 oz. per serving*

Prep. Time: 25–30 minutes
**Cooking/Baking Time: 45
minutes**

1 large onion, chopped
2 medium green bell
  peppers
2 Tbsp. canola oil
¼ cup flour
2 cups frozen *or* canned
  corn
2 cups cooked long-grain
  rice
14½-oz. can diced tomatoes
4 hard-cooked eggs, yolks
  removed
2 cups extra-sharp
  75%-less-fat shredded
  cheddar cheese
2 Tbsp. Worcestershire
  sauce
2 to 3 tsp. hot pepper sauce
¾ tsp. salt
1 tsp. pepper

1. In a large skillet, sauté chopped onion and green peppers in butter until tender.

2. Stir in flour. Remove from heat.

3. Add remaining ingredients except for ½ cup cheese. Pour into greased 2½-quart baking dish.

4. Bake, uncovered, at 350° for 45 minutes. Top with remaining cheese.

Exchange List Values
- Starch 1.0
- Vegetable 1.0
- Lean Meat 1.0
- Fat 0.5

Basic Nutritional Values
- Calories 180
  (Calories from Fat 45)
- Total Fat 5 gm
  (Saturated Fat 1.5 gm,
  Trans Fat 0.0 gm,
  Polyunsat Fat 1.0 gm,
  Monounsat Fat 2.3 gm)
- Cholesterol 10 mg
- Sodium 455 mg
- Potassium 320 gm
- Total Carb 23 gm
- Dietary Fiber 2 gm
- Sugars 4 gm
- Protein 11 gm
- Phosphorus 170 gm

I have always dreaded having to take a dish to a potluck. However, I finally decided such occasions were not contests or competitions. When I feel like preparing a nice dish, I use a recipe. Just as often I take a plate of fresh fruit or a simple relish plate. Many people seem to like fresh simple items. The kids love cupcakes, and angel food cakes and even something as simple as a bag of chips. Some people love to taste new dishes, but my kids belong to the group who needs to feed on more familiar fare.

Carol Friesen, Wallace, NE

Calico Corn

Linda Yoder
Fresno, OH

Makes 8 servings,
about 5 oz. per serving

Prep. Time: 10 minutes
Cooking Time: 10 minutes

¾ cup minced onion
⅓ cup finely chopped
  green bell pepper
⅓ cup finely chopped red
  bell pepper
1 medium garlic clove,
  minced
2 Tbsp. vegetable oil
2 pints frozen sweet corn,
  thawed
½ cup quick grits, uncooked
1½ cups water
1 tsp. salt
¼ tsp. white pepper

1. In 2-quart pan, sauté onion, peppers, and garlic in oil just until tender.
2. Stir in corn, grits, water, salt and pepper.
3. Bring mixture to a boil.
4. Reduce heat, cover, and cook, stirring occasionally for about 7 minutes more until grits are soft and water is absorbed.

Tip:
  If you're trying to reduce your stress by reducing the amount of last-minute preparation you do before serving a meal, you can prepare this dish in advance through Step 3. Refrigerate until it's nearly mealtime. Then begin with Step 3.

Exchange List Values
• Starch 1.5   • Fat 0.5

Basic Nutritional Values
• Calories 135   • Sodium 295 mg
  (Calories from Fat 35)   • Potassium 225 gm
• Total Fat 4 gm   • Total Carb 23 gm
  (Saturated Fat 0.4 gm,   • Dietary Fiber 2 gm
  Trans Fat 0.0 gm,   • Sugars 3 gm
  Polyunsat Fat 1.3 gm,   • Protein 3 gm
  Monounsat Fat 2.4 gm)   • Phosphorus 70 gm
• Cholesterol 0 mg

Corn Balls

Rhoda Nissley
Parkesburg, PA
Jeanette Oberholtzer
Lititz, PA

Makes 10 servings

Prep. Time: 20 minutes
Baking Time: 35 minutes

11-oz. pkg. soft bread cubes
1-lb. can crushed corn *or* 2
  cups fresh corn
3 eggs, beaten
½-1 chopped onion
½ tsp. salt
¼ tsp. pepper
⅓ cup no-trans-fat tub
  margarine

1. Combine bread cubes, corn, eggs, onion, salt and pepper in a large mixing bowl.
2. Form into balls, each about ⅓ cup in size. If balls are too dry to hold together, add 2 Tbsp. hot water to full mixture.
3. Place in greased 9×13 baking pan.
4. Pour melted margarine over balls.

5. Bake uncovered at 325° for 35 minutes.

Tip:
  I use about 3 cups of my home-frozen sweet corn for these. I like to put the corn in the blender with the eggs and onions before mixing with the bread and seasonings.
                    Rhoda Nissley
                    Parkesburg, PA

Exchange List Values
• Starch 1.5   • Fat 1.5

Basic Nutritional Values
• Calories 175   • Sodium 355 mg
  (Calories from Fat 65)   • Potassium 135 gm
• Total Fat 7 gm   • Total Carb 23 gm
  (Saturated Fat 1.5 gm,   • Dietary Fiber 2 gm
  Trans Fat 0.0 gm,   • Sugars 3 gm
  Polyunsat Fat 2.5 gm,   • Protein 6 gm
  Monounsat Fat 2.6 gm)   • Phosphorus 85 gm
• Cholesterol 55 mg

Stuffing Balls

Joan Brown
Warriors Mark, PA

Makes 8 servings

Prep. Time: 15 minutes
Baking Time: 20–25 minutes

1 lb. loaf whole wheat
  bread, stale
3 ribs celery, diced
1 medium, *or* small, onion,
  diced
2 eggs, beaten
10¾-oz. can lower-sodium,
  lower-fat cream of
  mushroom, *or* cream of
  chicken soup, *divided*

1. Tear bread in small pieces and place in large mixing bowl.

2. Add celery, onion, eggs, and half of soup. Mix together well.

3. Form into balls, each ⅓ cup in size. If too dry to hold together, add boiling water, 1–2 Tbsp. at a time to all of bread mixture.

4. Place balls in greased 9×13 baking.

5. Pour remaining soup over top.

6. Bake at 350° for 20–25 minutes.

Exchange List Values
- Starch 2.0
- Fat 0.5

Basic Nutritional Values
- Calories 185
  (Calories from Fat 30)
- Total Fat 4 gm
  (Saturated Fat 0.9 gm,
  Trans Fat 0.0 gm,
  Polyunsat Fat 0.9 gm,
  Monounsat Fat 1.5 gm)
- Cholesterol 45 mg
- Sodium 425 mg
- Potassium 485 gm
- Total Carb 29 gm
- Dietary Fiber 5 gm
- Sugars 5 gm
- Protein 10 gm
- Phosphorus 160 gm

Potato Corn Bake

Donna Treloar
Muncie, IN

*Makes 6 servings,
3½" square per serving*

Prep. Time: 15 minutes
Cooking/Baking Time: 20–25 minutes

¼ lb. bacon, cut in pieces
½ cup green bell pepper, diced
⅓ cup onion, diced
2½ cups 1% milk
14½-oz. can creamed corn
⅛ tsp. pepper
2 cups real, *or* instant, mashed potatoes, made with fat-free milk and minimal fat
¾ cup fat-free sour cream
¼ cup freshly grated Parmesan cheese
2 Tbsp. chopped green onion

1. In a sauté pan, cook bacon until crisp. Remove from pan and allow to drain on a paper towel. Discard drippings.

2. Add green pepper and onion to same pan. Cook until tender.

3. Add milk, corn, salt, and pepper to pan. Cook over medium heat until hot and bubbly.

4. Remove from heat. Stir in potatoes and sour cream until well blended.

5. Spoon into greased 7×11 baking dish.

6. Top with bacon, Parmesan cheese, and green onion.

7. Cover and bake at 375° for 20–25 minutes, or until heated through.

Exchange List Values
- Starch 1.5
- Fat 0.5
- Fat-Free Milk 1.0

Basic Nutritional Values
- Calories 225
  (Calories from Fat 55)
- Total Fat 6 gm
  (Saturated Fat 3.0 gm,
  Trans Fat 0.0 gm,
  Polyunsat Fat 0.8 gm,
  Monounsat Fat 2.1 gm)
- Cholesterol 20 mg
- Sodium 565 mg
- Potassium 545 gm
- Total Carb 33 gm
- Dietary Fiber 2 gm
- Sugars 12 gm
- Protein 10 gm
- Phosphorus 250 gm

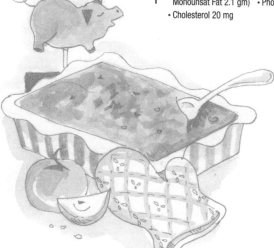

Stuffed Zucchini

Janet Batdorf
Harrisburg, PA

Makes 8 servings

Prep. Time: 25 minutes
Cooking/Baking Time: 35 minutes

1 large, *or* 2 medium, zucchini
2 tsp. no-trans-fat tub margarine
1 cup bread crumbs
2 Tbsp. chopped onion
½ cup marinara pasta sauce, light in sodium
¼ tsp. salt
¼ tsp. pepper
¼ tsp. dried oregano
¾ cup reduced-fat Italian shredded cheese blend

1. Parboil zucchini by submerging it/them in boiling salted water in large stockpot for 15 minutes (10 minutes for smaller size). Or cut in half lengthwise and cook in microwave until soft in center.

2. When cool enough to handle, scoop out pulp in the center, leaving ½" "shell" all around.

3. In a good-sized mixing bowl, mix pulp with butter, bread crumbs, onion, sauce, salt, pepper, and oregano.

4. Fill zucchini with mixture. Sprinkle with cheese.

5. Place zucchini "boats," stuffed side up and next to each other in a lightly greased baking dish. Bake at 350° until heated through, about 25 minutes.

6. Cut into 8 equal servings.

Tip:

I always use this recipe when I have oversized zucchini, especially at end of summer.

Exchange List Values
• Starch 1.0   • Fat 0.5

Basic Nutritional Values
• Calories 105   • Sodium 300 mg
  (Calories from Fat 30)   • Potassium 195 gm
• Total Fat 4 gm   • Total Carb 13 gm
  (Saturated Fat 1.5 gm,   • Dietary Fiber 1 gm
  Trans Fat 0.0 gm,   • Sugars 2 gm
  Polyunsat Fat 0.8 gm,   • Protein 6 gm
  Monounsat Fat 1.0 gm)   • Phosphorus 125 gm
• Cholesterol 5 mg

Stuffed Eggplant

Jean Harris Robinson
Pemberton, NJ

Makes 8 servings,
¼ eggplant per serving

Prep. Time: 30 minutes
Cooking/Baking Time: 30–45 minutes

2 large eggplants
1 medium onion, chopped
4 tomatoes, chopped
3 medium green bell peppers, chopped
1 rib celery, chopped
2 Tbsp. olive oil
½ cup egg substitute
1 tsp. salt
1 tsp. pepper
½ cup freshly grated Parmesan cheese
¼ tsp. cayenne pepper, *optional*
½ tsp. grated garlic, *optional*

1. Cut eggplants in half and scrape out seeds. Parboil* 15 minutes.

2. After eggplant halves have drained, remove pulp within ½" of outer "shell." Chop pulp. Set aside.

3. Place eggplant shells, cut side up, in 12×24 baking dish.

4. Empty stockpot of water. Place onion, tomatoes, peppers, and celery, and olive oil in stockpot. Cook until soft and almost a purée. Remove from heat.

5. Stir in eggplant pulp, beaten eggs, salt, and pepper.

6. Fill eggplant halves with the mixture. Sprinkle with cheese.

7. Distribute any leftover stuffing in baking dish around eggplant halves.

8. Bake at 350° for 30 minutes, or until eggplant is tender and cheese is brown.

* To parboil eggplants, submerge unpeeled halves in a stockpot of boiling water with a shake of salt added. Cook in boiling water for 15 minutes. Remove and drain.

Tip:

I have used 4–5 whole canned tomatoes when I haven't been able to find fresh tomatoes. Before adding them to the mixture (Step 4), I've chopped them, and drained off as much of their liquid as I could.

Exchange List Values
- Vegetable 4.0
- Fat 1.0

Basic Nutritional Values
- Calories 145
  (Calories from Fat 45)
- Total Fat 5 gm
  (Saturated Fat 1.3 gm,
  Trans Fat 0.0 gm,
  Polyunsat Fat 0.6 gm,
  Monounsat Fat 2.9 gm)
- Cholesterol 5 mg
- Sodium 405 mg
- Potassium 515 gm
- Total Carb 22 gm
- Dietary Fiber 6 gm
- Sugars 9 gm
- Protein 6 gm
- Phosphorus 90 gm

Pea Casserole

Janet Batdorf
Harrisburg, PA

*Makes 6 servings,
about 6 oz. per serving*

Prep. Time: 20 minutes
Baking Time: 25 minutes

1-lb. pkg. frozen peas
10¾-oz. can lower-sodium, lower-fat cream of mushroom soup
¼ cup fat-free milk
1 Tbsp. canola oil
⅓ cup diced celery
⅓ cup chopped onion
⅓ cup chopped green bell pepper
8-oz. can sliced water chestnuts, drained
¼ cup chopped pimento
¾ cup crushed cheese crackers, *or* other flavor of your choice

1. Cook peas as directed on package.

2. In a small bowl, mix milk and soup together. Stir into peas.

3. Sauté celery, onions and green pepper in oil in a small saucepan. Add to pea mixture.

4. Stir in water chestnuts and pimento. Mix well.

5. Place mixture in 1½-quart greased baking dish.

6. Sprinkle with cheese crackers.

7. Bake at 350° for 25 minutes, or until heated through.

Exchange List Values
- Starch 1.5
- Vegetable 1.0
- Fat 1.0

Basic Nutritional Values
- Calories 190
  (Calories from Fat 55)
- Total Fat 6 gm
  (Saturated Fat 1.5 gm,
  Trans Fat 0.0 gm,
  Polyunsat Fat 1.5 gm,
  Monounsat Fat 3.1 gm)
- Cholesterol 5 mg
- Sodium 380 mg
- Potassium 550 gm
- Total Carb 26 gm
- Dietary Fiber 6 gm
- Sugars 6 gm
- Protein 7 gm
- Phosphorus 120 gm

I remember a potluck meal I shared in Japan. Rice was prepared and each family brought something to go on top. The food committee served each person by putting rice in a bowl, adding seaweed, vegetables, eggs and whatever else was brought. In a few minutes a beautiful meal was prepared.
Betty J. Rosentrater, Nappanee, IN

Mushroom Casserole

Maryann Markano
Wilmington, DE

*Makes 12 servings,
about 6–7 oz. per serving*

Prep. Time: 40 minutes
Baking Time: 30 minutes

3 lbs. fresh mushrooms
⅓ cup no trans-fat tub
margarine
1 large onion, chopped
8 oz. 75%-less-fat shredded
cheddar cheese, *divided*
3 6-oz. boxes chicken-
flavor low-sodium
stuffing mix, *divided*
1 pint fat-free half-and-half

1. Be sure mushrooms are clean. If small, leave them whole. If large, cut in half. Place in 5-quart stockpot with margarine and chopped onion.

2. Cover and cook over low heat for about 30 minutes, until mushrooms are tender and have made their own juice.

3. Grease a 5-quart baking dish, or two 2½-3-quart baking dishes. Put in half the mushrooms, half the cheese, and half the stuffing mix.

4. Repeat layers, topping with remaining mushrooms and cheese. When spooning mushrooms into baking dish(es), use some of their juices, but not all because half-and-half must go in.

5. Pour half-and-half on top.

6. Bake at 350° for 30 minutes, or until set and cheese is melted. To test if mixture is done, insert blade of knife in center of dish. If knife comes out clean, the casserole is finished. If it doesn't, continue baking another 5 minutes. Test again. Continue baking and testing if needed.

Tips:

1. The dish may be done ahead of time, through Step 4. Pour half-and-half on just before baking. If baking dish was in refrigerator overnight, bring to room temperature and bake about 40 minutes.

2. This is a great alternative to traditional stuffing at holiday-time.

Exchange List Values

- Starch 2.5
- Vegetable 1.0
- Lean Meat 1.0
- Fat 0.5

Basic Nutritional Values

- Calories 295
  (Calories from Fat 70)
- Total Fat 8 gm
  (Saturated Fat 2.1 gm,
  Trans Fat 0.0 gm,
  Polyunsat Fat 2.0 gm,
  Monounsat Fat 2.3 gm)
- Cholesterol 10 mg
- Sodium 595 mg
- Potassium 590 gm
- Total Carb 42 gm
- Dietary Fiber 3 gm
- Sugars 8 gm
- Protein 15 gm
- Phosphorus 310 gm

Baked Rice with Spinach and Nuts

Carolyn Spohn
Shawnee, KS

*Makes 4 servings,
3½"×6" rectangle per serving*

Prep. Time: 20 minutes
Baking Time: 25–30 minutes

1–2 tsp. olive oil
2 garlic cloves, minced
1 medium onion, diced
14½-oz. can diced
tomatoes, drained
reserving ⅓ cup juice
1½ cups cooked rice
¼ tsp. salt
⅓ cup pine nuts, *or*
chopped walnuts, *or*
chopped pecans
half of 9-oz. pkg. fresh
spinach, chopped
¾ cup shredded reduced-
fat Colby Jack cheese,
divided
1 cup turkey *or* chicken,
cooked and cubed,
optional

1. Heat olive oil in large skillet over medium heat. Being careful not to splash yourself with hot oil, sauté garlic and onion until tender.

2. Add drained tomatoes and cook about 10 minutes, stirring frequently.

3. Stir cooked rice, salt, ⅓ cup reserved tomato juice, nuts, raw spinach, and meat if you wish into tomato mixture.

4. Spread half of mixture in greased 7×12 baking dish.

5. Sprinkle with half the cheese.

6. Repeat layers with cheese on top.

7. Cover and bake at 375° for about 25 minutes, or until bubbly.

8. Uncover for last few minutes of baking so cheese browns slightly.

Exchange List Values

- Starch 1.0
- Med-Fat Meat 1.0
- Vegetable 2.0
- Fat 1.5

Basic Nutritional Values

- Calories 270
  (Calories from Fat 115)
- Total Fat 13 gm
  (Saturated Fat 3.5 gm,
  Trans Fat 0.0 gm,
  Polyunsat Fat 4.3 gm,
  Monounsat Fat 4.1 gm)
- Cholesterol 10 mg
- Sodium 550 mg
- Potassium 580 gm
- Total Carb 29 gm
- Dietary Fiber 3 gm
- Sugars 5 gm
- Protein 11 gm
- Phosphorus 235 gm

Bounty Rice

Melissa Raber
Millersburg, OH

Makes 6 servings,
2"×4" rectangle per serving

Prep. Time: 30 minutes
Cooking/Baking Time: 30–60 minutes

½ lb. 90%-lean ground beef
1 cup chopped green bell pepper
1 cup chopped onion, chopped
1¼ cups long-grain rice, uncooked
3 cups water
4 cups diced canned tomatoes
4 cups shredded cabbage, shredded
½ tsp. salt
½ tsp. dried oregano
½ tsp. dried basil
½ tsp. garlic powder
¼ tsp. red, *or* black, pepper
1 cup shredded part-skim mozzarella cheese

1. In large skillet, sauté beef, peppers, and onion until meat is browned and vegetables are soft. Stir often to break up clumps of meat.

2. Meanwhile, place 3 cups water in good-sized saucepan. Cover. Cook over high heat until water boils.

3. Stir in rice. Cover. Reduce heat to low or medium so that rice simmers.

4. Check rice after 20 minutes. If water is absorbed, turn off heat. If not, continue cooking another 5–10 minutes.

5. While rice cooks, stir tomatoes, cabbage, salt, oregano, basil, garlic powder, and red pepper into skillet with beef and vegetables.

6. When rice is cooked, stir into skillet, too.

7. Spoon mixture into greased 8×8 casserole dish.

8. Bake at 325° for 30–60 minutes, or until cabbage is as tender as you like it and casserole is bubbly.

9. Top with cheese and let melt before serving.

Exchange List Values

- Starch 2.0
- Med-Fat Meat 1.0
- Vegetable 3.0

Basic Nutritional Values

- Calories 320
  (Calories from Fat 65)
- Total Fat 7 gm
  (Saturated Fat 3.3 gm,
  Trans Fat 0.2 gm,
  Polyunsat Fat 0.4 gm,
  Monounsat Fat 2.3 gm)
- Cholesterol 35 mg
- Sodium 585 mg
- Potassium 655 gm
- Total Carb 47 gm
- Dietary Fiber 4 gm
- Sugars 8 gm
- Protein 18 gm
- Phosphorus 260 gm

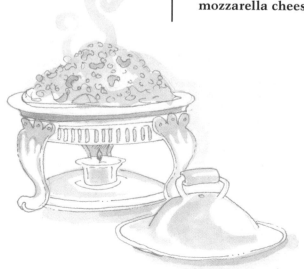

Hearty Spinach and Tofu Risotto

Julie Hurst
Leola, PA

*Makes 6 servings,
about ¾ cup per serving*

Prep. Time: 20 minutes
Baking Time: 30 minutes

8 oz. tofu, drained
1 medium onion, chopped
1 clove garlic, minced
2 Tbsp. canola oil
14-oz. can Italian tomatoes
1 tsp. dried oregano
2 cups cooked brown rice
10-oz. pkg. frozen spinach,
    thawed and drained
½ cup shredded Swiss
    cheese, *divided*
½ tsp. salt
¼ tsp. pepper
1 Tbsp. sesame seeds

1. Blend tofu until smooth.
Set aside.
2. In a large saucepan
sauté onion and garlic in
hot oil until onion is tender.
Add undrained tomatoes
and oregano. Bring to a full
boil; reduce heat. Simmer,
uncovered, about 3 minutes.
3. Stir in tofu and rice.
4. Add spinach, half of
cheese, salt and pepper. Mix
gently. Spoon mixture into
greased 1½-quart casserole
dish.
5. Bake, uncovered, at 350°
for 30 minutes. Top with
remaining cheese and sesame
seeds.

Exchange List Values
- Starch 1.0
- Vegetable 1.0
- Lean Meat 1.0
- Fat 1.5

Basic Nutritional Values
- Calories 215
  (Calories from Fat 90)
- Total Fat 10 gm
  (Saturated Fat 2.2 gm,
  Trans Fat 0.1 gm,
  Polyunsat Fat 2.6 gm,
  Monounsat Fat 4.3 gm)
- Cholesterol 10 mg
- Sodium 360 mg
- Potassium 395 gm
- Total Carb 24 gm
- Dietary Fiber 4 gm
- Sugars 4 gm
- Protein 9 gm
- Phosphorus 190 gm

J's Special Rice Dish

Joyce Bond
Stonyford, CA

Makes 6 servings, 4–5 oz. per serving

Prep. Time: 10–15 minutes
Cooking Time: 30 minutes

4 Tbsp. no-trans-fat tub
    margarine
1 cup long-grain rice,
    uncooked
3 cups water
2 chicken bouillon cubes
¼ tsp. salt
1 Tbsp. parsley flakes
1 Tbsp. chopped onion
1 tsp. minced garlic
¼ lb. fresh mushrooms,
    sliced, *or* 4-oz. can
    mushroom pieces
    mushrooms, drained
1 cup leftover cooked meat
    (lamb, beef, chicken *or*
    pork)

1. Melt butter in saucepan.
2. Stir in rice.

3. Stir in water, bouillon,
salt, parsley flakes, onion,
garlic, and mushrooms.
4. Cover and simmer over
low to medium heat for 20–30
minutes, or until liquid is
absorbed and rice is tender.
5. Stir in cooked meat.
Cover and cook over low heat,
just until meat is hot.

Exchange List Values
- Starch 2.0
- Lean Meat 1.0

Basic Nutritional Values
- Calories 200
  (Calories from Fat 45)
- Total Fat 5 gm
  (Saturated Fat 1.2 gm,
  Trans Fat 0.0 gm,
  Polyunsat Fat 1.7 gm,
  Monounsat Fat 1.7 gm)
- Cholesterol 20 mg
- Sodium 455 mg
- Potassium 165 gm
- Total Carb 28 gm
- Dietary Fiber 1 gm
- Sugars 1 gm
- Protein 10 gm
- Phosphorus 110 gm

Vietnam Fried Rice

Nancy Roth
Colorado Springs, CO
Mary Jane Miller
Wellman, IA

*Makes 6 servings,
about ¾ cup per serving*

Prep. Time: 15 minutes
Cooking Time: 15–20 minutes

1 Tbsp. canola oil
¼ lb. cooked beef, cut into
  strips
3 cloves garlic minced
1 large onion, chopped
½ tsp. salt
1 tsp. pepper
1 tsp. sugar
1 Tbsp. reduced-sodium
  soy sauce
3 cups cooked rice
1 cup leftover vegetables,
  such as peas, green
  beans, or carrots
2 eggs, beaten

1. Heat oil. Stir fry meat,
garlic, onion, salt, pepper,
sugar and soy sauce about 1–2
minutes.
2. Add cooked rice and stir
fry an additional 5 minutes.
3. Add any leftover
vegetables and stir well into
rice mixture.
4. Immediately before serving, add eggs. Over medium
heat stir eggs through rice
until eggs are cooked.

Exchange List Values
- Starch 1.5
- Vegetable 1.0
- Lean Meat 1.0
- Fat 1.0

Basic Nutritional Values
- Calories 225
  (Calories from Fat 70)
- Total Fat 8 gm
  (Saturated Fat 1.4 gm,
  Trans Fat 0.0 gm,
  Polyunsat Fat 1.8 gm,
  Monounsat Fat 4.0 gm)
- Cholesterol 70 mg
- Sodium 325 mg
- Potassium 215 gm
- Total Carb 30 gm
- Dietary Fiber 2 gm
- Sugars 3 gm
- Protein 9 gm
- Phosphorus 120 gm

Esther's Brown Rice

Esther Yoder
Hartville, OH

*Makes 6 servings,
about 5 oz. a serving*

Prep. Time: 10 minutes
Cooking Time: 1 hour

2 cups water
1 cup brown rice, uncooked
1 cup salsa

¼ cup chopped green
  pepper
½ cup chopped celery
½ cup chopped onion
1 tsp. reduced-sodium
  chicken bouillon
½ tsp. garlic salt
1 tsp. oil
½ tsp. sugar

1. Mix ingredients in a
4-quart saucepan.
2. Bring to boil. Turn heat
to low; cover and cook 1 hour.

Tip:
  Serve with more salsa at
the table.

Exchange List Values
- Starch 1.5
- Vegetable 1.0

Basic Nutritional Values
- Calories 145
  (Calories from Fat 20)
- Total Fat 2 gm
  (Saturated Fat 0.3 gm,
  Trans Fat 0.0 gm,
  Polyunsat Fat 0.6 gm,
  Monounsat Fat 0.8 gm)
- Cholesterol 0 mg
- Sodium 455 mg
- Potassium 225 gm
- Total Carb 29 gm
- Dietary Fiber 3 gm
- Sugars 3 gm
- Protein 4 gm
- Phosphorus 105 gm

One year we cooked for 35 persons at a weekend retreat. We asked each person to bring her or his own bowl, mug, and spoon. All the meals were one-dish meals which could be eaten with a spoon. On the side we served bread, muffins, fresh fruit, cookies, and other finger foods. To make sure no one was overwhelmed with the work, we assigned people to help with preparation and clean-up.

Elaine Gibble, Lititz, PA

Almond Rice

Dorothy VanDeest, Memphis, TN

Makes 8 servings,
about 5-6 oz. per serving

Prep. Time: 20 minutes
Cooking Time: 20 minutes

2 cups long-grain rice,
  uncooked
1 Tbsp. butter
3½ cups water
4 reduced-sodium beef
  bouillon cubes
½ cup slivered toasted
  almonds
6 green onions, chopped
2½ Tbsp. reduced-sodium
  soy sauce

1. Mix rice and butter in skillet. Sauté until rice begins to brown, stirring frequently to prevent burning.
2. In a small saucepan, bring water to a boil. Dissolve bouillon cubes in boiling water.
3. Add water to rice. Mix together. Cover and simmer until liquid disappears, 15–20 minutes.
4. Stir in almonds, chopped green onions, and soy sauce. Heat 1 minute longer.

Exchange List Values
- Starch 3.0
- Fat 0.5

Basic Nutritional Values
- Calories 250
  (Calories from Fat 45)
- Total Fat 5 gm
  (Saturated Fat 0.7 gm,
  Trans Fat 0.0 gm,
  Polyunsat Fat 1.5 gm,
  Monounsat Fat 2.8 gm)
- Cholesterol 0 mg
- Sodium 450 mg
- Potassium 145 gm
- Total Carb 43 gm
- Dietary Fiber 2 gm
- Sugars 1 gm
- Protein 6 gm
- Phosphorus 110 gm

Rice and Beans Bake

Jane Meiser
Harrisonburg, VA

Makes 8 servings,
2¼"×4½" rectangle per serving

Prep. Time: 20 minutes
Baking Time: 20–25 minutes

1 lb. 95%-lean ground beef
¾ cup onion, chopped
½ cup green pepper,
  chopped
2 cups low-sodium salsa,
  your choice of heat,
  divided
15-oz. can refried beans
1 Tbsp. ground cumin
2 cups cooked brown rice
¾ cup reduced-fat grated
  sharp cheddar cheese
tortilla chips, *optional*

1. Brown ground beef with onion and green pepper in large nonstick skillet. Stir frequently to break up clumps and until meat is no longer pink. Drain and discard any fat.
2. Stir in 1 cup salsa, beans, and cumin.
3. In a mixing bowl, combine rice and remaining cup salsa.
4. Place rice-salsa mixture in well-greased 9×9 baking dish.
5. Layer all of ground beef mixture over rice.
6. Top with cheese.
7. Bake at 350° for 20–25 minutes, or until cheese melts.
8. Serve with tortilla chips.

Exchange List Values
- Starch 1.0
- Vegetable 1.0
- Lean Meat 2.0

Basic Nutritional Values
- Calories 215
  (Calories from Fat 45)
- Total Fat 5 gm
  (Saturated Fat 2.5 gm,
  Trans Fat 0.1 gm,
  Polyunsat Fat 0.4 gm,
  Monounsat Fat 1.9 gm)
- Cholesterol 40 mg
- Sodium 555 mg
- Potassium 570 gm
- Total Carb 24 gm
- Dietary Fiber 4 gm
- Sugars 3 gm
- Protein 18 gm
- Phosphorus 240 gm

Red Beans and Rice

Rhoda Byler Yoder
Jackson, MS

Makes 20 servings, about ⅔ cup
rice and ⅔ cup beans per serving

Prep. Time: 20 minutes
Baking/Cooking Time: 2–10 hours

1 large onion, diced
1 Tbsp. canola oil
1¼ lbs. bulk lean turkey
  Italian sweet sausage
6 15-oz. cans red beans
1 tsp. pepper
½ tsp. red pepper
1 tsp. ground cumin
½ tsp. dried oregano
1 tsp. canola oil
4½ cups uncooked rice
¼ tsp. salt
9 cups water

1. Sauté onion in 1 Tbsp oil. Add sausage and brown. Drain excess fat.
2. Add beans, pepper, 1 tsp. salt, red pepper, cumin and oregano. Simmer at least

2 hours, stirring occasionally. Or simmer in slow cooker on low 8–10 hours.

3. Approximately ½ hour before mealtime stir 1 tsp. oil into rice in a large saucepan. Add salt and water. Bring to a rolling boil and stir well with a fork. Reduce heat to simmer. Cover and cook 20 minutes without lifting cover.

4. Serve beans and rice together. Offer hot sauce at the table.

Exchange List Values
- Starch 3.5
- Lean Meat 1.0

Basic Nutritional Values
- Calories 330
  (Calories from Fat 40)
- Total Fat 4.5 gm
  (Saturated Fat 1.0 gm,
  Trans Fat 0.1 gm,
  Polyunsat Fat 1.4 gm,
  Monounsat Fat 2.1 gm)
- Cholesterol 15 mg
- Sodium 585 mg
- Potassium 420 gm
- Total Carb 56 gm
- Dietary Fiber 8 gm
- Sugars 3 gm
- Protein 15 gm
- Phosphorus 210 gm

Lentil, Rice, and Veggie Bake
Andrea Zuercher
Lawrence, KS

*Makes 12 servings,
3" square per serving*

Prep. Time: 20 minutes
Cooking/Baking Time: 65–70 minutes

1 cup uncooked long-grain rice
5 cups water, *divided*
2 cups red lentils
2 tsp. vegetable oil

2 small onions, chopped
6 cloves garlic, minced
2 fresh tomatoes, chopped
⅔ cup chopped celery
⅔ cup chopped carrots
⅔ cup chopped summer squash
16-oz. can tomato sauce, *divided*
2 tsp. dried, *or* 2 Tbsp. fresh basil, *divided*
2 tsp. dried, *or* 2 Tbsp. fresh oregano, *divided*
2 tsp. ground cumin, *divided*
¾ tsp. salt, *divided*
½ tsp. pepper, *divided*

1. Cook rice according to package directions, using 2 cups water and cooking about 20 minutes. Set aside.

2. Cook lentils with remaining 3 cups water until tender, about 15 minutes. Set aside.

3. Heat oil in good-sized skillet over medium heat. Being careful not to splash yourself with hot oil, stir in onion and garlic. Sauté 5 minutes, or until just tender.

4. Stir in tomatoes, celery, carrots, squash, and half the tomato sauce.

5. Season with half the herbs, salt, and pepper.

6. Cook until vegetables are tender. Add water if too dry.

7. Place cooked, rice, lentils and vegetables in well-greased 9×13 baking pan, or equivalent-size casserole dish. Layer, or mix together, whichever you prefer.

8. Top with remaining tomato sauce and herbs.

9. Bake at 350° for 30 minutes, or until bubbly.

Tips:

1. As the vegetables cook in Step 6, keep checking that they are not getting too dry. Add water or tomato juice to vegetables if needed.

2. If you are not cooking for vegetarians or vegans, you can use broth or stock in place of water.

3. Substitute with other herbs if you wish.

4. If you don't have fresh tomatoes available, substitute canned tomatoes.

Exchange List Values
- Starch 2.0
- Vegetable 1.0

Basic Nutritional Values
- Calories 200
  (Calories from Fat 15)
- Total Fat 2 gm
  (Saturated Fat 0.2 gm,
  Trans Fat 0.0 gm,
  Polyunsat Fat 0.5 gm,
  Monounsat Fat 0.6 gm)
- Cholesterol 0 mg
- Sodium 355 mg
- Potassium 620 gm
- Total Carb 38 gm
- Dietary Fiber 9 gm
- Sugars 5 gm
- Protein 11 gm
- Phosphorus 215 gm

Sweet and Sour Lentil Bake

Helene Funk
Laird, Saskatchewan

*Makes 8 servings,
about ⅔ cup per serving*

***Prep. Time: 20 minutes
Cooking/Baking Time: 1 hour***

½ lb. 90%-lean ground
   beef
4 cups cooked lentils
2 Tbsp. no-trans-fat tub
   margarine
1 tsp. curry powder
¼ tsp. cayenne pepper
1 tsp. salt
1 large onion, chopped
1 large carrot, grated
1–2 cloves garlic, *optional*
1 tart apple, chopped
1 Tbsp. cornstarch
¼ cup brown sugar
¼ cup vinegar
2 tsp. Worcestershire sauce
½ cup lower-sodium non-
   fat chicken stock

1. Brown ground beef,
breaking it up. Drain and add
cooked lentils.
2. In separate skillet
melt margarine and sauté
curry, cayenne, salt, onion,
carrot, garlic and apple for 5
minutes.
3. In small bowl combine
cornstarch and brown sugar.
Slowly add vinegar, mixing
until smooth. Add Worcestershire sauce and chicken stock.
4. Combine all ingredients.
Spoon into greased casserole
dish.
5. Cover and bake at
325° for 45 minutes or until
bubbly. If mixture seems too
dry, add more chicken stock.

Exchange List Values

- Starch 1.5   • Lean Meat 2.0
- Carbohydrate 0.5

Basic Nutritional Values

- Calories 230   • Sodium 385 mg
  (Calories from Fat 45) • Potassium 580 gm
- Total Fat 5 gm   • Total Carb 32 gm
  (Saturated Fat 1.4 gm, • Dietary Fiber 9 gm
  Trans Fat 0.2 gm,   • Sugars 10 gm
  Polyunsat Fat 1.2 gm,   • Protein 15 gm
  Monounsat Fat 1.7 gm) • Phosphorus 245 gm
- Cholesterol 15 mg

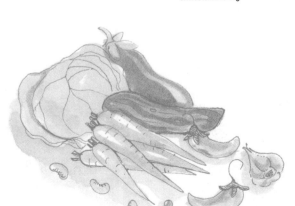

Middle Eastern Lentils

Judith Houser
Hershey, PA

*Makes 8 servings,
a serving of lentils is about 6 oz.
with ⅛ of the salad*

***Prep. Time: 20 minutes
Cooking/Baking Time: 50–60
minutes***

Lentils:
2 large onions, chopped
1 Tbsp. olive oil
¾ cup brown rice,
   uncooked
1½ tsp. salt
1½ cups lentils, rinsed
4 cups water

Salad:
1 bunch (about ½ lb.)
   leaf lettuce
2 medium tomatoes,
   diced
1 medium cucumber,
   peeled and sliced
2 green onions, chopped
1 red bell pepper, diced

Dressing:
2 Tbsp. olive oil
2 Tbsp. lemon juice
½ tsp. paprika
¼ tsp. dry mustard
1 garlic clove, finely
   minced
¼ tsp. salt
½ tsp. sugar

1. In a large kettle, prepare
lentils by sautéing onions in
olive oil until soft and golden.
2. Add rice and salt.

Continue cooking over medium heat for 3 minutes.

3. Stir in lentils and water. Bring to a simmer.

4. Cover and cook until rice and lentils are tender, 50–60 minutes.

5. While the lentil mixture cooks, prepare salad by tossing together lettuce, tomatoes, cucumber, onions, and pepper in a good-sized mixing bowl.

6. Place all dressing ingredients in a jar with a tight-fitting lid. Shake vigorously until well mixed.

7. Just before serving, shake dressing again to make sure it's thoroughly mixed. Then toss salad with dressing.

8. To serve each individual, place serving of lentil mixture on dinner plate and top with a generous serving of salad.

Tip:

This is a traditional, Middle East dish. As strange as it may sound, the combination of the salad on top of the hot lentil mixture is marvelous!

Exchange List Values
- Starch 2.0
- Vegetable 1.0
- Lean Meat 1.0
- Fat 1.0

Basic Nutritional Values
- Calories 270
  (Calories from Fat 55)
- Total Fat 6 gm
  (Saturated Fat 0.9 gm,
  Trans Fat 0.0 gm,
  Polyunsat Fat 1.0 gm,
  Monounsat Fat 4.0 gm)
- Cholesterol 0 mg
- Sodium 525 mg
- Potassium 685 gm
- Total Carb 43 gm
- Dietary Fiber 11 gm
- Sugars 7 gm
- Protein 12 gm
- Phosphorus 275 gm

Soybean Hamburger Casserole

Mary E. Martin
Goshen, IN

*Makes 8 servings,
about ¾ cup per serving*

**Prep. Time: 20 minutes
Cooking/Baking Time: 1 hour**

1½ Tbsp. canola oil
½ cup chopped onion
1 cup chopped celery
¼ cup chopped green
  peppers
¼ lb. 90%-lean ground
  beef
½ tsp. salt
⅛ tsp. pepper
½ tsp. seasoned salt
2½ cups cooked soybeans
1¼ cups lower-sodium,
  lower-fat cream of
  tomato soup
1 tsp. sodium-free beef
  bouillon powder
  dissolved in 1 cup hot
  water
2 cups cooked rice
⅓ cup freshly grated
  cheddar cheese

1. Heat cooking oil in large skillet. Sauté onion, celery, green peppers and ground beef.

2. When meat has browned, drain off any fat.

3. Add all other ingredients except cheese. Simmer a few minutes. Spoon into greased casserole dish.

4. Bake at 350° for 45 minutes. Remove from oven

and top with grated cheese. Return to oven only long enough to melt cheese.

Exchange List Values
- Starch 1.0
- Carbohydrate 0.5
- Lean Meat 2.0
- Fat 0.5

Basic Nutritional Values
- Calories 220
  (Calories from Fat 70)
- Total Fat 8 gm
  (Saturated Fat 1.9 gm,
  Trans Fat 0.1 gm,
  Polyunsat Fat 3.2 gm,
  Monounsat Fat 2.3 gm)
- Cholesterol 10 mg
- Sodium 420 mg
- Potassium 675 gm
- Total Carb 24 gm
- Dietary Fiber 4 gm
- Sugars 6 gm
- Protein 14 gm
- Phosphorus 215 gm

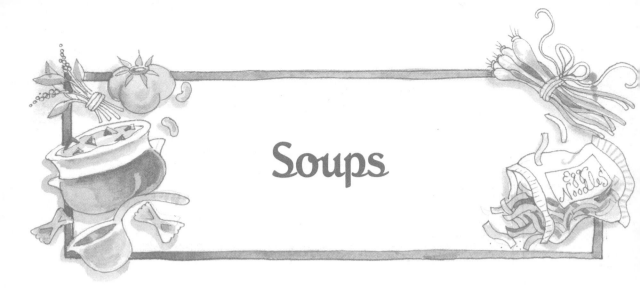

Soups

Tortellini Soup

Kim Rapp
Longmont, CO

Makes 8 servings

Prep. Time: 20 minutes
Cooking Time: 1 hour

12 oz. beef sausage,
    chopped *or* broken up
1 cup chopped onions
2 cloves garlic, chopped
2 cups chopped, peeled
    tomatoes
1 cup sliced carrots
8-oz. no-salt-added tomato
    sauce
5 cups lower-sodium, fat-
    free beef broth
½ cup water
½ cup dry red wine
1 tsp. dried basil
1 tsp. dried oregano
1½ cups sliced zucchini
8-oz. cheese tortellini
1 medium green pepper,
    chopped
3 Tbsp. chopped parsley

1. Combine sausage,
onions, garlic, tomatoes,
carrots, tomato sauce, broth,
water, wine, basil and
oregano in a pot.
2. Bring to a boil, then turn
down to a simmer.
3. Simmer uncovered, 30
minutes. Skim fat.
4. Stir in zucchini, tortellini, and pepper.
5. Simmer 30 minutes. Stir
in chopped parsley.

Warm Memories:

My friend, Nancy, had this
simmering on the stove when
I walked into her home for
a children/adult Christmas
party. It was a fun celebra-
tion making ornaments and
decorating cookies.

Good Go-Alongs:

Nice crusty bread and
green salad. I like to shred
Parmesan cheese over the top.

Exchange List Values
- Starch 1.0
- Vegetable 2.0
- High-Fat Meat 1.0

Basic Nutritional Values
- Calories 225
  (Calories from Fat 90)
- Total Fat 10 gm
  (Saturated Fat 3.6 gm,
  Trans Fat 0.0 gm,
  Polyunsat Fat 1.0 gm,
  Monounsat Fat 3.9 gm)
- Cholesterol 30 mg
- Sodium 565 mg
- Potassium 560 gm
- Total Carb 22 gm
- Dietary Fiber 4 gm
- Sugars 6 gm
- Protein 12 gm
- Phosphorus 160 gm

Use no-salt-added canned vegetables, soups,
and stocks, so that you can control the amount of
sodium in your cooking.

Andrea Zuercher, Lawrence, KS

Italian Sausage Soup

Mary Puskar
Forest Hill, MI

Makes 8 servings

Prep. Time: 30 minutes
Cooking Time: 1 hour

1 lb. lean sweet Italian turkey sausage
2 large onions, chopped
2 cloves garlic, minced
2 8-oz. cans Italian tomatoes and liquid
42-oz. low-sodium fat-free beef broth
1½ cups dry red wine
½ tsp. dry basil leaves
2 medium zucchini, cut in ¼" slices
2 cups shell pasta
1 medium green pepper, chopped
3 Tbsp. fresh parsley
grated Parmesan cheese, *optional*

1. Sauté sausage in large soup pot. Drain.
2. Add onions and garlic; sauté.
3. Stir in tomatoes, breaking them up.
4. Add broth, wine and basil. Simmer 30 minutes.
5. Add zucchini, pasta, pepper and parsley. Simmer 15 minutes.
6. Top with lots of grated Parmesan cheese if you wish.

Exchange List Values
- Starch 1.5
- Vegetable 2.0
- Med-Fat Meat 1.0

Basic Nutritional Values
- Calories 250
  (Calories from Fat 55)
- Total Fat 6 gm
  (Saturated Fat 1.5 gm,
  Trans Fat 0.2 gm,
  Polyunsat Fat 1.6 gm,
  Monounsat Fat 1.9 gm)
- Cholesterol 30 mg
- Sodium 595 mg
- Potassium 595 gm
- Total Carb 31 gm
- Dietary Fiber 4 gm
- Sugars 6 gm
- Protein 16 gm
- Phosphorus 185 gm

Broccoli Rabe & Sausage Soup

Carlene Horne
Bedford, NH

Makes 5 servings

Prep. Time: 15 minutes
Cooking/Baking Time: 15 minutes

1 Tbsp. olive oil
1 onion, chopped
5 cups chopped broccoli rabe, about 1 bunch
½ lb. lean fresh Italian turkey sausage, casing removed, sliced
32 oz. carton no-salt-added chicken broth
1 cup water
8-oz. frozen tortellini

1. Heat olive oil in a soup pot.
2. Add onions and sausage and sauté until tender.
3. Add broccoli rabe and sauté a few more minutes.
4. Pour broth and water into pan; bring to simmer.
5. Add tortellini and cook a few minutes until tender.

Variation:
Substitute any green such as Swiss chard, kale, or spinach for the broccoli rabe.

Exchange List Values
- Starch 1.0
- Vegetable 1.0
- Med-Fat Meat 1.0
- Fat 1.0

Basic Nutritional Values
- Calories 230
  (Calories from Fat 90)
- Total Fat 10 gm
  (Saturated Fat 2.9 gm,
  Trans Fat 0.1 gm,
  Polyunsat Fat 1.6 gm,
  Monounsat Fat 4.3 gm)
- Cholesterol 40 mg
- Sodium 505 mg
- Potassium 320 gm
- Total Carb 21 gm
- Dietary Fiber 2 gm
- Sugars 3 gm
- Protein 15 gm
- Phosphorus 185 gm

Mexican Beef and Barley Soup

Rebecca B. Stoltzfus
Lititz, PA

Makes 6 servings

Prep. Time: 10 minutes
Cooking Time: 35 minutes

1 lb. 90%-lean ground beef
1 small onion, chopped
1 Tbsp. olive oil
3 cups low-sodium beef
  broth
2 cups chunky salsa with
  the lowest sodium per
  serving you can find
½ cup quick-cooking
  barley
2 15-oz. cans red kidney
  beans, rinsed and
  drained
4 Tbsp. fat-free sour cream
paprika

1. In 12-inch skillet, brown beef and onion in oil, breaking up with a fork until no longer pink. Drain.
2. Add broth, salsa, and barley. Bring to a boil.
3. Reduce heat to medium and cook uncovered for 15 minutes.
4. Add beans and heat through.
5. Ladle into bowls. Garnish with dollops of sour cream dusted with paprika.

Tips:
1. To use pearl barley, add extra 1½ cups broth or water and cook an additional 40 minutes.

2. To increase Mexican flavor to your taste, add some cumin, chili powder, or cayenne.

Exchange List Values
- Starch 2.0
- Vegetable 2.0
- Lean Meat 3.0
- Fat 0.5

Basic Nutritional Values
- Calories 350
  (Calories from Fat 80)
- Total Fat 9 gm
  (Saturated Fat 2.9 gm,
  Trans Fat 0.4 gm,
  Polyunsat Fat 0.9 gm,
  Monounsat Fat 4.3 gm)
- Cholesterol 45 mg
- Sodium 555 mg
- Potassium 995 gm
- Total Carb 41 gm
- Dietary Fiber 9 gm
- Sugars 4 gm
- Protein 27 gm
- Phosphorus 335 gm

Springtime Soup

Clara L. Hershberger
Goshen, IN

Makes 12 servings,
about ¾ cup per serving

Prep. Time: 15 minutes
Cooking Time: about 1 hour

1 lb. 90%-lean ground beef
1 cup chopped onion
4 cups water
1 cup diced carrots
1 cup diced celery
1 cup diced potatoes
2 tsp. salt, *or less*
1 tsp. Worcestershire sauce
¼ tsp. pepper
1 bay leaf
⅛ tsp. dried basil
6 tomatoes, chopped
fresh parsley, to garnish

1. In large saucepan cook and stir ground beef until browned. Drain excess fat.

2. In large, heavy soup pot cook and stir onions with meat until onions are clear and tender, about 5 minutes.
3. Stir in all remaining ingredients except parsley. Bring to a boil.
4. Reduce heat, cover and simmer until vegetables are just tender.
5. Immediately before serving, add fresh parsley.

Exchange List Values
- Vegetable 1.0
- Lean Meat 1.0
- Fat 0.5

Basic Nutritional Values
- Calories 95
  (Calories from Fat 30)
- Total Fat 4 gm
  (Saturated Fat 1.3 gm,
  Trans Fat 0.2 gm,
  Polyunsat Fat 0.2 gm,
  Monounsat Fat 1.3 gm)
- Cholesterol 25 mg
- Sodium 435 mg
- Potassium 385 gm
- Total Carb 8 gm
- Dietary Fiber 2 gm
- Sugars 3 gm
- Protein 8 gm
- Phosphorus 95 gm

Wild Rice Soup

Elaine Unruh
Minneapolis, MN

Makes 10 servings,
about 1¼ cups per serving

Prep. Time: 15 minutes
Cooking Time: about 1 hour

1½ cups uncooked wild
  rice
3½ cups water
4 Tbsp. canola oil
2 Tbsp. minced onion
¾ cup flour
4 14½-oz. cans fat-free,
  lower-sodium chicken
  broth

⅔ cup minced ham
⅔ cup finely grated carrot
¼ cup slivered almonds
2 cups fat-free half-and-half

1. In a saucepan combine rice and water. Simmer for 45 minutes.

2. In a large soup kettle heat oil. Sauté onion until tender. With a wire whisk stir in flour.

3. Gradually add chicken broth and cook until mixture thickens, stirring constantly.

4. Stir in rice. Add ham, carrot and almonds. Simmer for 5 minutes.

5. Immediately before serving, blend in half-and-half.

Exchange List Values

- Starch 1.5
- Fat 1.0
- Fat-Free Milk 0.5

Basic Nutritional Values

- Calories 215
  (Calories from Fat 70)
- Total Fat 8 gm
  (Saturated Fat 1.0 gm,
  Trans Fat 0.0 gm,
  Polyunsat Fat 2.2 gm,
  Monounsat Fat 4.8 gm)
- Cholesterol 5 mg
- Sodium 580 mg
- Potassium 370 gm
- Total Carb 27 gm
- Dietary Fiber 2 gm
- Sugars 5 gm
- Protein 9 gm
- Phosphorus 195 gm

St. Paul Bean Pot

Jane Miller
Minneapolis, MN

*Makes 10 servings,
about ¾ cup per serving*

*Prep. Time: 15 minutes
Soaking Time: 12 hours or
  overnight
Cooking Time: 4–5 hours*

2½ cups dried white beans
2½ quarts water
2 Tbsp. reduced-sodium
  chicken bouillon
1 cup chopped onion
15-oz. can tomato sauce
1½ Tbsp. chili powder
2 tsp. garlic powder
pepper

1. Soak beans in water overnight.

2. Transfer to slow cooker and cook on high 4–5 hours.

3. Two hours into cooking time add all remaining ingredients to the slow cooker.

4. Serve with rice if you wish.

Exchange List Values

- Starch 2.0
- Lean Meat 1.0

Basic Nutritional Values

- Calories 195
  (Calories from Fat 10)
- Total Fat 1 gm
  (Saturated Fat 0.2 gm,
  Trans Fat 0.0 gm,
  Polyunsat Fat 0.3 gm,
  Monounsat Fat 0.1 gm)
- Cholesterol 0 mg
- Sodium 560 mg
- Potassium 875 gm
- Total Carb 35 gm
- Dietary Fiber 9 gm
- Sugars 6 gm
- Protein 13 gm
- Phosphorus 160 gm

Basic Bean Soup

Marjorie Weaver Nafziger
Harman, WV

*Makes 10 servings,
about ¾ cup per serving*

*Prep. Time: 10 minutes
Cooking Time: 9–13 hours*

2 cups dried white beans
1¾ -2 quarts water
8 oz. diced lean ham
1 onion, chopped
2–3 ribs celery, chopped
2–3 carrots, chopped
3–4 cups canned tomatoes
salt and pepper to taste

1. Bring the beans and water to a boil. Transfer to slow cooker turned on high.

2. Add all remaining ingredients and turn slow cooker on low overnight, or for 8–12 hours.

Exchange List Values

- Starch 1.5
- Lean Meat 1.0
- Vegetable 1.0

Basic Nutritional Values

- Calories 185
  (Calories from Fat 15)
- Total Fat 2 gm
  (Saturated Fat 0.3 gm,
  Trans Fat 0.0 gm,
  Polyunsat Fat 0.3 gm,
  Monounsat Fat 0.5 gm)
- Cholesterol 10 mg
- Sodium 415 mg
- Potassium 840 gm
- Total Carb 31 gm
- Dietary Fiber 8 gm
- Sugars 7 gm
- Protein 15 gm
- Phosphorus 195 gm

Gazpacho

Maxine Hershberger
Dalton, OH

*Makes 6 servings,
about 5 oz. per serving*

Prep. Time: 30 minutes
Chilling Time: 4 hours or more

1 cup finely chopped tomato
½ cup chopped green pepper
½ cup chopped celery
½ cup chopped cucumber
¼ cup finely chopped onion
2 tsp. snipped parsley
1 tsp. snipped chives
1 small clove garlic, minced
2–3 Tbsp. tarragon wine
** vinegar**
2 Tbsp. olive oil
½ tsp. salt
¼ tsp. black pepper
½ tsp. Worcestershire sauce
2 cups tomato juice
1 cup croutons

1. Combine all ingredients except croutons in a glass bowl. Toss to mix well.
2. Cover and chill at least 4 hours before serving.

3. Sprinkle croutons on top and serve. Serve as a salad or soup.

Exchange List Values
- Vegetable 2.0   • Fat 1.0

Basic Nutritional Values
- Calories 90
  (Calories from Fat 45)
- Total Fat 5 gm
  (Saturated Fat 0.7 gm,
  Trans Fat 0.0 gm,
  Polyunsat Fat 0.6 gm,
  Monounsat Fat 3.5 gm)
- Cholesterol 0 mg
- Sodium 365 mg
- Potassium 335 mg
- Total Carb 10 gm
- Dietary Fiber 1 gm
- Sugars 5 gm
- Protein 2 gm
- Phosphorus 35 gm

New Year's Soup

Rhoda M. Peachey
Reedsville, PA

*Makes 4 quarts,
1 cup per serving, 16 servings*

Prep. Time: 15 minutes
Soaking Time: overnight
Cooking Time: 3¼ hours

1 lb. dried white beans
2 tsp. salt
1½ lbs. ground turkey
2 quarts water

1 large onion, chopped
28-oz. can whole tomatoes
1 clove garlic, minced
juice of 1 lemon
1 tsp. chili powder,
** *optional***

1. Wash beans. Place in large kettle and cover with salt water to 2" above bean line. Soak beans overnight and drain in morning.
2. Brown ground turkey and add to beans. Add all remaining ingredients and simmer for 3 hours.
3. Serve hot and enjoy.

Variation:
To make in a slow cooker, instead of simmering on the stove for 3 hours, cook on high in a slow cooker for 3–4 hours.

Exchange List Values
- Starch 1.0   • Lean Meat 2.0

Basic Nutritional Values
- Calories 175
  (Calories from Fat 35)
- Total Fat 4 gm
  (Saturated Fat 1.0 gm,
  Trans Fat 0.0 gm,
  Polyunsat Fat 1.2 gm,
  Monounsat Fat 1.2 gm)
- Cholesterol 30 mg
- Sodium 400 mg
- Potassium 590 gm
- Total Carb 21 gm
- Dietary Fiber 5 gm
- Sugars 3 gm
- Protein 16 gm
- Phosphorus 170 gm

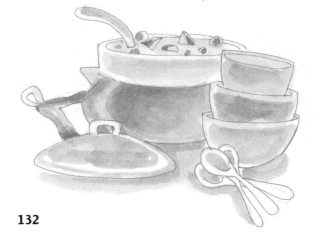

Tomato Basil Soup

Barbara Kuhns
Millersburg, OH

Makes 8 servings

Prep. Time: 15 minutes
Cooking Time: 25 minutes

¼ cup finely chopped onion
1 Tbsp. canola oil
2 10¾-oz. cans lower-sodium, lower-fat condensed tomato soup
2 cups no-added-salt tomato sauce
6-oz. can no-added-salt tomato paste
2⅔ cups low-sodium chicken broth
garlic cloves, minced, *optional*
2 Tbsp. Splenda Brown Sugar Blend
3 tsp. dried basil
1 cup fat-free half-and-half
⅓ cup flour

1. Heat oil in soup pot.
2. Add and sauté onion.
3. Add condensed soup, sauce, paste, broth, basil, Brown Sugar Blend, and garlic.
4. Cook, covered, until hot.
5. Whisk together flour and cream. Add and heat gently, stirring, until soup is steaming and thick. Do not boil.

Exchange List Values
- Carbohydrate 1.5
- Fat 0.5
- Vegetable 2.0

Basic Nutritional Values
- Calories 170 (Calories from Fat 30)
- Total Fat 4 gm (Saturated Fat 0.8 gm, Trans Fat 0.0 gm, Polyunsat Fat 0.9 gm, Monounsat Fat 1.3 gm)
- Cholesterol 5 mg
- Sodium 365 mg
- Potassium 1025 gm
- Total Carb 30 gm
- Dietary Fiber 4 gm
- Sugars 15 gm
- Protein 6 gm
- Phosphorus 125 gm

Cheeseburger Soup

Rebecca B. Stoltzfus
Lititz, PA

Makes 6 servings

Prep. Time: 35 minutes
Cooking Time: 1 hour

½ lb. extra-lean 90%-fat-free ground beef
1 cup chopped onion
¾ cup grated carrots
¾ cup chopped celery
1 tsp. dried basil
1 tsp. parsley flakes
3 cups no-added-salt chicken broth
4 cups diced potatoes
2 Tbsp. no-trans-fat tub margarine
¼ cup flour
1½ cups fat-free milk
4 oz. reduced-fat American cheese, sliced or cubed
¼ cup fat-free sour cream
¼ tsp. salt
¼ tsp. pepper

1. In a soup pot, fry the beef until almost browned.
2. Add onion, celery, carrots, basil, and parsley. Sauté for a few minutes.
3. Add broth, potatoes.
4. Simmer until tender, 20 minutes.
5. In another pot, melt margarine, add flour. Whisk vigorously.
6. Add milk, whisking constantly. Cook over low heat until thickened.
7. Add cheese, sour cream, salt, and pepper.
8. Pour the cheese sauce into the beef soup. Stir gently to combine.

Variation:
Put the recipe in the slow cooker on low 5 hours.

Exchange List Values
- Starch 1.5
- Med-Fat Meat 1.0
- Fat-Free Milk 0.5
- Fat 0.5
- Vegetable 1.0

Basic Nutritional Values
- Calories 295 (Calories from Fat 80)
- Total Fat 9 gm (Saturated Fat 3.4 gm, Trans Fat 0.2 gm, Polyunsat Fat 1.5 gm, Monounsat Fat 3.0 gm)
- Cholesterol 35 mg
- Sodium 515 mg
- Potassium 850 gm
- Total Carb 36 gm
- Dietary Fiber 3 gm
- Sugars 8 gm
- Protein 18 gm
- Phosphorus 375 gm

A fail-proof way to get the best recipes is to go to lots of potlucks. You get to try new recipes and ask for the ones you especially love.

Kathy Bless, Fayetteville, PA

Minestrone Soup

Lydia Konrad
Edmonton, Alberta

*Makes 12 servings,
about ¾ cup per serving*

Prep. Time: 15 minutes
Cooking Time: about 2 hours

1½ lbs. 90%-lean ground
  beef
1 cup diced onions
1 cup diced zucchini
1 cup cubed potatoes
1 cup sliced carrots
½ cup diced celery
1 cup shredded cabbage
15-oz. can tomatoes,
  chopped
1½ quarts water
1 bay leaf
½ tsp. dried thyme
2 tsp. salt
pepper to taste
1 tsp. Worcestershire sauce
¼ cup uncooked brown
  rice
½ cup freshly grated
  Parmesan cheese

1. Brown ground beef in
large soup kettle. Drain off
grease.
2. Add vegetables, water
and spice and bring to a boil.
3. Sprinkle rice into
mixture. Cover and simmer
for at least 1 hour.
4. Sprinkle with Parmesan
cheese and serve with brown
bread.

Exchange List Values
• Vegetable 2.0
• Lean Meat 1.0
• Fat 1.0

Basic Nutritional Values
• Calories 140
  (Calories from Fat 55)
• Total Fat 6 gm
  (Saturated Fat 2.4 gm,
  Trans Fat 0.3 gm,
  Polyunsat Fat 0.2 gm,
  Monounsat Fat 2.2 gm)
• Cholesterol 35 mg
• Sodium 525 mg
• Potassium 360 gm
• Total Carb 9 gm
• Dietary Fiber 1 gm
• Sugars 2 gm
• Protein 13 gm
• Phosphorus 145 gm

Hungry Man's Soup

Bernice Potoski
Riverton, Manitoba

*Makes 10 servings,
about 2 cups per serving*

Prep. Time: 20 minutes
Cooking Time: 1½ hours

2 lbs. 90%-lean ground
  beef
1 medium onion, diced
4 medium carrots, diced
2 cups diced turnips
4 cups diced cabbage
5 cups diced potatoes
10 cups water
¾ tsp. salt
½ tsp. pepper
19-oz. can tomatoes
2 10¾-oz. cans lower-
  sodium, lower-fat tomato
  soup
1 cup water
¾ cup flour

1. Brown ground beef
lightly. Drain excess fat.
2. In a large kettle combine
ground beef, onion, carrots,
turnips, cabbage, potatoes, 10
cups water, salt and pepper.
3. Cook on medium-low
heat until vegetables are
tender.
4. Add tomatoes and
tomato soup. Bring to a boil
and simmer on low boil for
30–45 minutes.
5. Combine 1 cup water
and flour to make a paste.
Thicken soup slightly with
paste.
6. Cook for 15 minutes
longer. Serve.

Exchange List Values
• Starch 2.0
• Vegetable 2.0
• Lean Meat 2.0
• Fat 0.5

Basic Nutritional Values
• Calories 320
  (Calories from Fat 80)
• Total Fat 9 gm
  (Saturated Fat 3.2 gm,
  Trans Fat 0.5 gm,
  Polyunsat Fat 0.7 gm,
  Monounsat Fat 3.2 gm)
• Cholesterol 55 mg
• Sodium 550 mg
• Potassium 1160 gm
• Total Carb 39 gm
• Dietary Fiber 5 gm
• Sugars 11 gm
• Protein 22 gm
• Phosphorus 250 gm

*Using leftover foods for a recipe saves time.
If the leftovers are seasoned, reduce the amount of
salt in the recipe.*

Healthy Hamburger Soup

Chris Peterson
Green Bay, WI

Makes 8 servings

Prep. Time: 20 minutes
Cooking Time: 1–2 hours

1¾ lbs. 90%-lean ground
   beef
14½-oz. can stewed
   tomatoes
1 cup sliced mushrooms
2 cups sliced cabbage
1 cup sliced carrots
2 cups chopped celery
2 cups fresh *or* frozen
   green beans
4 cups tomato juice
2 cups no-added salt
   tomato juice
2 tsp. dried basil
2 tsp. dried oregano
1 Tbsp. Worcestershire
   sauce

1. In a soup pot, fry beef until brown and drain.
2. Add rest of ingredients.
3. Simmer 1–2 hours.

Tips:
1. Use canned mushrooms (pieces and stems) and a 14½-oz. can green or wax beans, no need to drain. I also sometimes add ¾ cup barley, quinoa, or broken spaghetti.
2. This is a great recipe for cleaning out your refrigerator. Whatever leftover veggies you have in there – throw them in the soup. I've added broccoli or rice and it's great.

Exchange List Values
• Vegetable 3.0   • Med-Fat Meat 2.0

Basic Nutritional Values
• Calories 230
  (Calories from Fat 80)
• Total Fat 9 gm
  (Saturated Fat 3.3 gm,
  Trans Fat 0.5 gm,
  Polyunsat Fat 0.5 gm,
  Monounsat Fat 3.5 gm)
• Cholesterol 60 mg
• Sodium 560 mg
• Potassium 1055 gm
• Total Carb 18 gm
• Dietary Fiber 4 gm
• Sugars 11 gm
• Protein 22 gm
• Phosphorus 245 gm

Lentil Vegetable Soup

Mary C. Jungerman
Boulder, CO

*Makes 10 servings,
about ⅔ cup per serving*

Prep. Time: 15 minutes
Cooking Time: 2 hours

2 cups lentils
8 cups water
2 slices bacon, diced
½ cup chopped onion
½ cup chopped celery
¼ cup chopped carrots
3 Tbsp. snipped fresh
   parsley
1 clove garlic, minced
2 tsp. salt
¼ tsp. pepper
½ tsp. dried oregano
2 cups chopped tomatoes
2 Tbsp. wine vinegar

1. Rinse lentils. Drain and place in large soup kettle. Add water and all remaining ingredients except tomatoes and vinegar.

2. Cover and simmer 1½ hours.
3. Add tomatoes and vinegar. Cover and simmer for 30 minutes longer.
4. Adjust seasoning and serve.

Exchange List Values
• Starch 1.5   • Lean Meat 1.0

Basic Nutritional Values
• Calories 165
  (Calories from Fat 25)
• Total Fat 3 gm
  (Saturated Fat 1.1 gm,
  Trans Fat 0.0 gm,
  Polyunsat Fat 0.6 gm,
  Monounsat Fat 1.3 gm)
• Cholesterol 5 mg
• Sodium 510 mg
• Potassium 535 gm
• Total Carb 25 gm
• Dietary Fiber 9 gm
• Sugars 3 gm
• Protein 11 gm
• Phosphorus 215 gm

Soups

Adirondack Three Alarm Chili

Joanne Kennedy
Plattsburgh, NY

Makes 8 servings

Prep. Time: 25 minutes
Cooking Time: 3 hours

1¾ lbs. 90%-lean ground
   beef
3 medium onions, diced
4 garlic cloves, crushed
1 green pepper, chopped
28-oz. can crushed
   tomatoes
2 15½-oz. cans kidney
   beans, drained
16-oz. can no-added-salt
   tomato sauce
1 Tbsp. brown sugar
1 tsp. dried oregano
¼-1 tsp. crushed red
   pepper
3 Tbsp. chili powder
1 tsp. salt, *optional*

1. Brown ground beef in
large soup pot.
2. Add and sauté onion,
garlic, and green pepper.
3. Add the rest of ingredients. Simmer on low heat for
3 hours.

Variations:

Add a can of corn, or
replace some of the meat with
more beans. Simmer the chili
in a slow cooker instead of on
the stovetop.

Exchange List Values
- Starch 1.0   • Lean Meat 3.0
- Vegetable 4.0   • Fat 0.5

Basic Nutritional Values
- Calories 345   • Sodium 365 mg
  (Calories from Fat 80)   • Potassium 1255 gm
- Total Fat 9 gm   • Total Carb 39 gm
  (Saturated Fat 3.4 gm,   • Dietary Fiber 11 gm
  Trans Fat 0.5 gm,   • Sugars 12 gm
  Polyunsat Fat 0.9 gm,   • Protein 29 gm
  Monounsat Fat 3.6 gm)   • Phosphorus 350 gm
- Cholesterol 60 mg

Chick Pea Chili

Thelma Wolgemuth
Immokalee, FL

Makes 8 servings,
½ cup chili plus ¼ cup brown rice,
and 1 Tbsp. yogurt per serving

Prep. Time: 15 minutes
Cooking Time: 35–40 minutes

1 small onion, minced
2 cloves garlic, minced
15-oz. can garbanzo beans,
   drained
2 8-oz cans tomato sauce
1 Tbsp. chili powder
1 tsp. ground cumin
½ tsp. dried oregano
cayenne pepper to taste
⅔ cup fat-free plain yogurt
2 cups hot cooked brown
   rice

1. Sauté onion and garlic
over medium heat in a large
saucepan.
2. Stir in garbanzo beans,
tomato sauce, chili powder,
cumin, oregano and cayenne.
3. Simmer, uncovered,
about 30 minutes, stirring
occasionally. (If mixture
becomes too thick, add water.)
4. Pour into serving dish

and top with yogurt.
5. Serve with hot, cooked
rice on the side.

Exchange List Values
- Starch 1.5   • Vegetable 1.0

Basic Nutritional Values
- Calories 135   • Sodium 375 mg
  (Calories from Fat 15)   • Potassium 380 gm
- Total Fat 2 gm   • Total Carb 26 gm
  (Saturated Fat 0.2 gm,   • Dietary Fiber 5 gm
  Trans Fat 0.0 gm,   • Sugars 6 gm
  Polyunsat Fat 0.6 gm,   • Protein 6 gm
  Monounsat Fat 0.4 gm)   • Phosphorus 140 gm
- Cholesterol 0 mg

Three Bean Chili

Deb Kepiro
Strasburg, PA

Makes 8 servings

Prep. Time: 15 minutes
Cooking Time: 1 hour

1 large onion, chopped
2 Tbsp. oil
2 cups diced cooked
   chicken
15½-oz. can kidney beans,
   rinsed and drained
15½-oz. can pinto beans,
   rinsed and drained
15½-oz. can black beans,
   rinsed and drained
2 14½-oz. cans diced
   tomatoes
1 cup no-added-salt
   chicken broth
¾ cup salsa
1 tsp. cumin
shredded cheese, *optional*
green onions, *optional*
sour cream, *optional*

1. In a soup pot, sauté onion in oil until tender.

2. Add chicken, beans, tomatoes, broth, salsa, cumin, and salt.

3. Bring to a boil. Reduce heat and let simmer for 30–60 minutes.

4. If desired, garnish with shredded cheese, green onions and sour cream.

Go-Alongs:
Great with warm cornbread.

Exchange List Values
- Starch 1.5
- Vegetable 1.0
- Lean Meat 2.0
- Fat 0.5

Basic Nutritional Values
- Calories 270
  (Calories from Fat 65)
- Total Fat 7 gm
  (Saturated Fat 1.1 gm,
  Trans Fat 0.0 gm,
  Polyunsat Fat 1.9 gm,
  Monounsat Fat 3.3 gm)
- Cholesterol 30 mg
- Sodium 545 mg
- Potassium 820 gm
- Total Carb 33 gm
- Dietary Fiber 10 gm
- Sugars 5 gm
- Protein 21 gm
- Phosphorus 250 gm

Black Bean Pumpkin Soup

Bev Beiler
Gap, PA

Makes 8 servings

Prep. Time: 30 minutes
Cooking Time: 45 minutes

2 medium onions, chopped
½ cup minced shallots
4 cloves garlic, minced
4–5 tsp. ground cumin
2 Tbsp. canola oil
¼ tsp. salt

½ tsp. ground pepper
3 15½-oz. cans black beans, drained
1 cup chopped tomatoes
4 cups no-salt beef broth
1½ cups cooked pumpkin
½ lb. cooked low-sodium ham, diced
3 Tbsp. vinegar

1. In a large soup pot, sauté onion, shallot, garlic, cumin, salt, and pepper in oil.

2. Stir in beans, tomatoes, broth and pumpkin.

3. Simmer 25 minutes, uncovered, stirring occasionally.

4. Add ham and vinegar. Simmer until heated through.

Good Go-Alongs:
Warm, homemade, buttered bread

Exchange List Values
- Starch 1.5
- Vegetable 1.0
- Lean Meat 2.0
- Fat 0.5

Basic Nutritional Values
- Calories 255
  (Calories from Fat 55)
- Total Fat 6 gm
  (Saturated Fat 1.1 gm,
  Trans Fat 0.0 gm,
  Polyunsat Fat 1.4 gm,
  Monounsat Fat 3.2 gm)
- Cholesterol 15 mg
- Sodium 545 mg
- Potassium 735 gm
- Total Carb 34 gm
- Dietary Fiber 11 gm
- Sugars 7 gm
- Protein 17 gm
- Phosphorus 245 gm

Tater Soup

Suellen Fletcher
Noblesville, IN

Makes 6 servings

Prep. Time: 15 minutes
Cooking Time: 1 hour

3½ cups reduced-sodium, fat-free chicken broth
10¾-oz. can lower-sodium, lower-fat cream of celery soup
½ cup chopped celery
4 cups diced potatoes
1 Tbsp. onion powder
1 cup fat-free milk
1 Tbsp. flour

1. In a soup pot, bring to boil broth, soup, celery, potatoes and onion powder. Cook until potatoes are soft. Turn heat down to medium.

2. Whisk together milk and flour. Pour into soup pot. Cook and stir frequently until thick.

Good Go-Alongs:
Grilled ham and cheese sandwich

Exchange List Values
- Starch 1.5
- Carbohydrate 0.5

Basic Nutritional Values
- Calories 150
  (Calories from Fat 10)
- Total Fat 1 gm
  (Saturated Fat 0.3 gm,
  Trans Fat 0.0 gm,
  Polyunsat Fat 0.5 gm,
  Monounsat Fat 0.2 gm)
- Cholesterol 0 mg
- Sodium 525 mg
- Potassium 785 gm
- Total Carb 30 gm
- Dietary Fiber 3 gm
- Sugars 5 gm
- Protein 5 gm
- Phosphorus 125 gm

Beef and Bacon Chowder

Joan Dietrich
Kutztown, PA

Makes 10 servings

Prep. Time: 45 minutes
Cooking Time: 1 hour

12 bacon strips, cut in
  1-inch pieces
1 lb. 90%-lean ground beef
2–3 cups diced celery
½ cup diced onion
2 10-¾-oz. cans lower-
  sodium, lower-fat
  condensed cream of
  mushroom soup
4 cups fat-free milk
3- 4 cups diced, cooked
  potatoes
2 cups shredded carrots
¼ tsp. salt
1 tsp. pepper

1. In a large soup pot, cook bacon until crisp; pour off drippings and remove bacon to paper towel to drain.
2. In the same pot, sauté ground beef with celery and onion until the beef is browned and the vegetables are tender. Drain off the grease.
3. Add soup, milk, potatoes, carrots, salt and pepper.
4. Bring to a boil; reduce heat and simmer until heated through.
5. Add bacon.

Warm Memories:
There is never a drop of this soup left when I take it to a church supper.

Exchange List Values

- Starch 0.5
- Fat-Free Milk 0.5
- Carbohydrate 0.5
- Lean Meat 2.0
- Fat 0.5

Basic Nutritional Values

- Calories 235
  (Calories from Fat 70)
- Total Fat 8 gm
  (Saturated Fat 2.8 gm,
  Trans Fat 0.2 gm,
  Polyunsat Fat 1.1 gm,
  Monounsat Fat 3.3 gm)
- Cholesterol 40 mg
- Sodium 545 mg
- Potassium 1020 gm
- Total Carb 23 gm
- Dietary Fiber 2 gm
- Sugars 8 gm
- Protein 17 gm
- Phosphorus 270 gm

Harvest Corn Chowder

Flossie Sultzaberger
Mechanicsburg, PA

Makes 10 servings

Prep. Time: 20 minutes
Cooking/Baking Time:40 minutes

1 medium onion, chopped
1 Tbsp. no trans-fat tub
  margarine
2 14½-oz. cans no-salt-
  added cream-style corn
4 cups no-salt-added whole
  kernel corn
4 cups diced peeled
  potatoes
6-oz. jar sliced mushrooms,
  drained
½ medium green pepper,
  chopped

½-1 medium sweet red
  pepper, chopped
10¾-oz. can lower-sodium,
  lower-fat mushroom
  soup
3 cups fat-free milk
pepper, to taste
½ lb. bacon, cooked and
  crumbled

1. In a large saucepan, sauté onion in butter until tender.
2. Add cream-style corn, kernel corn, potatoes, mushrooms, peppers, and milk.
3. Simmer 30 minutes or until vegetables are tender.
4. To serve, garnish with bacon.

Exchange List Values

- Starch 2.5
- Carbohydrate 0.5
- Fat 0.5

Basic Nutritional Values

- Calories 265
  (Calories from Fat 45)
- Total Fat 5 gm
  (Saturated Fat 1.4 gm,
  Trans Fat 0.0 gm,
  Polyunsat Fat 1.5 gm,
  Monounsat Fat 2.0 gm)
- Cholesterol 10 mg
- Sodium 360 mg
- Potassium 850 gm
- Total Carb 46 gm
- Dietary Fiber 6 gm
- Sugars 14 gm
- Protein 11 gm
- Phosphorus 245 gm

Low-sodium, low-fat vegetable soups can be cooked down until thickened and used as a sauce.

Mom's Soup

Chrissy Baldwin
Mechanicsburg, PA

*Makes 10 servings,
about 8–9 oz. per serving*

Prep. Time: 20 minutes
**Cooking/Baking Time: 35
minutes**

3 cups diced potatoes
16-oz. frozen broccoli and
  cauliflower
1 cup chopped carrots
1 cup chopped onions
3 celery ribs, chopped
10 oz. low-sodium ham
  cubes
2 reduced-sodium chicken
  bouillon cubes
3 cups water
¼ tsp. pepper
⅓ cup no trans-fat tub
  margarine
½ cup flour
2 cups fat-free milk
1 cup reduced-fat shredded
  cheese

1. In soup pot, combine potatoes, broccoli, cauliflower, carrots, onions, celery, ham, bouillon, water, and pepper. Simmer for 20 minutes or until vegetables are tender.

2. In separate saucepan, make a white sauce. Melt butter over low heat and stir in flour to make a thick paste. Whisk in milk. Bring to a boil and stir for 2–3 minutes.

3. Add white sauce to soup pot and simmer for 10 minutes. Add shredded cheese and stir until melted.

Warm Memories:
  My mom would make this on cold snowy days.

Good Go-Alongs:
  Best served with a loaf of homemade bread

Exchange List Values
- Starch 1.0
- Vegetable 1.0
- Lean Meat 1.0
- Fat 1.5

Basic Nutritional Values
- Calories 220
  (Calories from Fat 80)
- Total Fat 9 gm
  (Saturated Fat 3.0 gm,
  Trans Fat 0.0 gm,
  Polyunsat Fat 2.2 gm,
  Monounsat Fat 2.8 gm)
- Cholesterol 20 mg
- Sodium 580 mg
- Potassium 505 gm
- Total Carb 23 gm
- Dietary Fiber 3 gm
- Sugars 5 gm
- Protein 13 gm
- Phosphorus 225 gm

Potato Soup

Dale Peterson
Rapid City, SD

*Makes 6 servings,
about 9 oz. per serving*

Prep. Time: 20 minutes
Cooking Time: 30 minutes

2 Tbsp. no trans-fat tub
  margarine
¼ cup diced onions
4 cups diced potatoes
1–2 carrots, grated
2 cups water
1 tsp. salt
½ tsp. pepper
1 tsp. dried dill weed
3 cups fat-free milk
2 Tbsp. fresh parsley,
  chopped

1. In a soup pot, sauté onions in butter until golden.

2. Bring potatoes, carrots, water, salt, pepper, and dill weed to boil.

3. Reduce heat to low and simmer with lid cocked until potatoes are tender.

4. Stir in milk and parsley and heat until hot.

Tip:
  If you like thicker soup, add in some instant potatoes.

Exchange List Values
- Starch 1.5
- Fat-Free Milk 0.5

Basic Nutritional Values
- Calories 165
  (Calories from Fat 25)
- Total Fat 3 gm
  (Saturated Fat 0.7 gm,
  Trans Fat 0.0 gm,
  Polyunsat Fat 1.2 gm,
  Monounsat Fat 1.0 gm)
- Cholesterol 0 mg
- Sodium 480 mg
- Potassium 590 gm
- Total Carb 29 gm
- Dietary Fiber 2 gm
- Sugars 8 gm
- Protein 6 gm
- Phosphorus 175 gm

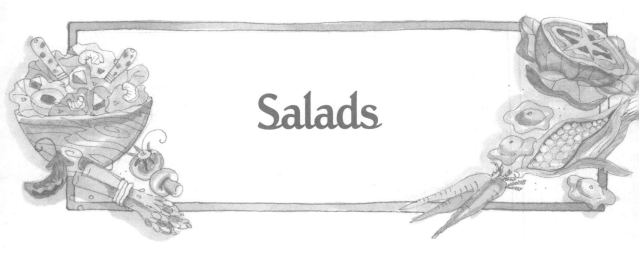

Salads

Festive Apple Salad

Susan Kasting
Jenks, OK

Makes 8 servings,
about 5 oz. per serving

Prep. Time: 15 minutes

Dressing:
  2 Tbsp. olive oil
  2 Tbsp. vinegar *or* lemon
    juice
  2 Tbsp. Dijon mustard
  1½ - 3 Tbsp. sugar
  salt and pepper

4–6 Tbsp. chopped walnuts
  or cashews
1 Granny Smith apple,
  chopped
1 large head Romaine
  lettuce, chopped
4 Tbsp. crumbled blue
  cheese, *or* shredded baby
  Swiss, *optional*

1. In the bottom of a large
salad bowl, make dressing
by mixing together the oil,
mustard, sugar, vinegar, salt,
and pepper.
  2. Add the apple and nuts
and stir to coat. Put lettuce
and blue cheese on top
without stirring.
  3. Mix it all together when
ready to serve.

Tips:
  1. This is so nice to bring
places because it has the
dressing in the bottom so the
salad doesn't wilt. You can also
serve the dressing on the side.
  2. You can add a little
chopped onion and 1 Tbs.
poppy seeds to the dressing.
Add ¼ cup craisins and one
diced pear to the salad.
Mary Ann Bowman, Ephrata, PA

Exchange List Values
• Fruit 0.5   • Fat 1.0
• Carbohydrate 0.5

Basic Nutritional Values
• Calories 115   • Sodium 95 mg
  (Calories from Fat 55) • Potassium 270 gm
• Total Fat 6 gm   • Total Carb 15 gm
  (Saturated Fat 0.7 gm, • Dietary Fiber 3 gm
  Trans Fat 0.0 gm,   • Sugars 10 gm
  Polyunsat Fat 2.3 gm, • Protein 2 gm
  Monounsat Fat 2.9 gm) • Phosphorus 45 gm
• Cholesterol 0 mg

Orange-Spinach Salad

Esther Shisler
Lansdale, PA

Makes 8 servings,
about 7 oz. per serving

Prep. Time: 25 minutes

10-oz. bag spinach *or*
  Romaine lettuce
1 medium head iceberg
  lettuce, shredded
2 Tbsp. diced onion
2 Tbsp. diced canned
  pimento *or* red pepper
2 large oranges, peeled and
  chopped
1 small cucumber, sliced

Honey-Caraway Dressing:
  ¾ cup low-fat
    mayonnaise
  2 Tbsp. honey
  1 Tbsp. lemon juice
  1 Tbsp. caraway seeds

1. In small bowl, whisk mayonnaise, honey, lemon juice, and caraway seeds until blended. Cover and refrigerate. Stir before using.

2. Into large salad bowl, tear spinach into bite-size pieces.

3. Add lettuce, onion, pimento, oranges, cucumber. Toss gently with dressing.

Tips:

A 15-oz. can mandarin oranges, drained, can be used instead of the 2 oranges. I use Romaine and spinach instead of the iceberg lettuce sometimes.

Good Go-Alongs:

Lasagna, calico bean bake, and pasta dishes go well with this salad.

Exchange List Values

- Fruit 0.5
- Vegetable 1.0
- Carbohydrate 0.5
- Fat 0.5

Basic Nutritional Values

- Calories 85
  (Calories from Fat 20)
- Total Fat 2 gm
  (Saturated Fat 0.3 gm,
  Trans Fat 0.0 gm,
  Polyunsat Fat 1.0 gm,
  Monounsat Fat 0.4 gm)
- Cholesterol 0 mg
- Sodium 240 mg
- Potassium 435 gm
- Total Carb 17 gm
- Dietary Fiber 3 gm
- Sugars 12 gm
- Protein 3 gm
- Phosphorus 55 gm

Spinach Salad

Ruth Zercher
Grantham, PA

Makes 15 servings
Prep. Time: 20 minutes

**1 lb. fresh spinach with
  stems discarded**
1 head Bibb lettuce
**¼ cup salted cashew nuts,
  *divided***
½ cup olive oil
1 tsp. celery seed
2 Tbsp. sugar
1 tsp. salt
1 tsp. dry mustard
1 tsp. grated onion
3 Tbsp. vinegar

1. Wash spinach and lettuce and tear into bite-sized pieces. Combine spinach, lettuce and nuts in serving bowl, reserving a few nuts for garnish.

2. Combine all other ingredients in blender and mix well.

3. Immediately before serving, pour dressing over greens and nuts. Sprinkle reserved nuts over top.

Exchange List Values

- Fat 2.0

Basic Nutritional Values

- Calories 95
  (Calories from Fat 70)
- Total Fat 8 gm
  (Saturated Fat 1.2 gm,
  Trans Fat 0.0 gm,
  Polyunsat Fat 1.0 gm,
  Monounsat Fat 5.9 gm)
- Cholesterol 0 mg
- Sodium 195 mg
- Potassium 215 gm
- Total Carb 4 gm
- Dietary Fiber 1 gm
- Sugars 2 gm
- Protein 1 gm
- Phosphorus 30 gm

BLT Salad

Alica Denlinger
Lancaster, PA

*Makes 12 servings,
about 3½ oz. per serving*
Prep. Time: 30 minutes

Salad:
**2 heads Romaine
  lettuce, torn**
2 cups chopped tomatoes
**4 bacon strips, cooked
  and crumbled**
**½ cup freshly grated
  Parmesan cheese**
1 cup croutons

Dressing:
¼ cup olive oil
½ tsp. salt
½ tsp. pepper
¼ cup fresh lemon juice
2 cloves garlic, crushed

1. Toss together salad ingredients in a large bowl.

2. Shake together dressing ingredients.

3. Pour dressing over salad immediately before serving.

Exchange List Values

- Vegetable 1.0
- Fat 1.5

Basic Nutritional Values

- Calories 90
  (Calories from Fat 65)
- Total Fat 7 gm
  (Saturated Fat 1.5 gm,
  Trans Fat 0.0 gm,
  Polyunsat Fat 0.7 gm,
  Monounsat Fat 4.0 gm)
- Cholesterol 5 mg
- Sodium 220 mg
- Potassium 250 gm
- Total Carb 6 gm
- Dietary Fiber 2 gm
- Sugars 2 gm
- Protein 3 gm
- Phosphorus 60 gm

Lettuce Salad with Hot Bacon Dressing

Mary B. Sensenig
New Holland, PA

*Makes 12 servings,
about 3 oz. lettuce and 2 Tbsp.
dressing per serving*

Prep. Time: 5 minutes
Cooking Time: 15 minutes

5 pieces bacon
¼ cup sugar
1 Tbsp. cornstarch
½ tsp. salt
1 beaten egg
1 cup fat-free milk
¼ cup vinegar
36 oz. ready-to-serve
   mixed lettuces, *or 2
   medium heads iceberg
   lettuce*

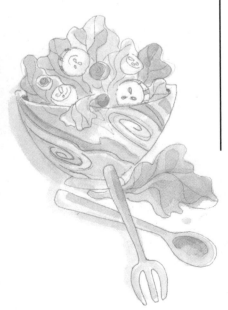

1. Sautée bacon in skillet until crisp.
2. Remove bacon from heat and drain. Chop. Discard drippings.
3. Add sugar, cornstarch, and salt to skillet. Blend together well.
4. Add egg, milk, and vinegar, stirring until smooth.
5. Cook over low heat, stirring continually until thickened and smooth.
6. When dressing is no longer hot, but still warm, toss with torn lettuce leaves and chopped bacon.
7. Serve immediately.

Exchange List Values
• Carbohydrate 0.5   • Fat 0.5

Basic Nutritional Values
• Calories 60
  (Calories from Fat 15)
• Total Fat 2 gm
  (Saturated Fat 0.5 gm,
  Trans Fat 0.0 gm,
  Polyunsat Fat 0.3 gm,
  Monounsat Fat 0.7 gm)
• Cholesterol 20 mg
• Sodium 180 mg
• Potassium 180 gm
• Total Carb 9 gm
• Dietary Fiber 1 gm
• Sugars 7 gm
• Protein 3 gm
• Phosphorus 60 gm

Italian Green Salad

Jane Geigley
Lancaster, PA

*Makes 4 servings,
about 7 oz. per serving*

Prep. Time: 10 minutes

16-oz. pkg. green salad mix
1 oz. pastrami, chopped in
   ½-inch pieces
¼ cup shredded part-skim
   mozzarella cheese
4 plum tomatoes, chopped
1 tsp. Italian herb
   seasoning
3 Tbsp. fat-free Italian
   salad dressing
¼ cup sliced ripe olives
1 cup seasoned croutons

1. Combine salad mix, pastrami or pepperoni, mozzarella, tomatoes, and seasoning.
2. Drizzle with salad dressing; toss to coat.
3. Before serving, top with olives and croutons. Serve immediately.

Warm Memories:
   It's a great dish on a hot day. People just love this salad when I take it to gatherings.

Good Go-Alongs:
   Great with a pizza party

Exchange List Values
• Starch 0.5   • Lean Meat 1.0
• Vegetable 1.0   • Fat 0.5

Basic Nutritional Values
• Calories 125
  (Calories from Fat 45)
• Total Fat 5 gm
  (Saturated Fat 1.7 gm,
  Trans Fat 0.0 gm,
  Polyunsat Fat 0.6 gm,
  Monounsat Fat 2.2 gm)
• Cholesterol 10 mg
• Sodium 455 mg
• Potassium 530 gm
• Total Carb 14 gm
• Dietary Fiber 4 gm
• Sugars 4 gm
• Protein 7 gm
• Phosphorus 120 gm

Tortellini Caesar Salad

Rebecca Meyerkorth
Wamego, KS

Makes 10 servings,
about 3 oz. per serving

Prep. Time: 30–35 minutes
Cooking Time: 15 minutes

9-oz. pkg. frozen cheese
 tortellini
½ cup low-fat mayonnaise
¼ cup fat-free milk
½ cup freshly shredded
 Parmesan cheese, *divided*
2 Tbsp. lemon juice
2 garlic cloves, minced
8 cups torn Romaine lettuce
1 cup seasoned croutons,
 optional
halved cherry tomatoes,
 optional

1. Cook tortellini according to package directions. Drain and rinse with cold water.
2. Meanwhile in a small bowl, combine mayonnaise, milk, ⅓ cup Parmesan cheese, lemon juice, and garlic. Mix well.
3. Put cooled tortellini in large bowl.
4. Add Romaine and remaining 2⅔ Tbsp. Parmesan.
5. Just before serving, drizzle with dressing and toss to coat. Top with croutons and tomatoes, if desired.

Tips:
 Tomatoes look great for color. Also, I don't always have seasoned croutons on hand. They are optional.

Warm Memories:
 Just plain delicious! This salad is especially good in hot summer weather. Our family loves it.

Exchange List Values
- Starch 0.5   • Fat 0.5
- Carbohydrate 0.5

Basic Nutritional Values
- Calories 95   • Sodium 225 mg
 (Calories from Fat 30)   • Potassium 120 gm
- Total Fat 4 gm   • Total Carb 12 gm
 (Saturated Fat 1.4 gm, • Dietary Fiber 1 gm
 Trans Fat 0.0 gm,   • Sugars 2 gm
 Polyunsat Fat 0.6 gm,   • Protein 5 gm
 Monounsat Fat 0.9 gm) • Phosphorus 85 gm
- Cholesterol 10 mg

Two-Cheese Tossed Salad

Elaine Hoover
Leola, PA

Makes 8 servings,
about 5 oz. per serving

Prep. Time: 20 minutes

10 cups spinach and
 Romaine lettuce,
 chopped
½ lb. mushrooms, sliced
8 oz. fat-free cottage cheese
10 strips bacon, fried and
 crumbled

Dressing:
 ¼ cup canola oil
 ½ cup minced red onion
 2 Tbsp. sugar
 ¼ cup vinegar
 1 tsp. poppy seed
 ½ tsp. prepared mustard
 ¼ tsp. salt

2 oz. reduced-fat shredded
 Swiss cheese

1. Layer in a large serving bowl: half of the spinach/lettuce, half mushrooms, half cottage cheese, and half bacon. Repeat layers.
2. Combine dressing ingredients together in a shaker or lidded jar and shake well.
3. Add dressing and Swiss cheese just before serving.

Exchange List Values
- Carbohydrate 0.5   • Fat 1.5
- Lean Meat 1.0

Basic Nutritional Values
- Calories 145   • Sodium 235 mg
 (Calories from Fat 90) • Potassium 345 gm
- Total Fat 10 gm   • Total Carb 9 gm
 (Saturated Fat 1.5 gm, • Dietary Fiber 2 gm
 Trans Fat 0.0 gm,   • Sugars 5 gm
 Polyunsat Fat 2.3 gm,   • Protein 8 gm
 Monounsat Fat 5.1 gm) • Phosphorus 155 gm
- Cholesterol 10 mg

Lettuce and Egg Salad

Frances Kruba & Cathy Kruba
Dundalk, MD

Makes 6 servings,
about 3½ oz. salad plus 2 Tbsp.
dressing per serving

Prep. Time: 25 minutes

⅔ cup low-fat mayonnaise
1⅓ Tbsp. vinegar
2 tsp. sugar
1 head lettuce, washed and
    dried, torn
2 hard-boiled eggs, chopped
1–4 green onions, chopped

1. In a jar, mix mayonnaise, vinegar, and sugar and shake well.
2. Just before serving, mix lettuce, eggs, and onion. Add dressing, a little at a time, to your taste preference.

Exchange List Values
• Carbohydrate 0.5   • Fat 0.5

Basic Nutritional Values
• Calories 70   • Sodium 265 mg
  (Calories from Fat 30) • Potassium 165 gm
• Total Fat 4 gm   • Total Carb 8 gm
  (Saturated Fat 0.8 gm, • Dietary Fiber 1 gm
  Trans Fat 0.0 gm,   • Sugars 4 gm
  Polyunsat Fat 1.4 gm, • Protein 3 gm
  Monounsat Fat 1.0 gm) • Phosphorus 60 gm
• Cholesterol 60 mg

Crunchy Romaine Toss

Jolene Schrock
Millersburg, OH

Jamie Mowry
Arlington, TX

Lucille Hollinger
Richland, PA

Makes 8 servings,
about 3 oz. per serving

Prep. Time: 20–30 minutes
Cooking Time: 10 minutes

Dressing:
  1 Tbsp. sugar
  2 Tbsp. canola oil
  2 Tbsp. cider vinegar
  1 tsp. reduced-sodium
      soy sauce
  salt and pepper to taste

3-oz. pkg. Ramen noodles,
  broken up, seasoning
  packets discarded
½ Tbsp. trans-fat-free tub
  margarine
1½ cups chopped broccoli
1 small head Romaine
  lettuce, torn up
4 green onions, chopped
½ cup chopped walnuts

1. In the blender, combine sugar, oil, vinegar, soy sauce, salt, and pepper. Blend until sugar is dissolved.
2. In a skillet, sauté Ramen noodles in margarine until golden brown.
3. In a large bowl, combine lettuce, broccoli, onions, and noodles.
4. Just before serving toss with nuts and dressing.

Tip:
Sometimes I like to set the dressing on the side and let everybody put their own dressing on. Plus, if you have any leftover salad it won't get soggy.

Variations:
1. Use 2 cups sliced fresh strawberries in place of broccoli. Increase walnuts to 1 cup.

Janice Nolt
Ephrata, PA

2. Add 1 small can mandarin oranges, drained.

Janet Derstine
Telford, PA

Exchange List Values
• Starch 0.5   • Fat 2.0
• Vegetable 1.0

Basic Nutritional Values
• Calories 150   • Sodium 75 mg
  (Calories from Fat 100) • Potassium 185 gm
• Total Fat 11 gm   • Total Carb 12 gm
  (Saturated Fat 1.5 gm, • Dietary Fiber 2 gm
  Trans Fat 0.0 gm,   • Sugars 3 gm
  Polyunsat Fat 5.6 gm, • Protein 3 gm
  Monounsat Fat 3.8 gm) • Phosphorus 60 gm
• Cholesterol 0 mg

Make your own salad dressing so you can use healthy oils, such as sunflower, canola, or soybean oil.

Our Favorite Dressing

Carol Eberly
Harrisonburg, VA

*Makes 3½ cups,
28 servings, 2 Tbsp. per serving*

Prep. Time: 10 minutes

1 cup granular Splenda
1 cup ketchup
1½ tsp. paprika
1½ tsp. salt
1½ tsp. celery seed
1½ tsp. grated onion, *optional*
1½ cups vegetable oil
½ cup vinegar

1. Shake ingredients together well in a quart jar. Keep in refrigerator.

Warm Memories:
This is our family's favorite salad dressing. I always have a jar in the refrigerator.

Good Go-Alongs:
This dressing is great on tossed salad or used as a dip for veggies.

Exchange List Values
• Fat 2.5

Basic Nutritional Values
• Calories 115   • Sodium 220 mg
 (Calories from Fat 110)   • Potassium 40 gm
• Total Fat 12 gm   • Total Carb 3 gm
 (Saturated Fat 0.9 gm,   • Dietary Fiber 0 gm
 Trans Fat 0.0 gm,   • Sugars 3 gm
 Polyunsat Fat 3.3 gm,   • Protein 0 gm
 Monounsat Fat 7.4 gm)   • Phosphorus 0 gm
• Cholesterol 0 mg

Very Good Salad Dressing

Lydia K. Stoltzfus
Gordonville, PA

*Makes 2⅔ cups,
24 servings, 2 Tbsp. per serving*

**Prep. Time: 10 minutes
Cooking/Baking Time:**

2 cups mayonnaise
½ cup granular Splenda
1 Tbsp. mustard
1 Tbsp. vinegar
¼ tsp. salt
¼ tsp. celery seed
¼ tsp. dried parsley
dash pepper
¼ cup pickle juice

1. Mix together mayonnaise, Splenda, mustard, vinegar, salt, celery seed, parsley, and pepper to taste.
2. Add pickle juice last to desired consistency.

Tip:
Use on tossed salad or coleslaw.

Exchange List Values
• Fat 0.5

Basic Nutritional Values
• Calories 25   • Sodium 235 mg
 (Calories from Fat 15)   • Potassium 10 gm
• Total Fat 2 gm   • Total Carb 3 gm
 (Saturated Fat 0.2 gm,   • Dietary Fiber 0 gm
 Trans Fat 0.0 gm,   • Sugars 1 gm
 Polyunsat Fat 0.8 gm,   • Protein 0 gm
 Monounsat Fat 0.3 gm)   • Phosphorus 5 gm
• Cholesterol 0 mg

Simple Salad Dressing

Cynthia Morris
Grottoes, VA

*Makes 1½ cups,
12 servings, 2 Tbsp. per serving*

Prep. Time: 5–10 minutes

¼ cup Splenda Brown Sugar Blend
½ cup oil
⅓ cup vinegar
⅓ cup ketchup
1 Tbsp. Worcestershire sauce

1. In a bottle or jar, combine ingredients. Cover and shake well to mix.

Tip:
I use an empty ketchup bottle to keep the salad dressing in. Shake well before each use.

Exchange List Values
• Carbohydrate 0.5 • Fat 1.5

Basic Nutritional Values
• Calories 105   • Sodium 90 mg
 (Calories from Fat 80)   • Potassium 45 gm
• Total Fat 9 gm   • Total Carb 6 gm
 (Saturated Fat 0.7 gm,   • Dietary Fiber 0 gm
 Trans Fat 0.0 gm,   • Sugars 3 gm
 Polyunsat Fat 2.6 gm,   • Protein 0 gm
 Monounsat Fat 5.8 gm)   • Phosphorus 0 gm
• Cholesterol 0 mg

145

Russian Dressing

Frances Schrag
Newton, KS

Makes 9 servings,
1 Tbsp. per serving

Prep. Time: 10 minutes

½ cup reduced-fat
  mayonnaise
1 Tbsp. chili sauce, *or*
  ketchup
1 tsp. finely chopped onion
½ tsp. horseradish
¼ tsp. Worcestershire
  sauce
1 Tbsp. finely chopped
  parsley

1. Combine all ingredients
and mix well.
2. Serve with choice of
tossed salad.

Exchange List Values
• Fat 0.5

Basic Nutritional Values
• Calories 35   • Sodium 140 mg
  (Calories from Fat 25) • Potassium 15 gm
• Total Fat 3 gm   • Total Carb 1 gm
  (Saturated Fat 0.4 gm, • Dietary Fiber 0 gm
  Trans Fat 0.0 gm,   • Sugars 1 gm
  Polyunsat Fat 1.8 gm, • Protein 0 gm
  Monounsat Fat 0.9 gm) • Phosphorus 5 gm
• Cholesterol 5 mg

Greek Pasta Salad

Edie Moran
West Babylon, NY
Judi Manos
West Islip, NY

Makes 8 servings,
about 4½ oz. per serving

Prep. Time: 15 minutes
Cooking Time for Pasta: 15
minutes

2 cups cooked pasta, rinsed
  and cooled (1 cup dry)
4 medium plum tomatoes,
  chopped
15-oz. can garbanzo beans,
  rinsed and drained
1 medium onion, chopped
6-oz. can pitted black
  olives, drained
1 oz. crumbled reduced-fat
  feta cheese
1 garlic clove, minced
¼ cup olive oil
2 Tbsp. lemon juice
½ tsp. salt
½ tsp. pepper

1. In a large bowl, combine
macaroni, tomatoes, garbanzo
beans, onion, olives, feta
cheese.
2. In a small bowl, whisk
together oil, lemon juice, salt
and pepper. Pour over salad
and toss to coat.

3. Cover and chill in
refrigerator. Stir before
serving.

Tips:
1. I like to serve it in a
clear glass salad bowl.
2. Add some baby spinach
leaves. Combine vegetables
with hot pasta right after
draining it. Kraft Greek
Vinaigrette is a good dressing
too.
Judi Manos
West Islip, NY

Warm Memories:
When visiting my hus-
band's family on the Island of
Samos, Greece, this was made
with all fresh ingredients
grown in their garden.
Judi Manos
West Islip, NY

Exchange List Values
• Starch 1.0   • Fat 2.0
• Vegetable 1.0

Basic Nutritional Values
• Calories 200   • Sodium 340 mg
  (Calories from Fat 90) • Potassium 220 gm
• Total Fat 10 gm   • Total Carb 23 gm
  (Saturated Fat 1.5 gm, • Dietary Fiber 4 gm
  Trans Fat 0.0 gm,   • Sugars 4 gm
  Polyunsat Fat 1.3 gm, • Protein 6 gm
  Monounsat Fat 6.1 gm) • Phosphorus 100 gm
• Cholesterol 0 mg

When I'm pressed for time, I contribute a big
dish of fresh celery to our church potluck. I buy it
at the local farmers' market.
Anne Wilson, Strasburg, PA

Macaroni Salad

**Frances L. Kruba and
Cathy C. Kruba**
Dundalk, MD
Marcia S. Myer
Manheim, PA

*Makes 12 servings,
about 7 oz. per serving*

*Prep. Time: 30 minutes
Cooking Time for Pasta: 15
minutes*

**1 lb. macaroni, cooked and
cooled
1 cup diced celery
1 cup diced onion
1 cup diced carrots
8 hard-boiled eggs, diced
3 Tbsp. sugar
3 Tbsp. vinegar
½ cup low-fat mayonnaise**

**1¼ cups egg substitute
1 Tbsp. mustard
1 Tbsp. trans-fat free tub
margarine
½ tsp. salt**

1. Mix together macaroni,
celery, onions, carrots, hard
boiled eggs, sugar, and
vinegar or lemon juice. Add
mayonnaise.
2. In a saucepan, mix egg
substitute, mustard, and
butter. Cook on medium heat
until thickened and steaming,
stirring constantly. Do not
boil.
3. Remove from heat
and cool 5 minutes. Add to
macaroni mixture.

Exchange List Values
• Starch 2.0   • Med-Fat Meat 1.0
• Carbohydrate 0.5

Basic Nutritional Values
• Calories 250
  (Calories from Fat 45)
• Total Fat 5 gm
  (Saturated Fat 1.5 gm,
  Trans Fat 0.0 gm,
  Polyunsat Fat 1.6 gm,
  Monounsat Fat 1.8 gm)
• Cholesterol 125 mg
• Sodium 315 mg
• Potassium 205 gm
• Total Carb 37 gm
• Dietary Fiber 2 gm
• Sugars 6 gm
• Protein 13 gm
• Phosphorus 140 gm

Chicken Pasta Salad

Esther Gingerich
Kalona, IA

*Makes 10 servings,
about 7 oz. per serving*

*Prep. Time: 15 minutes
Cooking Time for Pasta: 15
minutes*

**2¼ cups diced cooked
chicken
2 cups cooked small pasta
or macaroni (1 cup dry)
2 cups diced celery
2 cups seedless grape halves
4 hard boiled eggs, diced
15-oz. can pineapple
tidbits, drained**

**Dressing:
¾ cup low-fat
mayonnaise
½ cup fat-free sour cream
½ cup fat-free frozen
whipped topping,
thawed
1 Tbsp. lemon juice
1 Tbsp. sugar
½ tsp. salt**

½ cup cashew pieces

1. In a large bowl, combine
chicken, macaroni, celery,
grapes, eggs, and pineapple.
2. Whisk dressing ingre-
dients until smooth. Pour
dressing over salad; toss to
coat.
3. Chill at least one hour.
Just before serving, fold in
cashews.

Tip:
It's simple to put this
together if chicken is cooked
and diced, macaroni is cooked
and eggs are boiled ahead of
time.

Warm Memories:
I often take this to summer
potlucks for a "cooler" dish.
This could be a one-dish
meal.

Exchange List Values
• Starch 0.5   • Lean Meat 2.0
• Fruit 0.5   • Fat 0.5
• Carbohydrate 1.0

Basic Nutritional Values
• Calories 250
  (Calories from Fat 80)
• Total Fat 9 gm
  (Saturated Fat 2.2 gm,
  Trans Fat 0.0 gm,
  Polyunsat Fat 2.3 gm,
  Monounsat Fat 3.8 gm)
• Cholesterol 105 mg
• Sodium 360 mg
• Potassium 325 gm
• Total Carb 28 gm
• Dietary Fiber 2 gm
• Sugars 12 gm
• Protein 15 gm
• Phosphorus 185 gm

Creamy Pasta Salad

Irma Wengerd
Dundee, OH

*Makes 15 servings,
about 7 oz. per serving*

Prep. Time: 30 minutes
*Cooking Time for Pasta: 15
minutes*

1½ lbs. uncooked spiral
  pasta
½ cup chopped celery
2 tomatoes, chopped
1 small onion, chopped
1 green pepper, chopped
3-oz. can black olives,
  drained, sliced
10-oz. lower-sodium, lean
  ham, diced
8 oz. 75%-less fat cheddar
  cheese, diced

Dressing:
¾ cup reduced-fat
  Miracle Whip
1 Tbsp. spicy brown
  mustard
3 Tbsp. canola oil
1 Tbsp. vinegar
5 Tbsp. sugar
¼ tsp. onion salt
½ tsp. celery seed

1. Cook pasta in boiling,
unsalted water. Drain and rinse
with cold water. Set aside.
2. In large bowl, toss
together pasta, celery, tomatoes, onion, green pepper,
olives, ham, and cheese.
3. In a separate bowl, blend
the dressing ingredients together.
4. Pour dressing over pasta
and toss.

Good Go-Alongs:
  This salad is delicious with
grilled chicken.

Exchange List Values
- Starch 1.0   • Med-Fat Meat 1.0
- Carbohydrate 2.0

Basic Nutritional Values
- Calories 295   • Sodium 475 mg
  (Calories from Fat 70) • Potassium 190 gm
- Total Fat 8 gm   • Total Carb 42 gm
  (Saturated Fat 1.7 gm, • Dietary Fiber 2 gm
  Trans Fat 0.0 gm,   • Sugars 8 gm
  Polyunsat Fat 2.1 gm, • Protein 15 gm
  Monounsat Fat 3.0 gm) • Phosphorus 185 gm
- Cholesterol 20 mg

Spaghetti Salad

Lois Stoltzfus
Honey Brook, PA

*Makes 8 servings,
about 5 oz. per serving*

Prep. Time: 15 minutes
Cooking Time: 15 minutes
Cooling Time: 30 minutes

16 oz. angel hair pasta
¼ cup canola oil
¼ cup lemon juice
1 tsp. Accent
1 tsp. seasoned salt
¼ cup low-fat mayonnaise

1 green bell pepper, chopped
1 cup grape tomatoes
1 red onion, chopped
1 cup shredded 75%-less-
  fat cheddar cheese
½ cup sliced black olives
pepperoni, *optional*

1. Cook pasta according to
directions.

2. Mix oil, lemon juice,
Accent, seasoned salt, and
mayonnaise together. Add to
drained pasta while it is still
warm.
3. When pasta mixture has
cooled at least 30 minutes,
stir in pepper, tomatoes,
onion, cheese, olives, and
optional pepperoni. Chill.

Exchange List Values
- Starch 3.0   • Fat 1.5
- Lean Meat 1.0

Basic Nutritional Values
- Calories 335   • Sodium 420 mg
  (Calories from Fat 100) • Potassium 225 gm
- Total Fat 11 gm   • Total Carb 48 gm
  (Saturated Fat 1.6 gm, • Dietary Fiber 3 gm
  Trans Fat 0.0 gm,   • Sugars 4 gm
  Polyunsat Fat 2.7 gm, • Protein 12 gm
  Monounsat Fat 5.6 gm) • Phosphorus 170 gm
- Cholesterol 5 mg

Almond-Apricot Chicken Salad

Tracey Hanson Schramel
Windom, MN

*Makes 8 servings,
about 9 oz. per serving*

Prep. Time: 15 minutes
*Cooking Time for Pasta: 15
minutes*

Salad:
½ lb. bowtie pasta,
  cooked, rinsed, and
  drained
3 cups chopped broccoli
2½ cups chopped cooked
  chicken
1 cup chopped celery

1 cup dried apricots, cut into ¼-inch strips
¾ cup toasted whole almonds
½ cup finely chopped green onions

Dressing:
¾ cup low-fat mayonnaise
¾ cup fat-free sour cream
2 tsp. grated lemon peel
1 Tbsp. lemon juice
1 Tbsp. Dijon-style mustard
¾ tsp. salt
¼ tsp. pepper

1. In a large bowl, combine salad ingredients.
2. In another bowl, combine dressing ingredients.
3. Pour dressing over pasta mixture and toss.

Tips:
1. You can save the almonds out and sprinkle them on top if you like that look better.
2. Pass the dressing in a small pitcher so each person can put on the amount they like. The leftovers don't get soggy then either!

Exchange List Values
- Starch 1.5
- Lean Meat 2.0
- Fruit 1.0
- Fat 1.5
- Carbohydrate 0.5

Basic Nutritional Values
- Calories 370
  (Calories from Fat 110)
- Total Fat 12 gm
  (Saturated Fat 1.8 gm,
  Trans Fat 0.0 gm,
  Polyunsat Fat 3.6 gm,
  Monounsat Fat 5.8 gm)
- Cholesterol 40 mg
- Sodium 545 mg
- Potassium 635 gm
- Total Carb 46 gm
- Dietary Fiber 5 gm
- Sugars 15 gm
- Protein 22 gm
- Phosphorus 260 gm

Apple Chicken Salad

Marlene Fonken
Upland, CA

*Makes 6 servings,
about 6 oz. per serving*

Prep. Time: 30–40 minutes
Chilling Time: 2–12 hours

Dressing:
½ cup light mayonnaise
2 Tbsp. cider vinegar
2 Tbsp. lemon juice
2–3 Tbsp. Dijon mustard

2 cups chopped, cooked chicken breast
2 ribs celery, chopped
¼ cup diced onion
1 green apple, chopped
1 red apple, chopped
⅓ cup dried cranberries
salt and pepper to taste

1. Whisk together mayonnaise, vinegar, lemon juice, and mustard. Set aside.
2. Mix together chicken, celery, onion, apples, cranberries, salt, and pepper.
3. Pour on dressing and toss to mix. Refrigerate until serving. Flavor develops with longer chilling.

Tips:
1. Break up and soften a handful of rice sticks; drain and add to the finished salad. This salad is gluten-free!
2. If you're starting with raw chicken, chop it into bite-sized pieces. In a saucepan, cover the chicken pieces with water or chicken broth. Cover and cook on medium heat until the chicken pieces are white through, 10–20 minutes. Drain. This can be done ahead of time.
3. You can substitute 12.5-oz. can chicken, drained and broken up, for this salad.

Warm Memories:
At a church dinner, a man found out who had made my dish, found me, and asked for the recipe.

Exchange List Values
- Fruit 1.0
- Fat 1.0
- Lean Meat 2.0

Basic Nutritional Values
- Calories 190
  (Calories from Fat 65)
- Total Fat 7 gm
  (Saturated Fat 1.2 gm,
  Trans Fat 0.0 gm,
  Polyunsat Fat 3.2 gm,
  Monounsat Fat 2.0 gm)
- Cholesterol 45 mg
- Sodium 340 mg
- Potassium 270 gm
- Total Carb 17 gm
- Dietary Fiber 2 gm
- Sugars 13 gm
- Protein 15 gm
- Phosphorus 130 gm

You can reduce the amount of salt — or even eliminate it — in many recipes without changing the dish's taste.

Tomato Basil Couscous

Amber Martin
Mount Joy, PA

Makes 6 servings, 3½ oz. per serving

Prep. Time: 25 minutes
Cooking Time for Couscous: 10 minutes
Chilling Time: 2 hours or more

2 cups cooked couscous, cooled
1 cup chopped tomato
2 Tbsp. chopped basil
1 oz. reduced-fat feta cheese, crumbled fine
3 Tbsp. olive oil
2 Tbsp. lemon juice
1 tsp. Dijon mustard
1 clove garlic, crushed
fresh black pepper to taste

1. Mix together couscous, tomato, basil, and feta cheese.
2. In separate bowl, mix together olive oil, lemon juice, mustard, garlic, and black pepper. Pour over couscous mixture and toss.
3. Chill at least 2 hours before serving.

Tip:
To cook couscous, boil 1½ cups water and ½ tsp. salt. Remove from heat. Add 1 cup couscous, stir, and cover. Let stand 5 minutes. Fluff couscous lightly with fork. Cool before using in salad.

Exchange List Values
• Starch 1.0   • Fat 1.5

Basic Nutritional Values
• Calories 135   • Sodium 90 mg
  (Calories from Fat 70)   • Potassium 120 gm
• Total Fat 8 gm   • Total Carb 14 gm
  (Saturated Fat 1.4 gm,   • Dietary Fiber 1 gm
  Trans Fat 0.0 gm,   • Sugars 1 gm
  Polyunsat Fat 0.8 gm,   • Protein 3 gm
  Monounsat Fat 5.1 gm)   • Phosphorus 35 gm
• Cholesterol 0 mg

Chicken Salad with Blue Cheese

Susan Smith
Monument, CO

Makes 6 servings, about 5 oz. per serving

Prep. Time: 15 minutes

2½ cups cooked chicken breast, diced *or* julienned
6 cups shredded lettuce
¾ cup low-fat mayonnaise
2 Tbsp. tarragon vinegar
2½ Tbsp. chili sauce
2 Tbsp. chopped green pepper
1 oz. reduced-fat blue cheese, crumbled
whole lettuce leaves

1. Mix chicken with lettuce.
2. Mix mayonnaise, vinegar, chili sauce, and green pepper. Add crumbled cheese.
3. Gently combine chicken and mayonnaise mixtures.
4. Place salad in a bowl lined with lettuce or in individual lettuce cups.

Tip:
It is best made and eaten on the same day.

Exchange List Values
• Carbohydrate 0.5   • Lean Meat 3.0

Basic Nutritional Values
• Calories 155   • Sodium 470 mg
  (Calories from Fat 45)   • Potassium 275 gm
• Total Fat 5 gm   • Total Carb 7 gm
  (Saturated Fat 1.5 gm,   • Dietary Fiber 1 gm
  Trans Fat 0.0 gm,   • Sugars 2 gm
  Polyunsat Fat 1.7 gm,   • Protein 20 gm
  Monounsat Fat 1.4 gm)   • Phosphorus 175 gm
• Cholesterol 50 mg

If I don't have time to cook for a potluck, I take a tray with my home-canned pickled beets and dill pickles. To the tray I add a variety of fresh vegetables, whatever I have on hand.

Helen R. Goering, Moundridge, KS

Tortellini & Kidney Bean Salad

Mary C. Wirth
Lancaster, PA

Makes 6 servings,
about 3 oz. per serving

Prep. Time: 10–15 minutes
Cooking Time for Pasta: 9
minutes
Chilling Time: 2 hours or more

9 oz. frozen cheese
 tortellini
15½-oz. can kidney beans,
 rinsed and drained
1 cup sliced cucumber
¼ cup chopped red onion

Dressing:
 2 Tbsp. balsamic vinegar
 1 Tbsp. olive oil
 ½ tsp. sugar
 ½ tsp. Italian seasoning
 2 Tbsp. chopped fresh
  parsley

1. Cook tortellini according to package directions. Do not overcook. Rinse with cold water; drain.
2. Mix dressing ingredients in a small jar or bottle. Shake well.
3. In a large bowl, stir together tortellini, kidney beans, cucumber, and onion.
4. Add dressing and stir to coat.
5. Cover and refrigerate at least 2 hours.

Good Go-Alongs:
 This makes a good side dish at cook-outs, especially with grilled chicken.

Exchange List Values
• Starch 2.0   • Lean Meat 1.0

Basic Nutritional Values
• Calories 190   • Sodium 180 mg
 (Calories from Fat 45) • Potassium 260 gm
• Total Fat 5 gm   • Total Carb 28 gm
 (Saturated Fat 1.5 gm, • Dietary Fiber 4 gm
 Trans Fat 0.0 gm,   • Sugars 3 gm
 Polyunsat Fat 0.5 gm, • Protein 9 gm
 Monounsat Fat 2.3 gm) • Phosphorus 135 gm
• Cholesterol 10 mg

Broccoli, Cauliflower and Carrot Salad

Clara L. Yoder
Wadsworth, OH

Makes 8 servings,
about 6 oz. per serving

Prep. Time: 20 minutes
Cooking Time: 25 minutes
Chilling Time: 12 hours or
overnight

2 10-oz. pkgs. broccoli
 florets
10-oz. pkg. cauliflower
 florets
3 large carrots, chopped
1 cup diced celery
1 cup diced onion
1 green bell pepper, sliced
½ tsp. dry mustard
2 Tbsp. sugar
¼ cup granular Splenda
¾ Tbsp. cornstarch
½ cup vinegar
½ tsp. salt

1. Cook first three vegetables separately to a crisp stage. Drain each one and cool.
2. Combine all vegetables in large serving bowl.
3. In a saucepan combine mustard, sugar, cornstarch, vinegar and salt. Cook until clear. Pour over vegetables.
4. Cover and chill overnight or at least 12 hours before serving.

Exchange List Values
• Vegetable 3.0

Basic Nutritional Values
• Calories 75   • Sodium 210 mg
 (Calories from Fat 5) • Potassium 535 gm
• Total Fat 0.5 gm   • Total Carb 16 gm
 (Saturated Fat 0.1 gm, • Dietary Fiber 4 gm
 Trans Fat 0.0 gm,   • Sugars 9 gm
 Polyunsat Fat 0.2 gm, • Protein 4 gm
 Monounsat Fat 0.0 gm) • Phosphorus 85 gm
• Cholesterol 0 mg

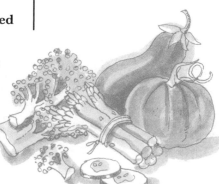

Salads

Broccoli, Cauliflower and Pea Salad

Virginia Graber
Freeman, SD

Makes 12 servings,
about ¾ cup per serving

Prep. Time: 25 minutes
Chilling Time: 8–12 hours or
overnight

2 cups chopped broccoli
2 cups chopped cauliflower
2 cups frozen peas, thawed
1 large onion, chopped
2 cups chopped celery
½ cup sour cream
½ cup low-fat mayonnaise
1½ Tbsp. sugar
2 Tbsp. vinegar
¼ tsp. salt

1. Combine all ingredients.
2. Refrigerate overnight
and serve.

Variation:
Add 1 can sliced water
chestnuts to ingredients.
Jeanne Heyerly
Reedley, CA

Exchange List Values
• Carbohydrate 0.5 • Vegetable 1.0

Basic Nutritional Values
• Calories 60   • Sodium 195 mg
(Calories from Fat 10) • Potassium 220 gm
• Total Fat 1 gm   • Total Carb 12 gm
(Saturated Fat 0.2 gm, • Dietary Fiber 2 gm
Trans Fat 0.0 gm,   • Sugars 5 gm
Polyunsat Fat 0.5 gm,   • Protein 3 gm
Monounsat Fat 0.2 gm)   • Phosphorus 60 gm
• Cholesterol 0 mg

Cauliflower Salad

Janice Deel
Paducah, KY

Makes 6 servings,
about 6 oz. per serving

Prep. Time: 20 minutes
Chilling Time: 1–2 hours

1 medium cauliflower, cut
into florets
2 cups frozen peas, thawed
and drained
3 ribs celery, chopped
3 eggs, hard-boiled and
chopped
¾ cup low-fat mayonnaise
3 Tbsp. onion, chopped
¼ tsp. seasoned salt
½ tsp. ground pepper
3 Tbsp. fat-free milk

1. In a large bowl, combine
cauliflower, peas, celery and
eggs.
2. Blend together mayon-
naise, onion, seasoned salt,
pepper and milk.
3. Pour over cauliflower
mixture and mix well. Chill
1–2 hours before serving.

Exchange List Values
• Starch 0.5   • Med-Fat Meat 1.0
• Vegetable 1.0

Basic Nutritional Values
• Calories 120   • Sodium 445 mg
(Calories from Fat 40) • Potassium 330 gm
• Total Fat 4.5 gm   • Total Carb 14 gm
(Saturated Fat 1.2 gm, • Dietary Fiber 3 gm
Trans Fat 0.0 gm,   • Sugars 6 gm
Polyunsat Fat 1.8 gm, • Protein 7 gm
Monounsat Fat 1.4 gm) • Phosphorus 130 gm
• Cholesterol 95 mg

Grape Broccoli Salad

Arianne Hochstetler
Goshen, IN

Makes 8 servings,
about 7 oz. per serving

Prep. Time: 15–20 minutes
Chilling Time: 1 hour

4 cups broccoli florets
3 cups halved seedless red
grapes
1⅓ cups celery, chopped
1 cup green onions,
chopped
1 cup raisins
4 tsp. honey
½ cup reduced-fat
mayonnaise
2 cups fat-free *or* light
plain yogurt
1 cup sliced water
chestnuts, *optional*

1. In a large bowl, combine
broccoli, grapes, celery,
onions, water chestnuts, and
raisins.
2. In a small bowl, combine
yogurt, mayonnaise, and honey.
3. Pour over broccoli
mixture and toss to coat.
4. Cover and refrigerate
for at least 1 hour or until
chilled.

Tip:
The broccoli, celery, and
green onions can be prepared
the night before. Putting the
salad together then is quick.

Exchange List Values
• Fruit 1.5   • Fat 0.5
• Carbohydrate 1.0

- Calories 185
  (Calories from Fat 35)
- Total Fat 4 gm
  (Saturated Fat 0.6 gm,
  Trans Fat 0.0 gm,
  Polyunsat Fat 2.1 gm,
  Monounsat Fat 1.1 gm)
- Cholesterol 5 mg
- Sodium 195 mg
- Potassium 580 gm
- Total Carb 36 gm
- Dietary Fiber 3 gm
- Sugars 28 gm
- Protein 5 gm
- Phosphorus 165 gm

Grandpa Steve's Potato Salad

Nanci Keatley
Salem, OR

*Makes 8 servings,
about 7 oz. per serving*

Prep. Time: 20 minutes
Cooking Time for Potatoes: 20 minutes

6 russet potatoes, peeled, cooked, and cubed
1 cup finely chopped onion
1 cup thinly sliced celery
1 cup sliced black olives (reserve 1 Tbsp. for top of salad)
1 large carrot, grated
6 hard boiled eggs (4 chopped, 2 sliced for top of salad)
1 cup low-fat mayonnaise
salt and pepper to taste
Tabasco, *optional*

1. Gently mix potatoes, onion, celery, olives, carrots, and chopped eggs together.
2. Add the mayonnaise and blend.
3. Season with salt and pepper to taste. Add Tabasco

sauce to taste. Garnish with egg slices and reserved olives.

Good Go-Alongs:
I helped Grandpa cater a few weddings with this recipe along with ham, beans, rolls, and green salad.

Exchange List Values
- Starch 1.0
- Carbohydrate 0.5
- Vegetable 1.0
- Fat 1.5

Basic Nutritional Values
- Calories 205
  (Calories from Fat 70)
- Total Fat 8 gm
  (Saturated Fat 1.8 gm,
  Trans Fat 0.0 gm,
  Polyunsat Fat 2.2 gm,
  Monounsat Fat 3.4 gm)
- Cholesterol 140 mg
- Sodium 455 mg
- Potassium 460 gm
- Total Carb 27 gm
- Dietary Fiber 3 gm
- Sugars 4 gm
- Protein 7 gm
- Phosphorus 135 gm

The Best Broccoli Salad

Sandra Haverstraw
Hummelstown, PA

*Makes 12 servings,
about 4 oz. per serving*

Prep. Time: 20–25 minutes
Cooking/Baking Time: 8–12 hours
Chilling Time: 8-12 hours

12 cups fresh broccoli florets, about 2 bunches broccoli, large stems discarded
1 cup golden raisins
1 small onion, chopped
6 slices bacon, fried and chopped
½ cup chopped cashews

Dressing:
¼ cup sugar
4 Tbsp. Splenda
2 Tbsp. vinegar
1 cup reduced-fat Miracle Whip dressing
2 Tbsp. horseradish
¼ tsp. salt
½ tsp. prepared mustard

1. Mix broccoli florets, raisins, chopped onion, and bacon.
2. Prepare dressing by blending sugar, Splenda, vinegar, Miracle Whip, horseradish, salt, and mustard until smooth.
3. Pour dressing over broccoli mix and toss gently until evenly coated.
4. Cover and refrigerate 8–12 hours. Add cashews just before serving.

Tip:
Precooked bacon works well.

Exchange List Values
- Fruit 0.5
- Carbohydrate 1.0
- Vegetable 1.0
- Fat 1.0

Basic Nutritional Values
- Calories 165
  (Calories from Fat 55)
- Total Fat 6 gm
  (Saturated Fat 1.4 gm,
  Trans Fat 0.0 gm,
  Polyunsat Fat 2.1 gm,
  Monounsat Fat 2.4 gm)
- Cholesterol 10 mg
- Sodium 375 mg
- Potassium 395 gm
- Total Carb 25 gm
- Dietary Fiber 3 gm
- Sugars 17 gm
- Protein 5 gm
- Phosphorus 110 gm

Unique Tuna Salad

Brenda J. Hochstedler
East Earl, PA

Makes 8 servings,
about 9 oz. per serving

Prep. Time: 10 minutes
Cooking Time (for potatoes and
eggs): 20–30 minutes
Cooling Time: 30 minutes

10 medium potatoes

Dressing:
¼ cup reduced-fat, light
mayonnaise
1¼ tsp. salt
¼ tsp. pepper
¼ tsp. paprika
2 Tbs. sweet pickle relish

4 eggs, hard boiled, chopped
6-oz. pouch water-packed
tuna, drained and flaked
½ cup chopped celery
½ head lettuce, torn

2 tomatoes, cut into wedges
Parmesan cheese, grated

1. Chop potatoes (peeled if you wish). Boil over medium heat until fork-tender but not mushy. Drain and cool.
2. Mix dressing ingredients. Stir gently into potatoes.
3. Add eggs, tuna, celery, and lettuce. Toss lightly.
4. Garnish with tomato wedges and Parmesan cheese.

Tips:
1. This is like a potato salad loaded, or a simplified salade necois.
2. If you already have potato salad in the refrigerator, use it instead of the potatoes and dressing. This transforms a leftover completely!

Exchange List Values
- Starch 2.0
- Lean Meat 1.0

Basic Nutritional Values
- Calories 210
  (Calories from Fat 40)
- Total Fat 4.5 gm
  (Saturated Fat 1.1 gm,
  Trans Fat 0.0 gm,
  Polyunsat Fat 1.7 gm,
  Monounsat Fat 1.5 gm)
- Cholesterol 105 mg
- Sodium 585 mg
- Potassium 695 gm
- Total Carb 31 gm
- Dietary Fiber 4 gm
- Sugars 4 gm
- Protein 11 gm
- Phosphorus 160 gm

Pink Potato Salad

Dawn Landowski
Eau Claire, WI

Makes 10 servings,
about 8 oz. per serving

Prep. Time: 30 minutes
Cooking Time: 20 minutes
Cooling Time: 1 hour

3 lbs. baby red potatoes
1 medium onion, diced
6 hard-boiled eggs, sliced,
divided
½ green pepper, diced
6 sliced radishes
1 cucumber, peeled and
diced
½ cup frozen peas, thawed
3 Tbsp. parsley

Dressing:
¼ cup chili sauce
1 cup light, reduced-fat
mayonnaise
½ cup light, reduced-fat
French dressing
3 tsp. onion powder
½ tsp. pepper
¼ tsp. garlic powder

paprika for garnish

1. Boil potatoes until tender but firm. Allow to cool. Peel and dice potatoes.
2. Mix dressing ingredients together and add to potatoes.
3. Fold in 5 sliced eggs, green pepper, radishes, cucumber, peas, and parsley.
4. Refrigerate. Garnish with reserved sliced egg and paprika.

Warm Memories:
My granny always made this for me.

Exchange List Values
- Starch 1.5
- Carbohydrate 0.5
- Fat 2.0

Basic Nutritional Values
- Calories 240
  (Calories from Fat 90)
- Total Fat 10 gm
  (Saturated Fat 1.9 gm,
  Trans Fat 0.0 gm,
  Polyunsat Fat 4.4 gm,
  Monounsat Fat 3.3 gm)
- Cholesterol 120 mg
- Sodium 470 mg
- Potassium 730 gm
- Total Carb 30 gm
- Dietary Fiber 4 gm
- Sugars 7 gm
- Protein 7 gm
- Phosphorus 165 gm

To peel cooked potatoes, use a butter knife and gently scrape across the surface.
Dawn Landowski, Eau Claire, WI

German Potato Salad

Rhonda Burgoon
Collingswood, NJ

Makes 4 servings,
about 6 oz. per serving

Prep. Time: 15 minutes
Cooking Time: 20 minutes

3 cups diced peeled potatoes
4 slices bacon
1 small onion, diced
¼ cup white vinegar
2 Tbsp. water
2 Tbsp. sugar
½ tsp. salt
⅛ tsp. ground black pepper
1 rib celery, chopped

1. Place potatoes in pot and just cover with water. Bring to boil and cook about 11 minutes or until tender. Drain and set aside to cool.
2. Fry bacon in a large skillet until browned and crisp. Remove from pan and set aside. Save 1 tsp. of bacon grease and discard the rest.
3. Add onion and celery to bacon grease and sauté for 5 minutes.
4. Mix together vinegar, water, sugar, salt, and pepper.
5. Over low heat, add vinegar mixture to the onion and celery in the skillet. Bring to a boil; pour over potatoes and stir gently to combine.

Tip:
My family prefers this cold, however you can serve right away warm.

Warm Memories:
This has been a family Easter tradition for over 50 years. My grandmother taught me how to make this when I was a teen.

Exchange List Values
- Carbohydrate 0.5   • Fat 0.5
- Vegetable 1.0

Basic Nutritional Values
- Calories 185   • Sodium 455 mg
  (Calories from Fat 35) • Potassium 490 gm
- Total Fat 4 gm   • Total Carb 32 gm
  (Saturated Fat 1.3 gm, • Dietary Fiber 3 gm
  Trans Fat 0.0 gm,   • Sugars 9 gm
  Polyunsat Fat 0.5 gm, • Protein 5 gm
  Monounsat Fat 1.7 gm) • Phosphorus 90 gm
- Cholesterol 10 mg

Red Bliss Potato Salad

Tim Smith
Wynnewood, PA

Makes 12 servings,
about 5½ oz. per serving

Prep. Time: 15 minutes
Cooking Time: 20–25 minutes
Chilling Time: 2½ hours

12 medium Red Bliss potatoes, about 5 oz. each
3 ribs celery, diced
2 hard boiled eggs, diced
¼ cup light, reduced-fat mayonnaise
2 Tbsp. white vinegar
1 Tbsp. Old English dry mustard
1 tsp. celery seed
1 tsp. white pepper
1 tsp. black pepper
salt to taste

1. Cook whole potatoes until medium soft, but still firm. Drain. Allow to cool, then dice.
2. Put diced potatoes in large bowl. Add rest of ingredients and stir gently.
3. Chill in refrigerator for 2 hours before serving.

Tip:
Do not overcook the potatoes! You want them soft but not soft like you're making mashed potatoes!

Warm Memories:
Everybody in my family loves this potato salad. My nieces and nephews always ask if I'm bringing it.

Exchange List Values
- Starch 2.0   • Fat 0.5

Basic Nutritional Values
- Calories 170   • Sodium 75 mg
  (Calories from Fat 20) • Potassium 650 gm
- Total Fat 2 gm   • Total Carb 33 gm
  (Saturated Fat 0.4 gm, • Dietary Fiber 3 gm
  Trans Fat 0.0 gm,   • Sugars 2 gm
  Polyunsat Fat 0.9 gm, • Protein 4 gm
  Monounsat Fat 0.6 gm) • Phosphorus 165 gm
- Cholesterol 30 mg

Summer Salad

June S. Groff
Denver, PA

Makes 8 servings,
about 6 oz. per serving

Prep. Time: 20 minutes
Cooking Time for Couscous: 10 minutes

Salad:
1½ cups cooked
    garbanzo beans
½ cup chopped onion
½ cup chopped celery
½ cup chopped
    cucumber
½ cup chopped red
    grapes
2 medium tomatoes,
    chopped
2.2-oz. can sliced black
    olives, drained
¾ cup couscous, cooked
    and cooled

Dressing:
½ cup olive oil
½ cup lemon juice *or*
    vinegar
⅛ tsp. minced garlic
1 Tbsp. Dijon mustard
¼ tsp. dried oregano
¼ tsp. dried basil
1 Tbsp. sugar
⅛ tsp. coriander
⅛ tsp. onion powder
1 tsp. dried parsley

2 Tbsp. freshly grated
    Parmesan cheese

1. Toss salad ingredients together.
2. Mix the dressing ingredients together. Pour dressing over salad mixture and toss.

3. Top with parmesan cheese.

Exchange List Values
- Starch 1.5   • Fat 3.0
- Carbohydrate 0.5

Basic Nutritional Values
- Calories 270   • Sodium 130 mg
  (Calories from Fat 145) • Potassium 285 gm
- Total Fat 16 gm   • Total Carb 28 gm
  (Saturated Fat 2.3 gm, • Dietary Fiber 4 gm
  Trans Fat 0.0 gm,   • Sugars 7 gm
  Polyunsat Fat 2.0 gm, • Protein 6 gm
  Monounsat Fat 10.9 gm) • Phosphorus 85 gm
- Cholesterol 0 mg

Marinated
Italian Salad

Tammy Smith
Dorchester, WI

Makes 8 servings,
about 6 oz. per serving

Prep. Time: 30 minutes
Chilling Time: 1 hour

Salad:
1 cup baby carrots,
    sliced lengthwise
1 cup chopped sweet red
    pepper
1 cup chopped celery
1 cup diced, peeled jicama
1 cup diced zucchini
1 cup small cauliflower
    florets
½ cup chopped red onion
½ cup sliced green onion
    tops
15-oz. can black beans,
    rinsed and drained
3 oz. turkey pepperoni
    slices, cut in half

3 oz. 75%-reduced-fat
    sharp cheddar cheese,
    diced *or* cubed

Dressing:
0.7-oz. packet Italian
    salad dressing mix, dry
¼ cup apple cider
    vinegar
3 Tbsp. water
⅓ cup olive oil

1. Place salad ingredients in large bowl.
2. Whisk together dressing mix, vinegar, water, and oil. Drizzle over salad. Toss to coat.
3. Chill at least 1 hour. Add cheese just before serving.

Tips:
1. You may use any vegetables you wish. Try to use 7–8 cups of vegetables for 1 recipe of dressing. Bacon bits, nuts and seeds also work well if added just before serving. Cubed pepperoni sticks or turkey ham can replace pepperoni slices.
2. For a change, serve this salad as a sauce over pasta.
3. Jicama is a Mexican vegetable with a mild sweet taste and a nice crunch. Look for it in the produce section of a big grocery store.

Exchange List Values
- Starch 0.5   • Lean Meat 1.0
- Vegetable 1.0   • Fat 2.0

Basic Nutritional Values
- Calories 205   • Sodium 600 mg
  (Calories from Fat 110) • Potassium 420 gm
- Total Fat 12 gm   • Total Carb 16 gm
  (Saturated Fat 2.4 gm, • Dietary Fiber 5 gm
  Trans Fat 0.0 gm,   • Sugars 5 gm
  Polyunsat Fat 1.4 gm, • Protein 10 gm
  Monounsat Fat 7.2 gm) • Phosphorus 190 gm
- Cholesterol 20 mg

Mexican Salad

Jan Pembleton
Arlington, TX

*Makes 10 servings,
about 6 oz. per serving*

Prep. Time: 20 minutes
Cooking Time: 15 minutes
Cooling Time: 30 minutes

1 head lettuce
¾ lb. 93%-lean ground
  beef
2 tomatoes, chopped
16-oz. can kidney beans,
  drained
¾ cup freshly grated
  cheddar cheese
¼ cup diced onion
¼ cup sliced black olives,
  sliced
1 avocado, diced
2 oz. taco chips, crushed

Sauce:
  8 oz. fat-free Thousand
    Island dressing
  1 Tbsp. dry low-sodium
    taco seasoning (see
    page 271)
  1 Tbsp. hot sauce
  1 Tbsp. sugar

1. Wash lettuce and tear
into bite-size pieces.
2. Brown, drain and cool
ground meat.
3. Combine all salad
ingredients except taco chips.
Set aside.
4. Combine all sauce
ingredients. Pour sauce over
salad and toss thoroughly.
5. Immediately before
serving, add taco chips.

Exchange List Values
• Starch 0.5   • Med-Fat Meat 1.0
• Carbohydrate 0.5   • Fat 0.5
• Vegetable 1.0

Basic Nutritional Values
• Calories 215   • Sodium 380 mg
  (Calories from Fat 70) • Potassium 495 gm
• Total Fat 8 gm   • Total Carb 23 gm
  (Saturated Fat 2.5 gm, • Dietary Fiber 5 gm
  Trans Fat 0.1 gm,   • Sugars 7 gm
  Polyunsat Fat 1.0 gm,   • Protein 13 gm
  Monounsat Fat 4.0 gm) • Phosphorus 180 gm
• Cholesterol 25 mg

Southwestern Bean Salad

Ellie Oberholtzer
Ronks, PA

Makes 7 cups, 1 cup per serving

Prep. Time: 20 minutes
Chilling Time: 2 hours

15-oz. can kidney beans,
  rinsed and drained
15-oz. can black beans,
  rinsed and drained
15-oz. can garbanzo beans,
  rinsed and drained
2 celery ribs, sliced
1 medium red onion, diced
1 medium tomato, diced
1 cup frozen corn, thawed

Dressing:
  ¾ cup thick and chunky
    salsa
  ¼ cup vegetable oil *or*
    olive oil
  ¼ cup lime juice
  1–2 tsp. chili powder
  ½ tsp. ground cumin

1. In a bowl, combine
beans, celery, onion, tomato,
and corn.
2. Mix together salsa, oil,
lime juice, chili powder, and
cumin.
3. Pour over bean mixture
and toss. Cover and chill 2
hours.

Tips:
  I like to serve this salad
with kale leaves lining the
bowl. It's also good with
a dollop of sour cream on
individual servings.

Exchange List Values
• Starch 2.0   • Fat 1.5
• Lean Meat 1.0

Basic Nutritional Values
• Calories 265   • Sodium 350 mg
  (Calories from Fat 80) • Potassium 645 gm
• Total Fat 9 gm   • Total Carb 37 gm
  (Saturated Fat 0.8 gm, • Dietary Fiber 10 gm
  Trans Fat 0.0 gm,   • Sugars 6 gm
  Polyunsat Fat 3.0 gm,   • Protein 11 gm
  Monounsat Fat 5.3 gm) • Phosphorus 205 gm
• Cholesterol 0 mg

Corn & Black Bean Salad

Jamie Mowry
Arlington, TX

*Makes 5 cups, 5 servings,
1 cup per serving*

Prep. Time: 15 minutes
Chilling Time: 30 minutes

4 medium ears sweet corn,
  kernels cut off (2 cups)
1 large red bell pepper,
  diced
½ cup thinly sliced green
  onions
½ cup chopped fresh
  cilantro
15½-oz. can black beans,
  rinsed and drained
¼ cup red wine vinegar
2 tsp. canola oil
1 tsp. sugar
½ tsp. garlic powder
½ tsp. ground cumin
½ tsp. freshly ground black
  pepper
salt to taste

1. Combine corn, bell
pepper, onions, cilantro, and
beans in a medium bowl.
2. Whisk together vinegar,
oil, sugar, garlic powder,
cumin, black pepper, and salt.
3. Stir dressing gently into
corn mixture.
4. Cover and chill for 30
minutes.

Good Go-Alongs:

This is wonderful alone or
especially good served with
fish. We enjoyed it with chips
sitting outside at the lake on
one Memorial Day in Texas.

Exchange List Values
- Starch 1.5   • Lean Meat 1.0

Basic Nutritional Values
- Calories 160   • Sodium 70 mg
  (Calories from Fat 25) • Potassium 435 gm
- Total Fat 3 gm   • Total Carb 29 gm
  (Saturated Fat 0.3 gm, • Dietary Fiber 7 gm
  Trans Fat 0.0 gm,   • Sugars 6 gm
  Polyunsat Fat 1.1 gm,   • Protein 7 gm
  Monounsat Fat 1.4 gm)   • Phosphorus 135 gm
- Cholesterol 0 mg

Chili Cornbread Salad

Marie Davis
Mineral Ridge, OH

*Makes 12 servings,
about 7 oz. per serving*

Prep. Time: 30 minutes
**Cooking/Baking Time: 20–25
minutes**
Chilling Time: 2 hours

Cornbread:
  8½-oz. pkg. corn bread
    mix
  4-oz. can chopped green
    chilies, undrained
  ⅛ tsp. ground cumin
  ⅛ tsp. dried oregano
  pinch of sage

Dressing:
  ½ cup low-fat mayonnaise
  1 cup fat-free sour cream
  1½ tsp. dried parsley
  ½ tsp. dried dill weed
  ½ tsp. onion powder
  ¼ tsp. garlic powder
  ½ tsp. dried minced
    garlic
  ⅛ tsp. black pepper

---

2 15-oz. cans pinto *or* black
  beans, drained
2 15¼-oz. cans whole
  kernel corn, drained
3 medium tomatoes,
  chopped
1 cup chopped green
  pepper
1 cup chopped green
  onions *or* red onion
1 cup 75%-reduced fat
  shredded cheddar cheese

1. Prepare corn bread
batter according to package
directions. Stir in chilies,
cumin, oregano, and sage.
Spread into greased 8" square
baking dish.
2. Bake at 400° for 20–25
minutes or until knife comes
out clean in center. Cool.
3. In a small bowl, combine
mayonnaise, sour cream, and
dressing mix; set aside.
4. Crumble half of corn-
bread into 9×13 baking dish.
5. Layer with half of the
beans, mayonnaise mixture,
corn, tomatoes, green pepper,
onions, and cheese.
6. Repeat layers (dish will
be very full).
7. Cover and refrigerate for
2 hours.

Tips:

1. If you want a less-full
serving dish, make it in a
9×13 plus an 8×8 pan.
2. The cornbread season-
ings are optional. Just use
regular cornbread if you
wish. The cheese is optional
as well. This really is almost
a meal in itself!

Karen Waggoner
Joplin, MO

Swedish Salad

Anne Townsend
Albuquerque, NM

Makes 6 cups, 1 cup per serving
Prep. Time: 20 minutes

14½-oz. can French style
  green beans, rinsed and
  drained
11-oz. can white shoepeg
  corn, rinsed and drained
1 cup frozen peas, thawed
2-oz. jar chopped pimento
  or half red bell pepper,
  chopped
1 cup chopped celery
1 cup chopped onion
⅛ tsp. salt
⅛ tsp. pepper

Dressing:
¼ cup sugar
¼ cup canola oil
¼ cup cider vinegar

1. In medium size bowl,
combine green beans, corn,
peas, pimento, celery, onion,
salt, and pepper.

2. Combine dressing
ingredients and mix well.
Pour on top of salad and stir.

Tip:
  It is best to use a slotted
spoon for serving.

Good Go-Alongs:
  Hamburgers and potato
salad go well with this
favorite salad.

Fresh Corn and Tomato Salad

Dawn Landowski
Eau Claire, WI

*Makes 12 servings,
about ⅔ cup per serving*

**Prep. Time: 20 minutes
Standing Time: 15 minutes-2
  hours**

4¼ cups fresh, raw corn
  cut off the cob (about
  6 medium ears corn,
  husked)
2 cups halved grape tomatoes
3 oz. fresh mozzarella, cut
  into small cubes

4–6 scallions, thinly sliced
3 Tbsp. white vinegar
2 tsp. salt
fresh ground pepper
¼ cup extra virgin olive oil
1½ cups fresh basil leaves,
  torn

1. Stir together corn,
tomatoes, mozzarella, and
scallions in a large bowl.
2. Whisk vinegar, salt, and
pepper together in a small
bowl. Gradually whisk in oil
to make a smooth dressing.
3. Pour vinaigrette over
salad and toss to coat.
4. Cover and let set for 15
minutes to 2 hours. Right
before serving, tear the basil
over the salad and stir.

Tip:
  For cutting corn off the
cob, I put the end of the cob
in a Bundt pan and cut down.
Kernels fall into pan.

Warm Memories:
  People can't believe the
corn is raw – there are always
discussions!

Asian Rice Salad

Lois Mae E. Kuh
Penfield, NY

*Makes 8 servings,
about 5½ oz. per serving*

Prep. Time: 15 minutes
Chilling Time: 12 hours

Salad:
- 3 cups cooked rice at room temperature
- 1 cup canned bean sprouts, drained
- 8-oz. fresh spinach, chopped
- 1 red pepper, sliced thin
- 1 cup thinly sliced mushrooms
- ½ cup diced shallots
- ½ cup cashews

Dressing:
- ¼ cup light soy sauce
- ⅓ cup canola oil
- 1 clove garlic, minced

1. Toss together rice, sprouts, spinach, pepper, mushrooms, and shallots.

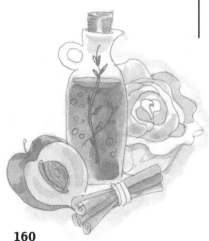

2. Mix soy sauce, oil, and garlic. Pour over salad ingredients and mix.

3. Refrigerate for at least 12 hours. Add cashews just before serving.

Exchange List Values
- Starch 1.5
- Vegetable 1.0
- Fat 2.0

Basic Nutritional Values
- Calories 235 (Calories from Fat 115)
- Total Fat 13 gm (Saturated Fat 1.5 gm, Trans Fat 0.0 gm, Polyunsat Fat 3.3 gm, Monounsat Fat 8.1 gm)
- Cholesterol 0 mg
- Sodium 360 mg
- Potassium 350 gm
- Total Carb 25 gm
- Dietary Fiber 2 gm
- Sugars 2 gm
- Protein 5 gm
- Phosphorus 115 gm

Picnic Pea Salad

Mary Kathryn Yoder
Harrisonville, MO

*Makes 6 servings,
about 3½ oz. per serving*

Prep. Time: 30 minutes
Chilling Time: 1 hour

- 10-oz. pkg. frozen peas, thawed
- ¼ cup chopped onion *or* green onions
- ½ cup chopped celery
- ½ cup fat-free sour cream
- 2 Tbsp. low-fat mayonnaise
- ¼ tsp. salt
- 1 tsp. dried dill weed
- ¼ tsp. pepper
- ⅓ cup Spanish peanuts
- ¼ cup fried and crumbled bacon
- 1 cup cherry tomatoes for garnish, *optional*

1. Mix peas, onion, celery, sour cream, mayonnaise, salt, dill weed, and pepper. Chill.

2. Just before serving, stir in peanuts. Garnish with bacon and tomatoes.

Tip:
Fry out bacon ahead of time and let cool.

Variation:
Omit celery, peanuts, and dill weed. Add a chopped hardboiled egg and a dash of garlic powder.

Dorothy VanDeest
Memphis, TN

Exchange List Values
- Starch 0.5
- Carbohydrate 0.5
- Med-Fat Meat 1.0

Basic Nutritional Values
- Calories 135 (Calories from Fat 65)
- Total Fat 7 gm (Saturated Fat 1.4 gm, Trans Fat 0.0 gm, Polyunsat Fat 1.9 gm, Monounsat Fat 2.7 gm)
- Cholesterol 5 mg
- Sodium 365 mg
- Potassium 230 gm
- Total Carb 13 gm
- Dietary Fiber 3 gm
- Sugars 4 gm
- Protein 8 gm
- Phosphorus 120 gm

Wash and dry whole lettuce leaves. Put a scoop of tuna or egg salad in each one. Enjoy your lettuce boats! You can also slip these into wraps or pitas.
Donna Conta, Saylorsburg, PA

Cherry Wild Rice Salad

Edie Moran
West Babylon, NY

Makes 8 servings,
about 1 cup per serving

Prep. Time: 20 minutes
Cooking Time (for rice): 35
minutes
Chilling Time: 30 minutes

2 cups snow peas, chopped
    in half
2 cups cooked wild rice,
    cooled
1 cup cooked long grain
    rice, cooled
8-oz. can sliced water
    chestnuts, drained
1 cup dried cherries
½ cup celery, sliced thin
¼ cup chopped green
    onions
¾ cup cashews, halved and
    toasted

Dressing:
    3 Tbsp. sugar
    3 Tbsp. cider vinegar
    4½ tsp. light soy sauce
    1 garlic clove, peeled
    ¾ tsp. minced fresh
        ginger root

1. Toast the cashews in
a medium oven or toaster
oven for 5 minutes or until
fragrant. Cool.
    2. In a large bowl, combine
peas, cooled rice, water
chestnuts, cherries, celery,
onions, and cashews.
    3. Combine dressing
ingredients in the blender and
process until well blended.

4. Pour dressing over rice
mixture and toss to coat.
Cover and refrigerate until
serving.

Tip:
    It can be made the day
before and add dressing an
hour before serving.

Warm Memories:
    We always serve it at our
annual cousins' reunion. I
double the recipe for that.

Exchange List Values
- Starch 1.0
- Fruit 1.0
- Carbohydrate 0.5
- Vegetable 1.0
- Fat 1.0

Basic Nutritional Values
- Calories 250
  (Calories from Fat 55)
- Total Fat 6 gm
  (Saturated Fat 1.2 gm,
  Trans Fat 0.0 gm,
  Polyunsat Fat 1.1 gm,
  Monounsat Fat 3.6 gm)
- Cholesterol 0 mg
- Sodium 205 mg
- Potassium 290 gm
- Total Carb 44 gm
- Dietary Fiber 4 gm
- Sugars 20 gm
- Protein 5 gm
- Phosphorus 235 gm

Tabouli

Ellen Helmuth
Debec, New Brunswick

Makes 8 servings,
about 4 oz. per serving

Prep. Time: 20 minutes
Standing Time: 30–40 minutes
Chilling Time: 8 hours or
overnight

1 cup dry bulgur wheat
1½ cups boiling water
1 tsp. salt
¼ cup lemon juice
¼ cup olive oil
1 cup chopped fresh parsley
1 cup chopped fresh mint
2–3 tomatoes, chopped
2 cloves garlic, crushed
½ cup chopped scallions,
    or onions, chopped
pepper to taste

1. Pour boiling water over
bulgur wheat and let stand
approximately ½ hour until
wheat is fluffy. Drain or
squeeze liquid from wheat
    2. Add all remaining
ingredients and mix well.
    3. Chill overnight before
serving.

Exchange List Values
- Starch 0.5
- Vegetable 1.0
- Fat 1.0

Basic Nutritional Values
- Calories 120
  (Calories from Fat 65)
- Total Fat 7 gm
  (Saturated Fat 1.0 gm,
  Trans Fat 0.0 gm,
  Polyunsat Fat 0.8 gm,
  Monounsat Fat 5.0 gm)
- Cholesterol 0 mg
- Sodium 305 mg
- Potassium 215 gm
- Total Carb 13 gm
- Dietary Fiber 4 gm
- Sugars 1 gm
- Protein 2 gm
- Phosphorus 40 gm

Carrot Raisin Salad

Shelia Heil
Lancaster, PA

Makes 6 servings,
about 4 oz. per serving

Prep. Time: 10 minutes
Chilling Time: 4–12 hours

5 large carrots, shredded
1 cup raisins
⅔ cup plain fat-free yogurt
4 Tbsp. reduced-fat
    mayonnaise
2 tsp. honey

1. Combine ingredients.
2. Chill for several hours or
overnight. Serve cold.

Warm Memories:

My mother often made a
recipe like this for guests in
our home. Adds color to a
meat and potato meal.

Exchange List Values
• Fruit 1.5   • Fat 0.5
• Vegetable 1.0

Basic Nutritional Values
• Calories 140   • Sodium 145 mg
  (Calories from Fat 20) • Potassium 440 gm
• Total Fat 2.5 gm   • Total Carb 29 gm
  (Saturated Fat 0.4 gm, • Dietary Fiber 3 gm
  Trans Fat 0.0 gm,   • Sugars 21 gm
  Polyunsat Fat 1.4 gm, • Protein 3 gm
  Monounsat Fat 0.7 gm) • Phosphorus 90 gm
• Cholesterol 5 mg

Pickled Beets, Sugar-Free

Sue Hamilton
Benson, AZ

Makes 4 cups,
½ cup per serving, 8 servings

Prep. Time: 5 minutes
Cooking Time: 2 minutes
Chilling Time: 24 hours

2 15-oz. cans sliced beets
⅔ cup vinegar
1 cup granular Splenda
½ tsp. pumpkin pie spice
1 tsp. vanilla
¼ tsp. butter powder
1 small onion, thinly sliced

1. Drain beets and save the
liquid.
2. Combine the liquid with
vinegar, Splenda, pumpkin
pie spice, vanilla, and butter
powder in a microwaveable
container. Heat on high for 2
minutes.
3. In a large jar or glass
dish, layer the beets and
onions. Pour hot liquid
mixture over top.
4. Refrigerate 24 hours or
longer. Drain and serve.

Tips:

1. Save the liquid when
you serve your beets. You
can bring it to a boil and then
pour it over new beets and
onions.
2. 1 cup sugar can be
substituted for the Splenda.

Exchange List Values
• Vegetable 1.0

Basic Nutritional Values
• Calories 30   • Sodium 140 mg
  (Calories from Fat 0) • Potassium 125 gm
• Total Fat 0 gm   • Total Carb 7 gm
  (Saturated Fat 0.0 gm, • Dietary Fiber 1 gm
  Trans Fat 0.0 gm,   • Sugars 5 gm
  Polyunsat Fat 0.0 gm, • Protein 1 gm
  Monounsat Fat 0.0 gm) • Phosphorus 15 gm
• Cholesterol 0 mg

Marinated Asparagus

Rebecca Meyerkorth
Wamego, KS

Makes 10 servings,
about 1¾ oz. per serving

Prep. Time: 20 minutes
Cooking Time: 5–10 minutes
Chilling Time: 2 -12 hours

½ cup brown sugar
½ cup cider vinegar
½ cup light soy sauce
½ cup vegetable oil
4 tsp. lemon juice
1 tsp. garlic powder
2 lbs. asparagus
¼ cup sliced almonds,
    optional

1. In saucepan, stir together
brown sugar, vinegar, soy sauce,
oil, juice, and garlic powder.
2. Bring to a boil and
simmer 5 minutes. Cool.
3. Meanwhile, microwave
or cook asparagus until just
crisp tender. Plunge it in cold
water to stop the cooking.
Drain well.
4. In large re-sealable
plastic bag, put asparagus and
marinade. Zip bag and turn to

coat asparagus.

5. Refrigerate at least 2 hours or overnight, turning occasionally.

6. Drain and discard marinade. Place asparagus on plate to serve. Sprinkle with sliced almonds, if desired.

Warm Memories:

A terrific way to use fresh asparagus in warm weather.

Exchange List Values
• Vegetable 1.0

Basic Nutritional Values
• Calories 30	• Sodium 60 mg
(Calories from Fat 15)	• Potassium 105 mg
• Total Fat 2 gm	• Total Carb 3 gm
(Saturated Fat 0.1 gm,	• Dietary Fiber 1 gm
Trans Fat 0.0 gm,	• Sugars 2 gm
Polyunsat Fat 0.4 gm,	• Protein 1 gm
Monounsat Fat 0.9 gm)	• Phosphorus 25 gm
• Cholesterol 0 mg	

Tangy Tomato Slices

Mary H. Nolt
East Earl, PA

*Makes 12 servings,
about 4 oz. per serving*

**Prep. Time: 20 minutes
Chilling Time: 2–4 hours**

Marinade:
1 cup olive oil
⅓ cup vinegar
¼ cup minced fresh
   parsley
3 Tbsp. minced fresh
   basil *or* 1 Tbsp. dried
   basil

1 Tbsp. sugar
½ tsp. pepper
1 tsp. salt
½ tsp. dry mustard
½ tsp. garlic powder

1 medium sweet onion,
   thinly sliced
6 large tomatoes, thinly
   sliced

1. Mix marinade in a shaker jar.
2. Layer onions and tomatoes in a shallow dish.
3. Pour the marinade over onions and tomatoes. Cover and refrigerate for several hours.
4. Lift tomatoes out of marinade with slotted spoon and serve.

Warm Memories:

Our daughter has a big greenhouse with tomatoes, and at picnics or gatherings when tomatoes are in season, she always brings this dish.

Exchange List Values
• Vegetable 1.0	• Fat 0.5

Basic Nutritional Values
• Calories 45	• Sodium 30 mg
(Calories from Fat 20)	• Potassium 245 gm
• Total Fat 2.5 gm	• Total Carb 5 gm
(Saturated Fat 0.3 gm,	• Dietary Fiber 1 gm
Trans Fat 0.0 gm,	• Sugars 4 gm
Polyunsat Fat 0.3 gm,	• Protein 1 gm
Monounsat Fat 1.7 gm)	• Phosphorus 30 gm
• Cholesterol 0 mg	

Salad Tomatoes

Lois Ostrander, Lebanon, PA

*Makes 6 servings,
about 3 oz. per serving*

**Prep. Time: 15 minutes
Cooking Time: 10 minutes**

3 medium tomatoes
1 Tbsp. instant minced onion
¼ cup chopped fresh
   parsley
½ cup water
½ tsp. salt
½ cup cider vinegar
2 Tbsp. granular Splenda
⅛ tsp. pepper

1. Peel tomatoes and slice. Overlap slices in a shallow serving bowl or pie plate.
2. Sprinkle with parsley and onion.
3. Combine vinegar, water, Splenda, salt and pepper in a small saucepan. Heat to boiling, stirring constantly.
4. Drizzle hot dressing over tomatoes. Chill until serving time.

Tip:

Use medium to firm tomatoes. Substitute ¼ cup fresh minced onion for instant.

Exchange List Values
• Vegetable 1.0

Basic Nutritional Values
• Calories 25	• Sodium 200 mg
(Calories from Fat 0)	• Potassium 205 gm
• Total Fat 0 gm	• Total Carb 4 gm
(Saturated Fat 0.0 gm,	• Dietary Fiber 1 gm
Trans Fat 0.0 gm,	• Sugars 3 gm
Polyunsat Fat 0.1 gm,	• Protein 1 gm
Monounsat Fat 0.0 gm)	• Phosphorus 20 gm
• Cholesterol 0 mg	

Marinated Carrots

Sarah Fisher
Christiana, PA

*Makes 12 servings,
about 3½ oz. per serving*

Prep. Time: 15 minutes
Cooking Time: 5–7 minutes
Chilling Time: 12 hours

2 lbs. carrots, sliced
1 large onion, diced
1 large green pepper,
    chopped
8-oz. can tomato sauce
1 cup granular Splenda
½ cup salad oil
¾ cup apple cider vinegar
1 tsp. salt
1 tsp. black pepper

1. Cook carrots in a little water until crisp-tender. Drain. Cool.

2. Combine cooled carrots, peppers, and onions in a bowl.

3. In a saucepan, mix tomato sauce, sugar, oil, vinegar, salt, and pepper. Bring to a boil, stirring constantly.

4. Pour hot mixture over vegetables and stir. Cool and refrigerate overnight.

5. Before serving, drain the carrots of any marinade that was not absorbed.

Tip:
    Using baby carrots for this recipe is great for saving chopping time, and is "extra delicious."

Exchange List Values
• Vegetable 2.0

Basic Nutritional Values
• Calories 50
    (Calories from Fat 15)
• Total Fat 2 gm
    (Saturated Fat 0.1 gm,
    Trans Fat 0.0 gm,
    Polyunsat Fat 0.4 gm,
    Monounsat Fat 0.8 gm)
• Cholesterol 0 mg
• Sodium 85 mg
• Potassium 280 gm
• Total Carb 9 gm
• Dietary Fiber 3 gm
• Sugars 5 gm
• Protein 1 gm
• Phosphorus 35 gm

Southwest Copper Pennies

Sue Hamilton
Benson, AZ

*Makes 8 servings,
about 4 oz. per serving*

Prep. Time: 10 minutes
Cooking Time: 3 minutes
Chilling Time: 12 hours

1 lb. carrots, peeled and
    sliced
1 small onion, diced
1 green pepper, diced
1 cup peach *or* pineapple
    salsa
½ cup granular Splenda
⅓ cup vinegar

1. In a glass bowl, combine the carrots, onion, and green pepper.

2. Heat the salsa, Splenda, and vinegar on stovetop or microwave until hot and steaming.

3. Pour over carrots. Stir. Allow to marinate 12 hours or more before serving.

Warm Memories:
    I took them to a gathering and I only told the person with diabetes that they were sugar-free. When they were all gone and people asked for the recipe, I had to tell them.

Exchange List Values
• Carbohydrate 0.5   • Vegetable 1.0

Basic Nutritional Values
• Calories 50
    (Calories from Fat 0)
• Total Fat 0 gm
    (Saturated Fat 0.0 gm,
    Trans Fat 0.0 gm,
    Polyunsat Fat 0.1 gm,
    Monounsat Fat 0.0 gm)
• Cholesterol 0 mg
• Sodium 185 mg
• Potassium 220 gm
• Total Carb 12 gm
• Dietary Fiber 2 gm
• Sugars 8 gm
• Protein 1 gm
• Phosphorus 25 gm

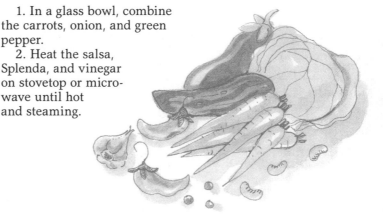

Sour Cream Cucumber Salad

Mary Jones
Marengo, OH

*Makes 6 servings,
about 5 oz. per serving*

Prep. Time: 20–30 minutes

3 medium cucumbers,
  about 9 oz. each,
  unpeeled and sliced
  thinly
½ tsp. salt
½ cup finely chopped
  green onions
1 Tbsp. white vinegar
dash pepper, *optional*
¼ cup fat-free sour cream

1. Sprinkle cucumber with salt. Let stand 15 minutes. Drain liquid.
2. Add onions, vinegar and pepper.
3. Just before serving, stir in sour cream.

Exchange List Values
• Vegetable 1.0

Basic Nutritional Values
• Calories 30
  (Calories from Fat 0)
• Total Fat 0 gm
  (Saturated Fat 0.1 gm,
  Trans Fat 0.0 gm,
  Polyunsat Fat 0.0 gm,
  Monounsat Fat 0.0 gm)
• Cholesterol 0 mg
• Sodium 110 mg
• Potassium 220 gm
• Total Carb 7 gm
• Dietary Fiber 1 gm
• Sugars 3 gm
• Protein 1 gm
• Phosphorus 45 gm

Mixed Vegetable Salad

Sharon Miller
Holmesville, OH

*Makes 8 servings,
about 4½ oz. per serving*

*Prep. Time: 15 minutes
Cooking Time: 10 minutes
Standing Time: 15 minutes
Chilling Time: 8–12 hours*

16-oz. frozen mixed
  vegetables, thawed
15-oz. can kidney beans,
  rinsed and drained
½ cup chopped celery
½ cup chopped onion
½ cup chopped green *or*
  red pepper
¾ cup granular Splenda
1 Tbsp. cornstarch
½ cup vinegar

1. Cook mixed vegetables until crisp-tender. Drain.
2. Add kidney beans, celery, onion, and pepper.
3. In saucepan, combine sugar and cornstarch. Add vinegar.
4. Cook over low heat until thick, stirring constantly. Or microwave uncovered until thickened, stirring once or twice.
5. Cool for 15 minutes. Pour over vegetables. Refrigerate overnight for best flavor.

Tips:
  The cornstarch-vinegar mix eliminates the oil usually used in a salad of this type. I use this same sauce in 3-bean salad recipes or other similar recipes.

Exchange List Values
• Starch 1.0

Basic Nutritional Values
• Calories 105
  (Calories from Fat 0)
• Total Fat 0 gm
  (Saturated Fat 0.1 gm,
  Trans Fat 0.0 gm,
  Polyunsat Fat 0.2 gm,
  Monounsat Fat 0.0 gm)
• Cholesterol 0 mg
• Sodium 80 mg
• Potassium 295 gm
• Total Carb 20 gm
• Dietary Fiber 5 gm
• Sugars 5 gm
• Protein 5 gm
• Phosphorus 85 gm

Try adding your favorite herbs and spices to your "tried and true" recipes, and you might come up with something even better.

Jeanne Heyerly, Shipshewana, IN

Green Bean and Walnut Salad

Mary Wheatley
Mashpee, MA

*Makes 4 servings,
about 3¼ oz. per serving*

Prep. Time: 20 minutes
Cooking Time: 5–7 minutes

¾ lb. fresh green beans, trimmed
¼ cup walnut pieces
3 Tbsp. finely chopped fresh parsley
3 Tbsp. finely chopped onion
1 Tbsp. walnut *or* olive oil
1½ tsp. red wine vinegar
1 tsp. Dijon mustard
salt, to taste
freshly ground pepper, to taste

1. Steam beans in basket over boiling water for 4 minutes. Transfer to a medium serving bowl.
2. Toast walnuts in a small dry skillet, stirring frequently until fragrant, 3–5 minutes. Chop the toasted walnuts finely.
3. Stir parsley and onion into walnuts.
4. Whisk together oil, vinegar, and mustard. Add to green beans. Season with salt and pepper and top with walnut mixture.
5. Serve warm or at room temperature.

Tips:
1. You'll want to double or triple the recipe, since people come back for more.
2. Pecans or almonds can be substituted for the walnuts.

Good Go-Alongs:
This is a good alternative to the soggy green bean casseroles so often used for holidays.

Exchange List Values
• Vegetable 2.0   • Fat 1.5

Basic Nutritional Values
• Calories 110   • Sodium 35 mg
 (Calories from Fat 80)   • Potassium 170 gm
• Total Fat 9 gm   • Total Carb 8 gm
 (Saturated Fat 0.8 gm,   • Dietary Fiber 3 gm
 Trans Fat 0.0 gm,   • Sugars 2 gm
 Polyunsat Fat 5.8 gm,   • Protein 3 gm
 Monounsat Fat 1.5 gm)   • Phosphorus 50 gm
• Cholesterol 0 mg

Five Bean Salad

Jeanne Heyerly
Shipshewana, IN

*Makes 10 servings,
about 6 oz. per serving*

Prep. Time: 20 minutes
Chilling Time: 12 hours

15-oz. can green beans
15-oz. can wax beans
15-oz. can lima beans
15-oz. can kidney beans
15-oz. can garbanzo beans
1 green *or* red pepper, chopped
1 medium onion, chopped
1 large clove garlic, minced
¼ cup canola *or* light olive oil
¼ cup apple cider vinegar
6 Tbsp. granular Splenda
½ tsp. salt
½ tsp. pepper
½ tsp. dry mustard
¾ tsp. celery seed

1. Drain all beans and combine in a large bowl.
2. Heat until hot (but do not boil) the oil, vinegar, sugar, salt, pepper, mustard, and celery seed.
3. Mix with bean mixture and let stand overnight.
4. Add onion, green pepper, and garlic about 1 hour before serving.

Tips:
1. Omit dry mustard, celery seed, and garlic. Serve with a slotted spoon. If there is another type of bean you like that's not listed, add it; or you could double up on the kinds you do like.
Jean Halloran
Green Bay, WI

2. Add ½ cup chopped celery and 2-oz jar pimento.
Joyce Kaut
Rochester, NY

Good Go-Alongs:
This always tastes so good along with casseroles that people bring to a church supper.

Exchange List Values
• Starch 1.5   • Fat 0.5
• Lean Meat 1.0

Basic Nutritional Values
• Calories 180   • Sodium 420 mg
 (Calories from Fat 55)   • Potassium 430 gm
• Total Fat 6 gm   • Total Carb 24 gm
 (Saturated Fat 0.5 gm,   • Dietary Fiber 7 gm
 Trans Fat 0.0 gm,   • Sugars 4 gm
 Polyunsat Fat 2.0 gm,   • Protein 8 gm
 Monounsat Fat 3.6 gm)   • Phosphorus 130 gm
• Cholesterol 0 mg

Sauerkraut Relish

Wilma Haberkamp
Fairbank, IA

Makes 24 cups, ¼ cup per serving
Prep. Time: 10–15 minutes

Dressing:
⅓ cup vinegar
1 cup granular Splenda
⅓ cup vegetable oil

1 quart jar sauerkraut,
  drained and rinsed
1 cup minced green pepper
1 cup minced celery
½ cup minced onion

1. Heat vinegar, Splenda, and oil to lukewarm so they dissolve and mix better. Cool.
2. Combine sauerkraut, green pepper, celery, and onion. Pour vinegar mixture over top and mix.

Tips:
This is better after it sets for a couple days and it keeps indefinitely in refrigerator. Serve it as salad, but it's also great on hot dogs or brats.

Exchange List Values
- Vegetable 1.0
- Fat 0.5

Basic Nutritional Values
- Calories 40
  (Calories from Fat 25)
- Total Fat 3 gm
  (Saturated Fat 0.2 gm,
  Trans Fat 0.0 gm,
  Polyunsat Fat 0.9 gm,
  Monounsat Fat 1.9 gm)
- Cholesterol 0 mg
- Sodium 155 mg
- Potassium 70 gm
- Total Carb 3 gm
- Dietary Fiber 1 gm
- Sugars 2 gm
- Protein 0 gm
- Phosphorus 10 gm

Going Away Salad

Judith Govotsos
Frederick, MD

*Makes 15 servings,
about 7 oz. per serving*
**Prep. Time: 30–45 minutes
Chilling Time: 8–12 hours**

15-oz. can kidney beans,
  drained
15-oz. can wax beans,
  drained
15-oz. can green beans,
  drained
15-oz. can garbanzo beans,
  drained
1 English cucumber, thinly
  sliced, 1 lb. total
2 carrots, thinly sliced
2–3 ribs celery, thinly
  sliced
1 medium to large onion,
  thinly sliced
1 medium cabbage
  shredded *or* 2 1 lb.
  packages coleslaw mix

Marinade:
1¾ tsp. salt
2 tsp. black pepper
⅔ cup white vinegar
½ cup canola oil
½ cup granular Splenda

1. Combine vegetables in a large lidded container.
2. In saucepan, combine salt, black pepper, vinegar, oil, and sugar. Bring to boil. Allow to cool.
3. Pour cooled marinade over vegetables.
4. Let the vegetables marinate in the refrigerator at least overnight before serving.

Tip:
I use a large orange Tupperware bowl with lid to take to church lunches (covered dish) or to family reunions.

Warm Memories:
My mom used to make this and it would last 1–2 weeks at home or we would take it to family reunions.

Good Go-Alongs:
Fried chicken or ham

Exchange List Values
- Starch 0.5
- Fat 1.5
- Vegetable 2.0

Basic Nutritional Values
- Calories 155
  (Calories from Fat 70)
- Total Fat 8 gm
  (Saturated Fat 0.6 gm,
  Trans Fat 0.0 gm,
  Polyunsat Fat 2.3 gm,
  Monounsat Fat 4.7 gm)
- Cholesterol 0 mg
- Sodium 440 mg
- Potassium 370 gm
- Total Carb 18 gm
- Dietary Fiber 5 gm
- Sugars 5 gm
- Protein 5 gm
- Phosphorus 90 gm

Chinese Cabbage Salad

Kim McEuen
Lincoln University, PA

*Makes 10 servings,
about 4 oz. per serving*

Prep. Time: 15–20 minutes
Cooking Time: 10 minutes

1 head bok choy, chopped
6 green onions, sliced
1 Tbsp. canola oil
1 pkg. Ramen noodles,
    crunched up, seasoning
    packs discarded
2 oz. slivered almonds
2 oz. sunflower seeds

Dressing:
    2 Tbsp. tarragon vinegar
    ½ Tbsp. light soy sauce
    2 Tbsp. canola oil
    2 Tbsp. granular Splenda

1. Mix bok choy and onions in a large bowl. Set aside.
2. In a frying pan, heat oil. Sauté noodles, almonds and sunflower seeds until lightly browned. Cool.
3. Mix dressing ingredients together.
4. Just before serving, mix together the bok choy mixture and noodle mixture.
5. Add the dressing, tossing to coat.

Exchange List Values
• Carbohydrate 1.0   • Fat 2.0

Basic Nutritional Values
• Calories 160
  (Calories from Fat 110)
• Total Fat 12 gm
  (Saturated Fat 1.5 gm,
  Trans Fat 0.0 gm,
  Polyunsat Fat 4.1 gm,
  Monounsat Fat 5.6 gm)
• Cholesterol 0 mg
• Sodium 110 mg
• Potassium 345 gm
• Total Carb 11 gm
• Dietary Fiber 3 gm
• Sugars 2 gm
• Protein 5 gm
• Phosphorus 140 gm

Creamy Coleslaw

Orpha M. Herr
Andover, NY

*Makes 10 servings,
about 4 oz. per serving*

Prep. Time: 15 minutes

1 head cabbage, shredded
1 medium carrot, shredded
3 Tbsp. low-fat mayonnaise
½ cup fat-free milk
1 tsp. prepared mustard
¼ cup vinegar
½ cup granular Splenda
⅛ tsp. salt

1. In a bowl, mix together cabbage and carrot. Set aside.
2. To make dressing, mix together mayonnaise, milk, mustard, vinegar, Splenda and salt.
3. Pour dressing over cabbage and carrots. Stir.

Good Go-Alongs:
    Bar-B-Q Chicken and baked beans

Exchange List Values
• Vegetable 1.0

Basic Nutritional Values
• Calories 40
  (Calories from Fat 0)
• Total Fat 0 gm
  (Saturated Fat 0.1 gm,
  Trans Fat 0.0 gm,
  Polyunsat Fat 0.2 gm,
  Monounsat Fat 0.1 gm)
• Cholesterol 0 mg
• Sodium 100 mg
• Potassium 200 gm
• Total Carb 8 gm
• Dietary Fiber 2 gm
• Sugars 5 gm
• Protein 2 gm
• Phosphorus 40 gm

We are a group of friends who meet once a week for quilting, embroidery, patchwork, or pottery. We usually carry bag lunches, but every now and then we have a potluck to celebrate a special occasion. One of our members takes cups and coffee pot into her house each week and puts them through her dishwasher. Any other dishes that we need, we bring and take home again. No disposables here! The key words at our potlucks are "ready-to-eat" dishes.

Jeanette Zacharias, Morden, Manitoba

Apple Coleslaw

Joy Uhler
Richardson, TX

Makes 9 servings,
about ½ cup per serving

Prep. Time: 20 minutes

2 cups coleslaw mix
1 unpeeled apple, cored
  and chopped
½ cup chopped celery
½ cup chopped green
  pepper
½ cup chopped broccoli,
  optional
¼ cup vegetable oil
2 Tbsp. lemon juice
1 Tbsp. honey

1. In a bowl, combine
coleslaw mix, apple, celery,
green pepper, and broccoli.
2. In a small bowl, whisk
together oil, lemon juice and
honey. Pour over coleslaw and
toss to coat evenly.

Tips:
1. This is a great recipe for
potlucks, as it doesn't contain
mayonnaise, so there's no
need to worry about it sitting
out.
2. Use red or yellow
peppers for even more color.

Good Go-Alongs:
It is perfect beside salmon.
It is a family must-have for
picnics!

Exchange List Values
- Fruit 0.5   • Fat 1.0

Basic Nutritional Values
- Calories 80
  (Calories from Fat 55)
- Total Fat 6 gm
  (Saturated Fat 0.5 gm,
  Trans Fat 0.0 gm,
  Polyunsat Fat 1.7 gm,
  Monounsat Fat 3.8 gm)
- Cholesterol 0 mg
- Sodium 10 mg
- Potassium 85 gm
- Total Carb 6 gm
- Dietary Fiber 1 gm
- Sugars 5 gm
- Protein 0 gm
- Phosphorus 10 gm

Cranberry Relish

Winifred Erb Paul
Scottdale, PA

Makes 7 cups,
28 servings, ¼ cup per serving

Prep. Time: 20 minutes
Chilling Time: at least a week

4 cups cranberries
2 apples, cored but not
  peeled, quartered
2 oranges, including rind,
  quartered
1 lemon, including rind,
  quartered
2 cups granular Splenda

1. Grind the whole fruit
together using meat grinder.
Alternatively, use a food
processor and pulse just until
most fruits are diced, but not
mushy.
2. Be sure to keep the juice
after fruits are ground. Add
sugar and let it set a week
in the refrigerator before
serving.

Tip:
To get a good grind from
a food processor, put in only
a few pieces of fruit – do not
fill up the processor bowl.
Push the pulse button once
and allow everything to come
to a stop before pushing the
button again. Look at the size
of the fruit carefully after
each pulse.

Warm Memories:
The Tillman Erb family
emigrated to Hesston, Kansas
in 1885. The brought this
recipe with them from
Lancaster County, PA. It was
always served at the Erb
Christmas get-together. My
husband makes it every year
and it goes well with turkey,
chicken or ham on Christmas
Day.

Exchange List Values
- Fruit 0.5

Basic Nutritional Values
- Calories 30
  (Calories from Fat 0)
- Total Fat 0 gm
  (Saturated Fat 0.0 gm,
  Trans Fat 0.0 gm,
  Polyunsat Fat 0.0 gm,
  Monounsat Fat 0.0 gm)
- Cholesterol 0 mg
- Sodium 0 mg
- Potassium 55 gm
- Total Carb 7 gm
- Dietary Fiber 2 gm
- Sugars 4 gm
- Protein 0 gm
- Phosphorus 5 gm

Thanksgiving Fruit Salad

Mary Vaughn Warye
West Liberty, OH

Makes 10 servings,
about 1 cup per serving

Prep. Time: 20 minutes
Chilling Time: 2½ hours

1 cup canned pineapple tidbits packed in juice, drained with ⅓ cup juice reserved
2 3-oz. pkgs. sugar-free cherry gelatin
2 cups hot water
1 cup cold water
2 Tbsp. lemon juice
¾ cup granular Splenda
1½ cups coarsely ground fresh cranberries
½ cup finely ground orange with peel
1 cup orange sections, halved
¾ cup diced celery
⅓ cup chopped walnuts

1. Drain pineapple, reserving ⅓ cup juice.
2. Dissolve gelatin in hot water. Stir in cold water, reserved pineapple juice, lemon juice and salt. Chill until partially set.
3. Meanwhile, stir Splenda into ground cranberries and orange.
4. Stir ground fruit mixture, pineapple, orange sections, celery and walnuts into partially set gelatin.
5. Pour into mold and chill until set, at least 2 hours.

Variation:
Add 1 cup red grapes to the partially set gelatin.
Betty Rutt
Elizabethtown, PA

Exchange List Values
• Fruit 1.0   • Fat 0.5

Basic Nutritional Values
• Calories 80   • Sodium 60 mg
  (Calories from Fat 20) • Potassium 150 gm
• Total Fat 2.5 gm   • Total Carb 13 gm
  (Saturated Fat 0.3 gm, • Dietary Fiber 2 gm
  Trans Fat 0.0 gm,   • Sugars 9 gm
  Polyunsat Fat 1.9 gm, • Protein 2 gm
  Monounsat Fat 0.4 gm) • Phosphorus 55 gm
• Cholesterol 0 mg

Cranberry Salad

Eileen M. Landis
Lebanon, PA

Makes 10 servings,
about 7 oz. per serving

Prep. Time: 15 minutes
Chilling Time: 2–4 hours

2 0.3-oz. pkgs. sugar-free cherry *or* raspberry gelatin
1½ cups boiling water
20-oz. can crushed pineapple, packed in juice, undrained
14-oz. can whole cranberry sauce
1½ cups halved red seedless grapes
½ cup chopped pecans *or* walnuts *(optional)*

1. Dissolve gelatin in hot water.

2. Add pineapple, cranberry sauce and grapes. Add nuts, if desired.
3. Chill until set.

Exchange List Values
• Fruit 1.0   • Carbohydrate 0.5

Basic Nutritional Values
• Calories 115   • Sodium 50 mg
  (Calories from Fat 0) • Potassium 115 gm
• Total Fat 0 gm   • Total Carb 26 gm
  (Saturated Fat 0.0 gm, • Dietary Fiber 1 gm
  Trans Fat 0.0 gm,   • Sugars 21 gm
  Polyunsat Fat 0.1 gm, • Protein 2 gm
  Monounsat Fat 0.0 gm) • Phosphorus 40 gm
• Cholesterol 0 mg

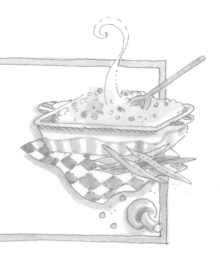

Vegetables

Donna's Baked Beans

Kathy Bless
Fayetteville, PA

*Makes 10 servings,
about 6½ oz. per serving*

Prep. Time: 15 minutes
**Cooking/Baking Time: 1 hour 15
 minutes**

2 oz. bacon, diced
1 Tbsp. canola oil
1 onion, diced
2 16-oz. cans pork and
 beans
2 16-oz. cans French-style
 green beans, drained
6-oz. can no-added-salt
 tomato paste
½ cup Splenda Brown
 Sugar Blend

1. Fry bacon until crisp and set aside. Discard drippings.
2. Heat the canola oil in the pan and fry the onion until soft.

3. Combine bacon, onion, beans, tomato paste, and brown sugar blend in a large bowl. Mix well.
4. Pour into a 2½-quart baking dish. Bake at 375° for 1 hour.

Exchange List Values

- Starch 1.0
- Carbohydrate 0.5
- Vegetable 1.0
- Fat 0.5

Basic Nutritional Values

- Calories 175
  (Calories from Fat 25)
- Total Fat 3 gm
  (Saturated Fat 0.6 gm,
  Trans Fat 0.0 gm,
  Polyunsat Fat 0.7 gm,
  Monounsat Fat 1.5 gm)
- Cholesterol 10 mg
- Sodium 590 mg
- Potassium 540 gm
- Total Carb 33 gm
- Dietary Fiber 6 gm
- Sugars 13 gm
- Protein 7 gm
- Phosphorus 145 gm

*If you don't cook but you want to contribute
to the church supper, arrange fresh green and red
seedless grapes in a beautiful glass dish.*

Pearl Zehr, New Wilmington, PA

Baked Navy Beans

Gloria Julien
Cornell, MI

*Makes 20 servings,
about ½ cup per serving*

Prep. Time: 20 minutes
Soaking Time: 8 hours or
overnight
Cooking Time: 9–11 hours

2 lbs. navy beans
¼ lb. bacon, cut up
1 cup ketchup
2 tsp. vinegar
1 onion, chopped
6 Tbsp. Splenda Brown
Sugar Blend
salt and pepper to taste

1. Wash and sort beans. Soak beans overnight or at least 8 hours. Bring beans to a boil in same liquid and cook until slightly tender, approximately ¾ hour.

2. Spoon beans into a 5-quart slow cooker and add all remaining ingredients.

3. Cook on low for 8–10 hours.

Exchange List Values
- Starch 2.0
- Lean Meat 1.0

Basic Nutritional Values
- Calories 215
  (Calories from Fat 35)
- Total Fat 4 gm
  (Saturated Fat 1.3 gm,
  Trans Fat 0.0 gm,
  Polyunsat Fat 0.9 gm,
  Monounsat Fat 1.7 gm)
- Cholesterol 5 mg
- Sodium 175 mg
- Potassium 495 gm
- Total Carb 36 gm
- Dietary Fiber 12 gm
- Sugars 5 gm
- Protein 10 gm
- Phosphorus 170 gm

Baked Beans

Barbara Hershey
Lititz, PA

*Makes 10 servings,
about 6½ oz. per serving*

Prep. Time: 30 minutes
Soaking Time: overnight
Cooking/Baking Time: 2½ hours

1 lb. dry northern beans
1 tsp. salt
½ tsp. baking soda
2 cups low-sodium V8 juice
1 small onion, minced
2 Tbsp. molasses
1 tsp. dry mustard
7 pieces bacon, fried and
drained
½ cup ketchup
¼ cup Splenda Brown
Sugar Blend

1. Cover beans with about 3" water and allow to soak overnight.

2. In morning, add salt and baking soda.

3. Bring to boil. Cook about 20–25 minutes until beans are soft. Drain.

4. Pour beans into large baking dish.

5. Add juice, onion, molasses, mustard, bacon, ketchup, and Splenda. Mix.

6. Bake at 325° for 2 hours or on low in slow cooker for 5–6 hours.

Tip:
If you don't have time to soak dry beans, you could purchase 6 16-oz. cans of northern beans and drain before adding other ingredients.

Good Go-Alongs:
Hamburgers, hot dogs, coleslaw

Exchange List Values
- Starch 1.5
- Carbohydrate 0.5
- Lean Meat 1.0

Basic Nutritional Values
- Calories 215
  (Calories from Fat 20)
- Total Fat 2.5 gm
  (Saturated Fat 0.8 gm,
  Trans Fat 0.0 gm,
  Polyunsat Fat 0.4 gm,
  Monounsat Fat 0.9 gm)
- Cholesterol 5 mg
- Sodium 565 mg
- Potassium 685 gm
- Total Carb 37 gm
- Dietary Fiber 9 gm
- Sugars 11 gm
- Protein 12 gm
- Phosphorus 225 gm

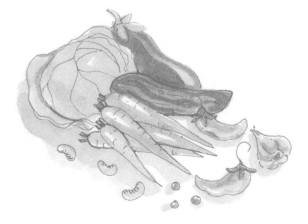

Best-in-the-West Beans

Lorraine Martin
Dryden, MI

*Makes 10 servings,
about ⅔ cup per serving*

Prep. Time: 20 minutes
Baking Time: 1½-5 hours

½ lb. ground beef
5 slices bacon, chopped
½ cup chopped onion
¼ cup brown sugar
¼ cup white sugar
¼ cup no-salt ketchup
¼ cup low-sodium,
    low-carb barbecue sauce
    (see page 270)
2 Tbsp. mustard
2 Tbsp. molasses
½ tsp. chili powder
½ tsp. pepper
1-lb. can kidney beans
1-lb. can butter beans
1-lb. can pork and beans

1. Brown ground beef and bacon. Drain. Add onion and cook until tender. Add all other ingredients except beans and mix well.
2. Drain kidney beans and butter beans. Add all beans to meat mixture. Pour into slow cooker or 3-quart casserole dish.
3. To prepare in slow cooker, cook on high for 1 hour. Reduce heat to low and cook for 4 hours.
4. To prepare in oven bake at 350° for 1 hour.

Exchange List Values
• Starch 1.5   • Lean Meat 1.0
• Carbohydrate 1.0

Basic Nutritional Values
• Calories 225   • Sodium 470 mg
  (Calories from Fat 35) • Potassium 615 gm
• Total Fat 4 gm   • Total Carb 37 gm
  (Saturated Fat 1.3 gm, • Dietary Fiber 6 gm
  Trans Fat 0.1 gm,   • Sugars 17 gm
  Polyunsat Fat 0.5 gm, • Protein 13 gm
  Monounsat Fat 1.6 gm) • Phosphorus 190 gm
• Cholesterol 20 mg

Triple Bean Bake

Phyllis Eller
LaVerne, CA

*Makes 10 servings,
about ⅔ cup per serving*

Prep. Time: 15 minutes
Baking Time: about 1 hour

1 cup chopped onion
½ cup chopped celery
1 Tbsp. canola oil
1 lb. pork and beans
1 lb. kidney beans rinsed
    and drained
2 10-oz. pkgs. lima beans,
    thawed
½ cup no-salt-added
    ketchup
1 Tbsp. brown sugar
1 Tbsp. vinegar
1½ tsp. dry mustard
¼ tsp. salt
⅛ tsp. garlic powder
¾ cup shredded reduced-
    fat Monterey Jack
    cheese, *divided*

1. Sauté onions and celery in oil until tender, about 5 minutes.
2. Add pork and beans, kidney beans, lima beans, ketchup, brown sugar, vinegar, mustard, salt, garlic powder and ¼ cup cheese.
3. Pour into 2-quart casserole dish.
4. Bake, uncovered at 350° for 40–50 minutes or until hot and bubbly. Remove from oven.
5. Sprinkle with remaining ½ cup cheese. Let stand 5 minutes before serving.

Exchange List Values
• Starch 2.0   • Lean Meat 1.0

Basic Nutritional Values
• Calories 210   • Sodium 430 mg
  (Calories from Fat 35) • Potassium 555 gm
• Total Fat 4 gm   • Total Carb 35 gm
  (Saturated Fat 1.4 gm, • Dietary Fiber 8 gm
  Trans Fat 0.0 gm,   • Sugars 9 gm
  Polyunsat Fat 0.7 gm, • Protein 11 gm
  Monounsat Fat 1.5 gm) • Phosphorus 205 gm
• Cholesterol 10 mg

Lima Bean Supreme

Lizzie Ann Yoder
Hartville, OH

Jean Butzer
Batavia, NY

Makes 9 servings,
about 6 oz. per serving

Prep. Time: 20 minutes
Soaking Time: 8 hours or
overnight
Cooking/Baking Time: 3 hours

1 lb. lima beans, dry
⅓ cup trans-fat free tub
    margarine
1 cup fat-free sour cream
¼ cup Splenda Brown
    Sugar Blend
1 Tbsp. dry mustard
1 tsp. molasses *or* 1 Tbsp.
    light corn syrup

1. Soak the dried beans
overnight covered in water.
Drain.
2. Cook until almost tender
in salted water. Drain, rinse,
and place in a deep casserole.
3. Mix well the butter, sour
cream, sugar, mustard, and
molasses. Pour over beans
and mix well.
4. Bake at 300° for 2
hours, stirring several times.

Mixture will be thin when
you take it from the oven, but
thickens as it cools.

Variations:
    Bake at 350° for 1 hour.
Joanne Warfel
Lancaster, PA

Tips:
    1. To speed up this
preparation, bring the beans
to a boil in the salted water.
Let stand a couple of hours
vs. overnight. Then proceed
to cook (boil) until almost
tender.
    2. May be served warm or
cold.

Warm Memories:
    This recipe was shared
many years ago by a friend
and is always a hit at potlucks
because it's different and
delicious. It's "comfort" food.

Exchange List Values
- Starch 1.5
- Lean Meat 1.0
- Carbohydrate 0.5
- Fat 0.5

Basic Nutritional Values
- Calories 235
- (Calories from Fat 55)
- Total Fat 6 gm
- (Saturated Fat 1.3 gm,
- Trans Fat 0.0 gm,
- Polyunsat Fat 2.3 gm,
- Monounsat Fat 1.6 gm)
- Cholesterol 5 mg
- Sodium 375 mg
- Potassium 700 gm
- Total Carb 36 gm
- Dietary Fiber 9 gm
- Sugars 8 gm
- Protein 11 gm
- Phosphorus 170 gm

Green Beans and Bacon

Millie Glick
Edmonton, Alberta

Makes 8 servings, 1 cup per serving

Prep. Time: 10 minutes
Cooking Time: 20–30 minutes

2 quarts fresh green beans,
    trimmed
5 slices bacon

1. Cook green beans in
small amount of water until
tender. Drain.
2. In large skillet fry bacon
pieces. Save 1 Tbsp. bacon
grease and drain off the rest.
3. Add green beans and stir
occasionally until beans are
heated through.

Variation:
    Substitute 1 lb. smoked
turkey sausage for bacon. Cut
smoked sausage into ½" slices
and put into slow cooker in
alternating layers with green
beans. Heat 2 hours on high.
Eva Blosser
Dayton, OH

Exchange List Values
- Vegetable 2.0
- Fat 0.5

Basic Nutritional Values
- Calories 80
- (Calories from Fat 30)
- Total Fat 4 gm
- (Saturated Fat 1.2 gm,
- Trans Fat 0.0 gm,
- Polyunsat Fat 0.5 gm,
- Monounsat Fat 1.4 gm)
- Cholesterol 5 mg
- Sodium 90 mg
- Potassium 205 gm
- Total Carb 10 gm
- Dietary Fiber 4 gm
- Sugars 2 gm
- Protein 4 gm
- Phosphorus 55 gm

When I come home from grocery-shopping, I like to clean and cut up the fresh veggies and store them in air-tight containers. Meal prep is faster later.
Edwina Stoltzfus, Narvon, PA

Green Beans Caesar

Carol Shirk
Leola, PA

Makes 8 servings,
3 oz. per serving, a generous ½ cup

Prep. Time: 10 minutes
Cooking/Baking Time: 30
minutes

1½ lbs. green beans,
   trimmed
2 Tbsp. oil
1 Tbsp. vinegar
1 Tbsp. minced onion
salt and pepper, to taste
2 Tbsp. bread crumbs
2 Tbsp. freshly grated
   Parmesan cheese
1 Tbsp. trans-fat free tub
   margarine, melted

1. Cook the green beans
until barely tender. Drain.
2. Toss with oil, vinegar,
onion, salt, and pepper.
3. Pour into an ungreased
2-quart casserole.
4. Mix bread crumbs,
Parmesan cheese, and butter.
Sprinkle over beans.
5. Bake at 350° for 20
minutes.

Exchange List Values
• Vegetable 1.0   • Fat 1.0

Basic Nutritional Values
• Calories 80   • Sodium 45 mg
  (Calories from Fat 45) • Potassium 115 gm
• Total Fat 5 gm   • Total Carb 7 gm
  (Saturated Fat 0.8 gm, • Dietary Fiber 2 gm
  Trans Fat 0.0 gm,   • Sugars 1 gm
  Polyunsat Fat 1.6 gm, • Protein 2 gm
  Monounsat Fat 2.7 gm) • Phosphorus 30 gm
• Cholesterol 0 mg

Sweet & Sour Green Beans

Meredith Miller
Dover, DE

Makes 8 servings,
about ⅓ cup per serving

Prep. Time: 15 minutes
Cooking/Baking Time: 30
minutes

4 strips bacon
1 medium onion, diced
4 cups green beans,
   trimmed
1 Tbsp. flour
½ cup granular Splenda
2 Tbsp. vinegar
¼ cup water
1 tsp. dry mustard
½ tsp. salt

1. Fry the bacon. Cool and
crumble. Discard drippings.
2. Spray the pan lightly
with cooking spray. Sauté the
onion. Set aside.
3. Meanwhile put the
green beans in a pot with a
little water. Cover and cook
until beans are tender, 10–15
minutes.
4. Combine flour, Splenda,
vinegar, water, mustard and
salt.
5. In a small saucepan, stir
and cook flour mixture until
thick thickened, then add the
sautéed onions.
6. Put the drained, cooked
beans in a serving dish. Pour
the sauce over the beans
and sprinkle with crumbled
bacon.

Tips:
   1. To evenly distribute the
bacon, stir it into the sauce
along with the onions then
pour over beans and toss
gently.
   2. The sauce can be made
ahead of time, then added to
beans when ready.

Exchange List Values
• Vegetable 1.0   • Fat 0.5

Basic Nutritional Values
• Calories 50   • Sodium 220 mg
  (Calories from Fat 15) • Potassium 110 gm
• Total Fat 2 gm   • Total Carb 7 gm
  (Saturated Fat 0.5 gm, • Dietary Fiber 2 gm
  Trans Fat 0.0 gm,   • Sugars 3 gm
  Polyunsat Fat 0.2 gm, • Protein 2 gm
  Monounsat Fat 0.6 gm) • Phosphorus 35 gm
• Cholesterol 5 mg

175

Tasty Beans

Linda Yoder
Fresno, OH

*Makes 6 servings,
about 4½ oz. per serving*

Prep. Time: 5 minutes
Cooking Time: 10 minutes

1 cup thinly sliced onion
1 clove garlic, minced
4-oz. fresh *or* canned
   mushrooms, sliced
1 Tbsp. olive oil
2 pints (4 cups) frozen
   green beans, partially
   thawed
½ tsp. salt
1 Tbsp. dill seeds
dash of cayenne pepper
¾ cup water

1. Sauté onions and garlic, plus fresh mushrooms if using, in olive oil just until tender but not brown.

2. Add green beans, salt, dill seeds, cayenne pepper and water and bring to boil.

3. Reduce heat; cover. Simmer until beans are crisp-tender.

Tips:
1. May be doubled. Best if it can be cooked just before the meal.
2. Garnish with sliced almonds for more color and crunch.

Exchange List Values
• Vegetable 2.0   • Fat 0.5

Basic Nutritional Values
• Calories 60   • Sodium 195 mg
  (Calories from Fat 20) • Potassium 235 gm
• Total Fat 2.5 gm   • Total Carb 8 gm
  (Saturated Fat 0.4 gm, • Dietary Fiber 3 gm
  Trans Fat 0.0 gm,   • Sugars 2 gm
  Polyunsat Fat 0.3 gm,   • Protein 2 gm
  Monounsat Fat 1.7 gm)   • Phosphorus 50 gm
• Cholesterol 0 mg

Barbecued Green Beans

Naomi Ressler
Harrisonburg, VA

*Makes 8 servings,
about 4½ oz. per serving*

Prep. Time: 15 minutes
Cooking/Baking Time: 20 minutes

4 slices bacon, chopped
   into small pieces
½ cup sliced *or* chopped
   onions
½ cup no-added-salt
   ketchup
2 Tbsp. Splenda Brown
   Sugar Blend
1 Tbsp. Worcestershire
   sauce
1½ quarts (3 lb. 2-oz. can)
   green beans, drained

1. Fry bacon and set aside. Discard drippings. Spray pan lightly with cooking spray and sauté onions.

2. Add ketchup, Splenda, and Worcestershire sauce. Simmer several minutes.

3. Add to drained beans in a 1½-quart casserole dish.

4. Bake at 350° for 20 minutes or until heated throughout.

Tip:
I often double the recipe and put in the slow cooker on low for 3 hours. This is a favorite at our church suppers.

Warm Memories:
My elderly aunt introduced me to this recipe so I often think of her with gratitude.

Exchange List Values
• Carbohydrate 0.5   • Vegetable 2.0

Basic Nutritional Values
• Calories 80   • Sodium 365 mg
  (Calories from Fat 15) • Potassium 240 gm
• Total Fat 2 gm   • Total Carb 14 gm
  (Saturated Fat 0.5 gm, • Dietary Fiber 3 gm
  Trans Fat 0.0 gm,   • Sugars 7 gm
  Polyunsat Fat 0.2 gm,   • Protein 3 gm
  Monounsat Fat 0.6 gm)   • Phosphorus 45 gm
• Cholesterol 5 mg

Squash Apple Bake

Ruth Ann Swartzendruber
Hydro, OK

Makes 8 servings,
about 3 oz. per serving

Prep. Time: 20 minutes
Baking Time: 45–60 minutes

4 cups cubed, peeled
butternut squash
2 Tbsp. honey
⅓ cup orange, *or* apple juice
2 apples, thinly sliced
¼ cup raisins
cinnamon

1. Slice butternut squash into ¾" rounds. Peel and remove any seeds. Cut into cubes.
2. Combine honey and juice.
3. In a greased 2-quart casserole dish make 2 layers of squash, apples and raisins. Sprinkle generously with cinnamon and pour juice mixture over layers.
4. Cover and bake at 350° for 45–60 minutes or until tender.

Exchange List Values
- Starch 0.5
- Fruit 1.0

Basic Nutritional Values
- Calories 75
  (Calories from Fat 0)
- Total Fat 0 gm
  (Saturated Fat 0.0 gm,
  Trans Fat 0.0 gm,
  Polyunsat Fat 0.0 gm,
  Monounsat Fat 0.0 gm)
- Cholesterol 0 mg
- Sodium 0 mg
- Potassium 270 gm
- Total Carb 20 gm
- Dietary Fiber 3 gm
- Sugars 13 gm
- Protein 1 gm
- Phosphorus 25 gm

Orange-Glazed Sweet Potatoes

Annabelle Kratz
Clarksville, MD

Makes 12 servings,
a 3" square per serving

Prep. Time: 20 minutes
Cooking/Baking Time: 1 hour

8 medium sweet potatoes,
6 oz. each
½ tsp. salt
¼ cup Splenda Brown
Sugar Blend
2 Tbsp. cornstarch
½ tsp. shredded orange peel
2 cups orange juice
½ cup raisins
2 Tbsp. no-trans-fat tub
margarine
¼ cup chopped walnuts

1. Cook potatoes in boiling, salted water until just tender. Drain.
2. Peel potatoes and cut lengthwise into ½" slices. Arrange in 9×13 baking dish. Sprinkle with salt.
3. In a saucepan combine brown sugar and cornstarch. Blend in orange peel and juice. Add raisins. Cook and stir over medium heat until thickened and bubbly. Cook 1 minute longer.
4. Add margarine and walnuts, stirring until butter has melted. Pour sauce over sweet potatoes.
5. Bake at 325° for 30 minutes or until sweet potatoes are well-glazed. Baste occasionally.

Variation:
Immediately before pouring sauce over sweet potatoes, fold in 2 cups apricot halves
Dorothy Shank
Goshen, IN

Exchange List Values
- Starch 1.5
- Fruit 0.5
- Fat 0.5

Basic Nutritional Values
- Calories 160
  (Calories from Fat 25)
- Total Fat 3 gm
  (Saturated Fat 0.5 gm,
  Trans Fat 0.0 gm,
  Polyunsat Fat 1.8 gm,
  Monounsat Fat 0.7 gm)
- Cholesterol 0 mg
- Sodium 140 mg
- Potassium 375 gm
- Total Carb 32 gm
- Dietary Fiber 3 gm
- Sugars 15 gm
- Protein 2 gm
- Phosphorus 55 gm

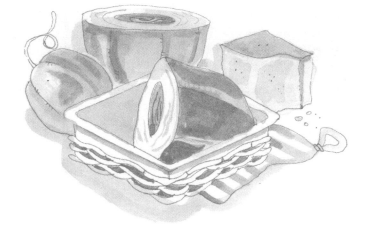

Ranch Potato Cubes

Charlotte Shaffer
East Earl, PA

Makes 8 servings,
about 6 oz. per serving

Prep. Time: 20 minutes
Cooking/Baking Time: 1 hour

6 medium potatoes, cut
　into ½" cubes
4 Tbsp. trans-fat free tub
　margarine
1 cup fat-free sour cream
1-oz. packet Ranch salad
　dressing mix
1 cup (4-oz.) 75%-less-fat
　shredded cheddar cheese

1. Place potatoes in a
greased 11×7 baking dish.
Dot with margarine.

2. Cover. Bake at 350° for
1 hour.

3. Combine sour cream and
salad dressing mix.

4. Spoon over potatoes.
Sprinkle with cheese.

5. Bake uncovered 10
minutes until cheese is
melted.

Exchange List Values

- Starch 2.0   • Fat 0.5
- Fat-Free Milk 0.5

Basic Nutritional Values

- Calories 215   • Sodium 450 mg
  (Calories from Fat 55) • Potassium 675 gm
- Total Fat 6 gm   • Total Carb 33 gm
  (Saturated Fat 1.8 gm, • Dietary Fiber 3 gm
  Trans Fat 0.0 gm,   • Sugars 2 gm
  Polyunsat Fat 1.8 gm, • Protein 9 gm
  Monounsat Fat 1.6 gm) • Phosphorus 180 gm
- Cholesterol 10 mg

Baked German Potato Salad

Bernice Hertzler
Phoenix, AZ

Makes 12 servings,
about 6 oz. per serving

Prep. Time: 30 minutes
Baking/Cooking Time: 50 minutes

8 strips bacon
1 cup chopped celery
1 cup chopped onion
3 Tbsp. flour
1⅓ cups water
1 cup cider vinegar
⅔ cup granular Splenda
1 tsp. salt
¼ tsp. pepper
8 cups cooked potatoes,
　cubed
1 cup sliced radishes,
　optional

1. Fry, drain and crumble
bacon. Drain all bacon drippings from skillet, reserving
1½ Tbsp. Set bacon pieces
aside.

2. Sauté celery and onion
in bacon drippings for 1 minute. Blend in flour, stirring
until bubbly. Add water and
vinegar, stirring constantly
until mixture is thick and
bubbly. Stir in sugar, salt and
pepper, cooking until sugar
dissolves.

3. Cube cooked potatoes
into greased 3-quart casserole
dish. Pour sauce over potatoes
and mix lightly. Fold in bacon
pieces.

4. Cover and bake at 350°
for 30 minutes.

5. Remove from oven
and stir in radishes. Serve
immediately.

Exchange List Values

- Starch 1.5   • Fat 0.5

Basic Nutritional Values

- Calories 150   • Sodium 305 mg
  (Calories from Fat 30) • Potassium 420 gm
- Total Fat 4 gm   • Total Carb 25 gm
  (Saturated Fat 1.2 gm, • Dietary Fiber 2 gm
  Trans Fat 0.0 gm,   • Sugars 3 gm
  Polyunsat Fat 0.4 gm, • Protein 4 gm
  Monounsat Fat 1.5 gm) • Phosphorus 70 gm
- Cholesterol 5 mg

When choosing high-fat ingredients, such as
cheese, pick the most flavorful option and use less.

Cottage Potatoes

Janice Yoskovich
Carmichaels, PA

Makes 8 servings,
about 5 oz. per serving

Prep. Time: 15 minutes
Baking Time: 45 minutes

3 Tbsp. + 2 tsp. trans-fat
free tub margarine
6 boiled potatoes, diced
½ onion, diced
½ green pepper, diced
3 1-oz. slices Italian bread,
broken in pieces
3 oz. 75%-less fat cheddar
cheese, cubed

1. Melt margarine in the
microwave.
2. Mix melted margarine
with potatoes, onion, green
pepper, bread, and cheese.
3. Put mixture in greased
2-quart casserole dish.
4. Bake at 350° for 45
minutes.

Warm Memories:
This is an old recipe and
good one of my mother's best
friend who has been deceased
25 years.

Exchange List Values
• Starch 2.0   • Fat 1.0

Basic Nutritional Values
• Calories 195   • Sodium 170 mg
(Calories from Fat 45) • Potassium 530 gm
• Total Fat 5 gm   • Total Carb 31 gm
(Saturated Fat 1.5 gm, • Dietary Fiber 3 gm
Trans Fat 0.0 gm,   • Sugars 2 gm
Polyunsat Fat 1.8 gm,   • Protein 7 gm
Monounsat Fat 1.5 gm)   • Phosphorus 175 gm
• Cholesterol 5 mg

Rosemary Roasted Potatoes

Pamela Pierce
Annville, PA

Makes 8 servings,
6 wedges per serving

Prep. Time: 10 minutes
Baking Time: 45–60 minutes

8 medium red potatoes,
scrubbed, dried, and cut
into 6 wedges each
3 Tbsp. olive oil
1 tsp. dried rosemary
1 tsp. dried thyme
½ tsp. salt
⅛ tsp. pepper

1. Toss potato wedges in oil.
2. Place in shallow roasting
pan in single layer. Sprinkle
evenly with seasonings. Stir.
3. Roast in 375° oven for
45–60 minutes, stirring and
flipping every 10–15 minutes,
until wedges are golden and
fork-tender.

Good Go-Alongs:
Great with roast pork.

Exchange List Values
• Starch 2.0   • Fat 1.0

Basic Nutritional Values
• Calories 195   • Sodium 155 mg
(Calories from Fat 45) • Potassium 825 gm
• Total Fat 5 gm   • Total Carb 34 gm
(Saturated Fat 0.8 gm, • Dietary Fiber 4 gm
Trans Fat 0.0 gm,   • Sugars 2 gm
Polyunsat Fat 0.6 gm,   • Protein 4 gm
Monounsat Fat 3.7 gm)   • Phosphorus 110 gm
• Cholesterol 0 mg

Shredded Baked Potatoes

Alice Miller
Stuarts Draft, VA

Makes 6 servings,
about 7½ oz. per serving

Prep. Time: 35 minutes
Cooking/Baking Time: 1 hour

6 medium potatoes
1 cup fat-free sour cream
6–8 green onions, chopped
1 cup 75%-less-fat
shredded cheddar cheese
½ tsp. salt
2 Tbsp. trans-fat-free tub
margarine

1. Cook, cool, peel, and
shred potatoes.
2. Combine potatoes, sour
cream, onions, cheese, and
salt.
3. Spoon into 2-quart
casserole dish.
4. Melt margarine and pour
over top of casserole.
5. Bake at 400° for 45
minutes, until light brown
and bubbly.

Exchange List Values
• Starch 1.5   • Fat 0.5
• Fat-Free Milk 0.5

Basic Nutritional Values
• Calories 200   • Sodium 430 mg
(Calories from Fat 45) • Potassium 745 gm
• Total Fat 5 gm   • Total Carb 30 gm
(Saturated Fat 1.8 gm, • Dietary Fiber 3 gm
Trans Fat 0.0 gm,   • Sugars 4 gm
Polyunsat Fat 1.3 gm,   • Protein 11 gm
Monounsat Fat 1.2 gm)   • Phosphorus 220 gm
• Cholesterol 10 mg

Aunt Jean's Potatoes

Jen Hoover
Akron, PA

*Makes 8 servings,
about 5½ oz. per serving*

Prep. Time: 30 minutes
Cooking/Baking Time: 1 hour
Cooling Time: 1 hour

6 medium potatoes
½ Tbsp. canola oil
⅓ cup onions, chopped fine
1 cup shredded 75%-reduced-fat cheddar cheese
1 cup fat-free sour cream
½ tsp. salt
¼ tsp. pepper
1 Tbsp. trans-fat free tub margarine
4 slices bacon, fried and crumbled
paprika

1. Microwave, cook, or bake potatoes in skins; cool at least an hour.
2. Peel and shred coarsely.
3. In saucepan over low heat, sauté onion in canola oil, about 8 minutes. Do not brown!
4. Add cheese and stir until almost melted.
5. Remove from heat. Blend in sour cream, salt, and pepper.

6. Fold in shredded potatoes.
7. Put in greased casserole.
8. Dot with margarine, and sprinkle with paprika and bacon.
9. Bake at 350° for 30 minutes or until heated through.

Tips:

1. Can be made the day before baking or frozen for later use.
2. Great dish for pot luck picnics.
3. Use frozen shredded potatoes instead – this is more costly but quicker to prepare.

Warm Memories:

Mom brings these potatoes to our Diener family gatherings. She is *not* allowed to *not* bring them!

Exchange List Values
- Starch 2.0
- Lean Meat 1.0

Basic Nutritional Values
- Calories 205
  (Calories from Fat 45)
- Total Fat 5 gm
  (Saturated Fat 1.6 gm,
  Trans Fat 0.0 gm,
  Polyunsat Fat 0.9 gm,
  Monounsat Fat 1.7 gm)
- Cholesterol 10 mg
- Sodium 370 mg
- Potassium 565 gm
- Total Carb 32 gm
- Dietary Fiber 3 gm
- Sugars 3 gm
- Protein 10 gm
- Phosphorus 230 gm

Sour Cream Potatoes

Renee Baum
Chambersburg, PA

*Makes 8 servings,
about 7½ oz. per serving*

Prep. Time: 30 minutes
Baking/Cooking Time: 1 hour

3½ lbs. potatoes, about 10 medium
4 oz. fat-free cream cheese
4 oz. Neufchatel (⅓-less-fat) cream cheese
8 oz. fat-free sour cream
¼ cup fat-free milk
2 Tbsp. trans-fat-free tub margarine, *divided*
2 Tbsp. chopped fresh parsley *or* 1 Tbsp. dried parsley
1¼ tsp. garlic salt
¼ tsp. paprika

1. Peel and quarter potatoes. Place in a large saucepan and cover with water. Bring to a boil
2. Reduce heat, cover partially, and cook 15–20 minutes until tender. Drain.
3. Mash the potatoes.
4. Add cream cheese, Neufchatel cheese, sour cream, milk, 1 Tbsp. margarine, parsley and garlic salt. Beat until smooth.
5. Spoon mixture into a greased 2-quart baking dish.
6. Dot with remaining margarine. Sprinkle with paprika.
7. Bake, uncovered, at 350° for 30–40 minutes or until heated through.

Use low-fat ingredients, such as low-fat yogurt or milk, in recipes whenever possible.

Scalloped Corn

Rhonda Freed
Croghan, NY

Makes 6 servings,
3½" square per serving

Prep. Time: 15 minutes
Baking Time: 30–50 minutes

2 eggs
1 cup fat-free milk
⅔ cup cracker crumbs,
   Ritz *or* Club crackers
2 cups canned creamed corn
⅓ cup 75%-less-fat
   shredded cheddar cheese
1 Tbsp. trans-fat free tub
   margarine, melted
1 tsp. dried minced onion
1 Tbsp. sugar
¼ tsp. salt
⅛ tsp. pepper

1. In a medium bowl, beat eggs with a whisk.
2. Add milk and cracker crumbs. Whisk again.
3. Add the rest of the ingredients. Stir together well.
4. Pour into greased 7×11 casserole dish.

5. Bake at 350° for 30–50 minutes, checking at 30 minutes. If center is still jiggly, bake for 5–10 more minutes. Check again. Repeat checking and baking until center is firm.

Sweet Onion Corn Bake

Rebecca B. Stoltzfus
Lititz, PA
Sherry Mayer
Menomonee Falls, WI

Makes 12 servings,
3" square per serving

Prep. Time: 30 minutes
Baking Time: 45–50 minutes

2 large sweet onions,
   thinly sliced
2 Tbsp. canola oil
1 cup fat-free sour cream
½ cup fat-free milk
½ tsp. dill weed
¼ tsp. salt
1 cup 75%-reduced-fat
   shredded cheddar
   cheese, *divided*

¼ cup egg substitute
14¾-oz. can cream style
   corn
8½-oz. pkg. corn bread
   muffin mix
4 drops hot pepper sauce,
   or to taste

1. In a large skillet, sauté onions in oil until tender.
2. In a small bowl, combine sour cream, milk, dill, and salt until blended.
3. Stir in ½ cup cheese.
4. Stir cheese mixture into onion mixture; remove from heat and set aside.
5. In a bowl, combine egg substitute, corn, corn bread mix, and hot pepper sauce.
6. Pour into a greased 9×13 baking dish.
7. Spoon onion mixture over top. Sprinkle with remaining cheese.
8. Bake at 350° for 45–50 minutes or until top is set and lightly browned.
9. Let stand 10 minutes before cutting and serving.

Grandma's Baked Corn

Jen Hoover
Akron, PA

*Makes 6 servings,
about 5 oz. per serving*

Prep. Time: 15 minutes
Baking Time: 45 minutes

3 cups corn
½ tsp. salt
1½ Tbsp. flour
2 Tbsp. melted trans-fat
   free tub margarine
3 eggs
1 cup fat-free milk
1 tsp. sugar

1. Place all ingredients in blender and blend.
2. Pour into 1½-quart greased baking dish.
3. Bake at 350° for 45 minutes.

Tip:
This is extra-yummy when made with frozen sweet corn from the summer.

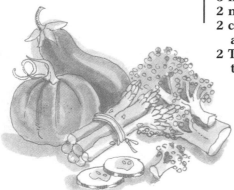

Warm Memories:
I got this from my mother-in-law and it is a favorite of my husband and 3 boys, especially when served with a Mexican dish such as tacos, taco salad, or bean and cheese tortillas.

Exchange List Values
• Starch 1.0   • Med-Fat Meat 1.0

Basic Nutritional Values
• Calories 140   • Sodium 275 mg
  (Calories from Fat 55)   • Potassium 260 gm
• Total Fat 6 gm   • Total Carb 18 gm
  (Saturated Fat 1.5 gm,   • Dietary Fiber 2 gm
  Trans Fat 0.0 gm,   • Sugars 5 gm
  Polyunsat Fat 1.9 gm,   • Protein 6 gm
  Monounsat Fat 2.0 gm)   • Phosphorus 145 gm
• Cholesterol 95 mg

Asparagus Bake

Leona M. Slabaugh
Apple Creek, OH

Makes 6 servings

Prep. Time: 20 minutes
Baking Time: 45–60 minutes

5 medium potatoes, sliced
2 medium onions, diced
2 cups fresh, chopped
   asparagus
2 Tbsp. tub margarine,
   trans-fat free
     salt and pepper
     3 oz. 75%-less-fat
       cheddar cheese

1. Lay potatoes in greased 2-quart casserole dish. Sprinkle with salt and pepper.
2. Sprinkle diced onions over potatoes.
3. Add asparagus.
4. Add salt and pepper to taste.
5. Dot top with pieces of margarine.
6. Cover tightly.
7. Bake at 325° for 45–60 minutes, or until potatoes are tender when poked with a fork.
8. Remove from oven and lay sliced cheese over hot vegetables to melt.

Tip:
Experiment with adding garlic, fresh parsley or other herbs, or even a dash of cayenne.

Good Go-Alongs:
Meat loaf, corn, apple crisp – a meal made entirely in the oven.

Exchange List Values
• Starch 1.5   • Lean Meat 1.0
• Vegetable 1.0   • Fat 0.5

Basic Nutritional Values
• Calories 195   • Sodium 150 mg
  (Calories from Fat 40)   • Potassium 820 gm
• Total Fat 4.5 gm   • Total Carb 32 gm
  (Saturated Fat 1.4 gm,   • Dietary Fiber 5 gm
  Trans Fat 0.0 gm,   • Sugars 4 gm
  Polyunsat Fat 1.3 gm,   • Protein 9 gm
  Monounsat Fat 1.2 gm)   • Phosphorus 195 gm
• Cholesterol 5 mg

Baked Asparagus Roll-Ups

Peggy C. Forsythe
Memphis, TN

Makes 12 servings,
1 roll-up per serving

Prep. Time: 20 minutes
Baking Time: 15 minutes

12 slices white bread,
  crusts removed
½ cup reduced-fat
  crumbled blue cheese
1–2 Tbsp. mayonnaise
12 asparagus spears,
  canned and patted dry,
  ***or* fresh and lightly**
  steamed, dried, and
  cooled
2 Tbsp. tub margarine,
  trans-fat free, melted
paprika
4 Tbsp. freshly grated
  Parmesan cheese

1. Flatten bread with a rolling pin. Set aside.

2. In a small bowl, mix blue cheese and mayonnaise to a spreading consistency, stating with 1 Tbsp. mayonnaise and adding by teaspoons as needed. Set aside.

3. Divide cheese mixture among bread slices and spread evenly.

4. Place an asparagus spear on one end of a bread slice. Starting with the spear end, roll up with the bread with the spear inside. Pinch seam a little bit to hold in place.

5. Place roll-up seam side down on greased cookie sheet. Roll up remaining bread and asparagus.

6. Brush each roll-up with melted butter. Sprinkle each roll-up with 1 tsp. Parmesan cheese and a sprinkle of paprika.

7. Bake for 15 minutes at 375° or until golden brown.

Exchange List Values
• Starch 0.5   • Fat 0.5

Basic Nutritional Values
• Calories 85   • Sodium 240 mg
  (Calories from Fat 30) • Potassium 65 gm
• Total Fat 4 gm   • Total Carb 10 gm
  (Saturated Fat 1.3 gm, • Dietary Fiber 1 gm
  Trans Fat 0.0 gm,   • Sugars 1 gm
  Polyunsat Fat 0.9 gm, • Protein 3 gm
  Monounsat Fat 1.0 gm) • Phosphorus 55 gm
• Cholesterol 5 mg

Glazed Carrot Coins

Dorothy Lingerfelt
Stonyford, CA

Makes 6 servings,
about 4 oz. per serving

Prep. Time: 20 minutes
Cooking/Baking Time: 30
  minutes

12 medium carrots, cut
  into 1-inch pieces
¼ cup Splenda Brown
  Sugar Blend
2 Tbsp. trans-fat free
  margarine
1 Tbsp. grated lemon peel
¼ tsp. vanilla

1. In saucepan, cook carrots in a small amount of water until crisp-tender; drain. Remove and keep warm.

2. In the same pan, heat Splenda and margarine until bubbly. Stir in lemon peel.

3. Return carrots to pan; cook and stir over low heat for 10 minutes or until glazed.

4. Remove from heat; stir in vanilla.

Variation:
Substitute 2 Tbsp. Dijon mustard for the lemon peel and vanilla.

Joette Droz
Kalona, IA

Exchange List Values
• Carbohydrate 0.5   • Fat 0.5
• Vegetable 2.0

Basic Nutritional Values
• Calories 105   • Sodium 115 mg
  (Calories from Fat 25) • Potassium 405 gm
• Total Fat 3 gm   • Total Carb 20 gm
  (Saturated Fat 0.6 gm, • Dietary Fiber 4 gm
  Trans Fat 0.0 gm,   • Sugars 9 gm
  Polyunsat Fat 1.3 gm, • Protein 1 gm
  Monounsat Fat 0.9 gm) • Phosphorus 45 gm
• Cholesterol 0 mg

Crisp Carrot Casserole

Jan McDowell
New Holland, PA

Makes 8 servings,
3¼"×4½" rectangle per serving

Prep. Time: 30 minutes
Cooking/Baking Time: 50 minutes

6 cups sliced carrots
1 large onion, chopped
2 Tbsp. trans-fat free tub margarine
1 cup shredded 75%-reduced fat cheddar cheese
1 oz. lightly crumbled baked potato chips

1. In a covered saucepan, cook carrots and onions in small amount of water until barely crisp-tender. Drain.
2. Place carrots and onions in a greased 9×13 baking dish.
3. Slice margarine into pieces and layer over top of carrots and onions in dish.
4. Sprinkle with cheese. Top with potato chips.
5. Bake at 350° for 30–40 minutes, until casserole is hot through and bubbling at edges.

Warm Memories:
I always have an empty dish to take home from potlucks!

Exchange List Values
• Starch 0.5   • Fat 0.5
• Vegetable 2.0

Basic Nutritional Values
• Calories 115
(Calories from Fat 35)
• Total Fat 4 gm
(Saturated Fat 1.2 gm,
Trans Fat 0.0 gm,
Polyunsat Fat 1.1 gm,
Monounsat Fat 1.0 gm)
• Cholesterol 5 mg
• Sodium 210 mg
• Potassium 385 gm
• Total Carb 15 gm
• Dietary Fiber 3 gm
• Sugars 6 gm
• Protein 6 gm
• Phosphorus 115 gm

Mercy Home Medley

Esther H. Becker
Gordonville, PA

Makes 8 servings,
about 5 oz. per serving

Prep. Time: 25–30 minutes
Cooking Time: 20–30 minutes

1 medium onion, chopped
2 garlic cloves, minced, *optional*
2 Tbsp. oil
3 tomatoes, chopped
2 cups finely shredded cabbage
2 cups diced potatoes, peeled, or unpeeled
5 cups finely shredded kale
pepper, *optional*
hot pepper flakes, *optional*

1. In a large pan, sauté onions and garlic until translucent.
2. Add tomatoes. Cover and cook 5 minutes.
3. Add cabbage and potatoes. Simmer gently, covered, for 10 minutes, or until vegetables are nearly tender.
4. Stir in kale. Continue cooking, covered, for about 10 minutes, or just until kale is tender but not mushy.
5. Stir in hot pepper flakes if you like.

Warm Memories:
This dish was served every day when we visited Mercy Home in Maseno, Kenya, a girl's orphanage. The cooks there used only salt for seasoning, but I like the zip that pepper, pepper flakes, and minced garlic add.

Good Go-Alongs:
Chapati

Exchange List Values
• Starch 0.5   • Fat 0.5
• Vegetable 2.0

Basic Nutritional Values
• Calories 115
(Calories from Fat 35)
• Total Fat 4 gm
(Saturated Fat 0.3 gm,
Trans Fat 0.0 gm,
Polyunsat Fat 1.2 gm,
Monounsat Fat 2.3 gm)
• Cholesterol 0 mg
• Sodium 25 mg
• Potassium 530 gm
• Total Carb 18 gm
• Dietary Fiber 3 gm
• Sugars 6 gm
• Protein 3 gm
• Phosphorus 85 gm

Cabbage Casserole

Cova Rexroad
Baltimore, MD

Makes 8 servings,
3¼"×4½" rectangle per serving

Prep. Time: 20 minutes
Cooking/Baking Time: 45 minutes

1½ cups crushed corn flakes, *divided*
2 Tbsp. tub margarine, trans-fat free

10¾-oz. can lower-sodium,
  lower-fat cream of celery
  soup
¼ cup low-fat mayonnaise
6–7 cups shredded cabbage
1 cup 75%-less fat sharp
  cheddar cheese, *divided*

1. Put 1 cup corn flakes in
bottom of 9×13 baking dish.

2. Heat together margarine,
soup, mayonnaise and ¾ cup
cheese until the cheese is
melted.

3. Add to cabbage and mix.

4. Pour and spread the
cabbage mixture over the
cornflakes in the baking dish.
Pat it down to fill the baking
dish.

5. Sprinkle ½ cup corn
flakes on top.

6. Cover with foil and bake
at 350° for 30 minutes.

7. Remove cover, sprinkle
on remaining cheese. Bake 15
minutes longer to finish.

Tips:
  Chopped red sweet pepper
added to the cabbage gives
a festive look. I use frozen
peppers from my freezer.

Exchange List Values
• Starch 0.5   • Fat 1.0
• Carbohydrate 0.5

Basic Nutritional Values
• Calories 120   • Sodium 380 mg
  (Calories from Fat 40) • Potassium 300 gm
• Total Fat 4.5 gm   • Total Carb 15 gm
  (Saturated Fat 1.4 gm, • Dietary Fiber 2 gm
  Trans Fat 0.0 gm,   • Sugars 3 gm
  Polyunsat Fat 1.5 gm, • Protein 6 gm
  Monounsat Fat 1.2 gm) • Phosphorus 100 gm
• Cholesterol 5 mg

German Red Cabbage

Annie C. Boshart
Lebanon, PA

*Makes 12 servings,
about 5 oz. per serving*

Prep. Time: 30–40 minutes
Cooking/Baking Time: 3–4 hours

1 large red cabbage,
  shredded
3 apples, peeled and cored,
  sliced thin
1 medium onion, chopped
  or sliced
4 tsp. sugar
salt to taste
2 bay leaves
10 whole cloves
½ lb. bacon
2 Tbsp. white vinegar, or
  more to taste

1. Place water in bottom
of Dutch oven or 4 quart pot.
Put in half the apples, half
the onions, half the sugar, and
some salt to taste.

2. Put in all the cabbage.

3. Top with the rest of the
apples, onions, sugar, and any
more salt desired. Add bay
leaves and cloves.

4. Cover and cook on low
heat.

5. Meanwhile, fry bacon
until brown. Remove bacon
and set aside on paper towels.
Pat it dry. Chop.

6. Reserve 1½ Tbsp. bacon
grease and discard the rest.

7. Add the chopped bacon
and the reserved grease on
top of the cabbage.

8. Add vinegar. Simmer
3–4 hours on low. Add more
vinegar to your taste.

9. Remove bay leaves and
cloves and discard.

Tips:
  1. This could be cooked to
completion in a slow cooker
if desired to serve at a buffet
meal.

  2. To shred the cabbage
efficiently and with less mess,
use a food processor with a
slicer blade. You can run the
apples and onions through as
well.

  3. This dish improves with
age and reheating!

Warm Memories:
  Originally a German
immigrant cooked and served
us this delicious dish.

Good Go-Alongs:
  Sausage and hot German
potato salad

Exchange List Values
• Fruit 0.5   • Fat 1.0
• Vegetable 1.0

Basic Nutritional Values
• Calories 100   • Sodium 150 mg
  (Calories from Fat 35) • Potassium 305 gm
• Total Fat 4 gm   • Total Carb 14 gm
  (Saturated Fat 1.4 gm, • Dietary Fiber 3 gm
  Trans Fat 0.0 gm,   • Sugars 9 gm
  Polyunsat Fat 0.5 gm, • Protein 4 gm
  Monounsat Fat 1.7 gm) • Phosphorus 65 gm
• Cholesterol 5 mg

Cheesy Zucchini

Louise Stackhouse
Benton, PA

Makes 6 servings,
about 3 oz. per serving

Prep. Time: 10 minutes
Cooking/Baking Time: 20
minutes

2 small to medium size
zucchini, peeled, sliced
1 large onion, sliced
3 Tbsp. no trans-fat tub
margarine, sliced
salt and pepper to taste
2 slices (¾-oz. each)
reduced-fat American
cheese
basil, fresh *or* dry

1. Spray casserole bowl with non-stick cooking spray.
2. Layer zucchini and onion in bowl, adding slices of butter, salt and pepper as you go.
3. Lay cheese on top. Sprinkle with basil.
4. Cover and microwave approximately 20 minutes until zucchini is tender when tested with a fork.

Variation:

Sauté onion and zucchini in margarine in a large skillet. Add cheese and basil on top. Cover and cook on low until tender.

Exchange List Values
• Vegetable 1.0   • Fat 1.0

Basic Nutritional Values
• Calories 75
  (Calories from Fat 45)
• Total Fat 5 gm
  (Saturated Fat 1.4 gm,
  Trans Fat 0.0 gm,
  Polyunsat Fat 1.8 gm,
  Monounsat Fat 1.6 gm)
• Cholesterol 5 mg
• Sodium 145 mg
• Potassium 185 gm
• Total Carb 6 gm
• Dietary Fiber 1 gm
• Sugars 3 gm
• Protein 2 gm
• Phosphorus 85 gm

Oven Roasted Vegetables

Martha G. Zimmerman
Lititz, PA

Makes 4 servings

Prep. Time: 20 minutes
Baking Time: 30 minutes

1 medium zucchini
1 medium summer squash
**   *or* another zucchini**
1 medium red bell pepper
1 medium yellow bell
**   pepper**
1 lb. fresh asparagus
1 sweet potato, *optional*
1 red onion
1–3 garlic cloves, minced
3 Tbsp. olive oil
salt and pepper, to taste
Italian herb seasoning, to
**   taste**

1. Cut vegetables into bite-sized pieces.
2. Place on two large rimmed baking sheets.
3. Drizzle olive oil evenly over vegetables. Sprinkle evenly with garlic, salt, pepper, and Italian seasoning.
4. Mix well. (Hands work well for this!)
5. Bake at 400° for 25–35 minutes, stirring and flipping every 5–10 minutes. Test a few vegetables at 25 minutes to see if they are done to your preference. Keep roasting and stirring until soft to your liking.

Exchange List Values
• Vegetable 3.0   • Fat 2.0

Basic Nutritional Values
• Calories 155
  (Calories from Fat 100)
• Total Fat 11 gm
  (Saturated Fat 1.5 gm,
  Trans Fat 0.0 gm,
  Polyunsat Fat 1.3 gm,
  Monounsat Fat 7.5 gm)
• Cholesterol 0 mg
• Sodium 15 mg
• Potassium 595 gm
• Total Carb 14 gm
• Dietary Fiber 4 gm
• Sugars 7 gm
• Protein 4 gm
• Phosphorus 95 gm

Oven Brussels Sprouts

Gail Martin
Elkhart, IN

Makes 8 servings

Prep. Time: 15 minutes
Baking Time: 15–20 minutes

1½ lbs. Brussels sprouts, halved
¼ cup plus 2 Tbsp. olive oil
juice of 1 lemon
½ tsp. salt
½ tsp. pepper
½ tsp. crushed red pepper flakes

1. In a large bowl, toss halved sprouts with 2 Tbsp. olive oil.
2. Place them on a single layer on a rimmed cookie sheet.
3. Roast sprouts in the oven at 450°, stirring twice, until crisp and lightly browned, about 15–20 minutes.
4. Whisk together in a large bowl ¼ cup oil, lemon juice, salt, pepper, and red pepper flakes.
5. Toss sprouts with dressing and serve.

Tip:
Don't overcook the sprouts.

Warm Memories:
This is a lovely dish for any meal but especially nice at Easter.

Good Go-Alongs:
Sliced ham and new potatoes

Exchange List Values
- Vegetable 1.0
- Fat 2.0

Basic Nutritional Values
- Calories 120 (Calories from Fat 100)
- Total Fat 11 gm (Saturated Fat 1.5 gm, Trans Fat 0.0 gm, Polyunsat Fat 1.3 gm, Monounsat Fat 7.4 gm)
- Cholesterol 0 mg
- Sodium 165 mg
- Potassium 280 gm
- Total Carb 7 gm
- Dietary Fiber 2 gm
- Sugars 2 gm
- Protein 2 gm
- Phosphorus 50 gm

Creamed Peas and Mushrooms

Diena Schmidt
Henderson, NE

Makes 8 servings, about 4 oz. per serving

Prep. Time: 15 minutes
Cooking Time: 25 minutes

20-oz pkg. frozen peas
½ cup mushroom caps
1 Tbsp. minced onion
2 Tbsp. trans-fat-free tub margarine
2 Tbsp. flour
1½ cups fat-free half-and-half
3 Tbsp. reduced-fat Velveeta cheese
¼ tsp. salt

1. Cook peas in boiling salted water until tender.
2. Sauté mushrooms and onion in oil until lightly browned. Add to peas.
3. Stir flour into remaining drippings. Add half-and-half gradually, cooking and stirring until slightly thickened.
4. Turn heat to low and add cheese. Stir until dissolved. Combine with peas and mushrooms.

Exchange List Values
- Starch 1.0
- Fat 0.5

Basic Nutritional Values
- Calories 115 (Calories from Fat 30)
- Total Fat 4 gm (Saturated Fat 1.2 gm, Trans Fat 0.0 gm, Polyunsat Fat 1.0 gm, Monounsat Fat 1.0 gm)
- Cholesterol 5 mg
- Sodium 280 mg
- Potassium 195 gm
- Total Carb 15 gm
- Dietary Fiber 4 gm
- Sugars 6 gm
- Protein 6 gm
- Phosphorus 185 gm

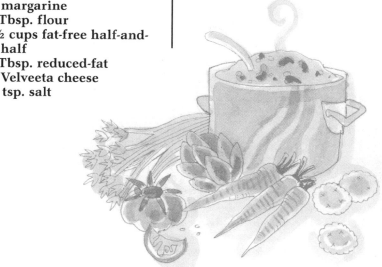

Garlic Mushrooms

Lizzie Ann Yoder
Hartville, OH

Makes 4 servings,
about ½ cup per serving

Prep. Time: 20 minutes
Cooking Time: 15–20 minutes

3 Tbsp. trans-fat free tub
  margarine
2 cloves garlic, minced
1 lb. mushrooms, sliced
4 scallions, chopped
1 tsp. lemon juice

1. In a skillet, melt the
butter and sauté the garlic
briefly.
2. Add mushrooms,
scallions, and lemon juice
and cook, stirring, about 10
minutes.

Good Go-Alongs:
  A nice side dish for meat.

Exchange List Values
• Vegetable 1.0   • Fat 1.5

Basic Nutritional Values
• Calories 90   • Sodium 75 mg
  (Calories from Fat 65) • Potassium 400 gm
• Total Fat 7 gm   • Total Carb 5 gm
  (Saturated Fat 1.4 gm, • Dietary Fiber 2 gm
  Trans Fat 0.0 gm,   • Sugars 2 gm
  Polyunsat Fat 2.8 gm, • Protein 4 gm
  Monounsat Fat 2.0 gm) • Phosphorus 105 gm
• Cholesterol 0 mg

Grilled Onions

Loretta Weisz
Auburn, WA

Makes 4 servings,
2 wedges per serving

Prep. Time: 5 minutes
Grilling Time: 35–45 minutes

2 medium white, *or* yellow,
  sweet onions
butter-flavored cooking
  spray
¼ tsp. pepper
¼ tsp. salt

1. Slice each onion into 4
wedges, but without slicing
through the bottom, so that
each onion stays whole.
2. Spray each onion with
one spray of cooking spray.
Sprinkle evenly with salt
and pepper, being sure it gets
down between each wedge.
3. Wrap stuffed onions
tightly in foil.
4. Grill until soft and
tender, 35–45 minutes.

Tip:
  These onions are delicious
with grilled steaks and
chicken.

Exchange List Values
• Vegetable 2.0

Basic Nutritional Values
• Calories 40   • Sodium 155 mg
  (Calories from Fat 0) • Potassium 145 gm
• Total Fat 0 gm   • Total Carb 9 gm
  (Saturated Fat 0.0 gm, • Dietary Fiber 1 gm
  Trans Fat 0.0 gm,   • Sugars 6 gm
  Polyunsat Fat 0.0 gm, • Protein 1 gm
  Monounsat Fat 0.1 gm) • Phosphorus 35 gm
• Cholesterol 0 mg

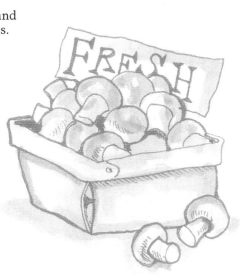

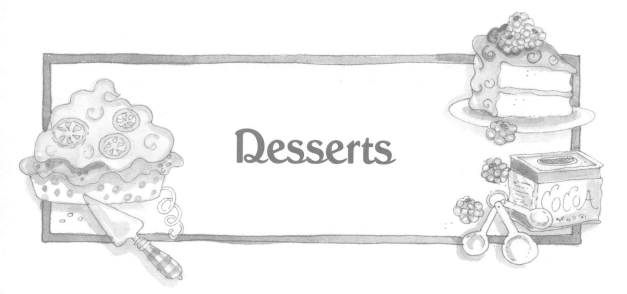

Desserts

Jumbleberry Crumble

Joanna Harrison
Lafayette, CO

Makes 10 servings,
2"×3½" rectangle per serving

Prep. Time: 20 minutes
Baking Time: 50 minutes

3 cups strawberries
1½ cups blueberries
1½ cups raspberries
⅓ cup Splenda Blend for
   Baking
3 Tbsp. quick-cooking
   tapioca
½ cup flour
½ cup quick oats
¼ cup Splenda Brown
   Sugar Blend
1 tsp. cinnamon
5 Tbsp. trans-fat-free tub
   margarine

1. In large bowl, combine berries, tapioca, and Splenda Blend for Baking.

2. Pour into a greased 11×7 baking dish. Let stand 15 minutes.

3. Combine flour, oats, brown sugar blend, and cinnamon in small bowl.

4. Stir in melted margarine.

5. Sprinkle over berry mixture.

6. Bake at 350° for 45–50 minutes or until filling is bubbly and topping is golden brown. Serve warm.

Tips:

I've used fresh or frozen berries depending on the season. Yummy with vanilla ice cream.

Exchange List Values
- Carbohydrate 2.0   • Fat 1.0

Basic Nutritional Values
- Calories 165
  (Calories from Fat 45)
- Total Fat 5 gm
  (Saturated Fat 1.0 gm,
  Trans Fat 0.0 gm,
  Polyunsat Fat 2.0 gm,
  Monounsat Fat 1.5 gm)
- Cholesterol 0 mg
- Sodium 45 mg
- Potassium 145 gm
- Total Carb 30 gm
- Dietary Fiber 3 gm
- Sugars 14 gm
- Protein 2 gm
- Phosphorus 45 gm

Keep a notebook of when you have guests over for a meal. List how many people attended, the weather, menus, how much you made, and how much was left over. This is handy to look at when you are planning for new guests.

Jane Geigley, Lancaster, PA

Blackberry Rolypoly

Elaine Gibbel
Lititz, PA

Makes 12 servings, 1 slice per serving

Prep. Time: 30 minutes
Baking Time: 30 minutes

2 cups flour
2 tsp. baking powder
½ tsp. salt
1 Tbsp. sugar
dash nutmeg
4 Tbsp. trans-fat-free tub
     margarine
¾ cup milk
3–4 sprays of cooking spray
6 cups blackberries
1 cup granular Splenda
½ tsp. salt
whipped topping, *optional*

1. Combine flour, baking powder, ½ tsp. salt, sugar and nutmeg. Work 4 Tbsp. butter into dry ingredients with fingers. Gradually stir in milk until dough holds together but is soft. Turn out onto floured board and roll into a ½" thick rectangle
2. Spray with cooking spray.
3. Combine berries, sugar and ½ tsp. salt. Sprinkle ½ fruit mixture over dough. Roll up like a jelly roll.
4. Place in greased 8×12 pan, seam side down. Spoon remaining fruit mixture around roll.
5. Bake at 425° for 30 minutes. Cut into 12 slices. Serve with whipped topping if your diet allows.

Exchange List Values
- Carbohydrate 2.0   • Fat 0.5

Basic Nutritional Values
- Calories 150
  (Calories from Fat 30)
- Total Fat 4 gm
  (Saturated Fat 0.7 gm,
  Trans Fat 0.0 gm,
  Polyunsat Fat 1.5 gm,
  Monounsat Fat 1.0 gm)
- Cholesterol 0 mg
- Sodium 290 mg
- Potassium 165 gm
- Total Carb 27 gm
- Dietary Fiber 4 gm
- Sugars 8 gm
- Protein 4 gm
- Phosphorus 130 gm

Fruit Cobbler

Verna Birky
Albany, OR

Makes 15 servings,
a 2⅗"×3" rectangle per serving

Prep. Time: 20 minutes
Baking Time: 45–55 minutes

4 cups fresh fruit
½ cup granular Splenda
½ tsp. cinnamon
1 egg, beaten
½ cup fat-free milk
⅓ cup canola oil
1 cup flour
½ cup Splenda Blend for
     Baking
1 tsp. baking powder
¼ tsp. salt
1–2 Tbsp. minute tapioca,
     optional

1. Arrange choice of fruit in lightly greased 9×13 pan. Sprinkle with ½ cup Splenda and cinnamon.
2. Combine egg, milk and oil.
3. Combine dry ingredients, add minute tapioca only if the fruit is quite juicy. Stir egg mixture into dry ingredients. Pour over layer of fruit.
4. Bake at 325° for 45 minutes until fruit is bubbling or soft. May need to bake longer, depending on choice of fruit.

Exchange List Values
- Carbohydrate 1.0   • Fat 1.0

Basic Nutritional Values
- Calories 130
  (Calories from Fat 45)
- Total Fat 5 gm
  (Saturated Fat 0.5 gm,
  Trans Fat 0.0 gm,
  Polyunsat Fat 1.5 gm,
  Monounsat Fat 3.2 gm)
- Cholesterol 15 mg
- Sodium 70 mg
- Potassium 75 gm
- Total Carb 19 gm
- Dietary Fiber 1 gm
- Sugars 12 gm
- Protein 2 gm
- Phosphorus 60 gm

If you've invited guests who have diabetes, call them ahead of time and tell them what recipes you're making and the nutritional information if you have it.

Zucchini Strudel

Judith Houser
Hershey, PA

Makes 20 servings,
2½" square per serving

Prep. Time: 30 minutes
Cooking/Baking Time: 50
minutes

Dough part:
  4 cups flour
  ¾ cup Splenda Blend for
    Baking
  ½ tsp. salt
  1 cup trans-fat-free tub
    margarine

Filling part:
  4 cups peeled and cubed
    zucchini
  ½ to ⅔ cup lemon juice
  ¾ cup granular Splenda
  ¼ tsp. nutmeg
  ½ tsp. cinnamon

1. Cut together flour, Splenda, salt, and margarine until crumbly.
2. Press half of the mixture into a 9×13 baking pan to make a crust.
3. Bake at 375° for 10 minutes.
4. Combine zucchini and lemon juice in saucepan. Bring to a boil, covered.
5. Add Splenda and nutmeg. Simmer 5 minutes.
6. Add ½ cup reserved crumbs and stir over low heat until thickened.
7. Spread zucchini mixture over baked dough.
8. Cover with remaining crumbs. Sprinkle with cinnamon.
9. Bake at 375° for 30 minutes.

Tips:
  Use smaller amount of lemon juice if you want a less tart dessert. A great way to use extra zucchini – people will think it's an apple strudel.

Good Go-Alongs:
  This is delicious served warm with vanilla ice cream.

Exchange List Values
• Carbohydrate 2.0   • Fat 1.0

Basic Nutritional Values
• Calories 190   • Sodium 135 mg
  (Calories from Fat 65) • Potassium 100 gm
• Total Fat 7 gm   • Total Carb 28 gm
  (Saturated Fat 1.5 gm, • Dietary Fiber 1 gm
  Trans Fat 0.0 gm, • Sugars 9 gm
  Polyunsat Fat 2.9 gm, • Protein 3 gm
  Monounsat Fat 2.2 gm) • Phosphorus 40 gm
• Cholesterol 0 mg

Peach Crumble

Nathan LeBeau
Rapid City, SD

Makes 8 servings,
2"×4" rectangle per serving

Prep. Time: 10 minutes
Baking Time: 20–30 minutes

4 cups peeled, sliced fresh
  peaches
6 Tbsp. Splenda Brown
  Sugar Blend
⅓ cup (5⅓ Tbsp.) trans-fat-
  free tub margarine
¾ tsp. nutmeg
¾ tsp. cinnamon
1 cup crushed graham
  cracker

1. Mix Splenda and peaches together.
2. Place in a greased 8-inch pan.
3. Combine margarine, nutmeg, cinnamon and graham crackers.
4. Sprinkle mixture over top of peaches.
5. Bake at 375° for 20–30 minutes until bubbling.

Variation:
  Use apples instead of peaches.

Exchange List Values
• Carbohydrate 2.0   • Fat 1.0

Basic Nutritional Values
• Calories 165   • Sodium 125 mg
  (Calories from Fat 65) • Potassium 195 gm
• Total Fat 7 gm   • Total Carb 26 gm
  (Saturated Fat 1.4 gm, • Dietary Fiber 2 gm
  Trans Fat 0.0 gm, • Sugars 15 gm
  Polyunsat Fat 2.8 gm, • Protein 2 gm
  Monounsat Fat 2.3 gm) • Phosphorus 30 gm
• Cholesterol 0 mg

Sunflower Cookies

Anna Kathryn Reesor
Markham, Ontario

*Makes 5 dozen cookies,
1 cookie per serving*

Prep. Time: 30 minutes
***Baking Time: 10 minutes per
cookie sheet***

½ cup trans-fat-free tub
  margarine
6 Tbsp. Splenda Brown
  Sugar Blend
6 Tbsp. Splenda Blend for
  Baking
1 egg, beaten
½ tsp. vanilla
½ tsp. baking soda
2 tsp. hot water
1 cup shelled, unsalted
  sunflower seeds
½ cup all-purpose flour
½ cup rolled oats
½ cup chocolate chips
½ cup raisins
⅓ cup natural wheat bran
⅓ cup wheat germ
1 tsp. salt

1. In large bowl cream
margarine and Splenda until
fluffy. Stir in egg, vanilla
and baking soda dissolved
in hot water. Add all other
ingredients and mix thor-
oughly.
2. Drop by spoonfuls onto
lightly greased cookie sheet.
3. Bake at 350° for approximately 10 minutes.

Exchange List Values
• Carbohydrate 0.5 • Fat 0.5

Basic Nutritional Values
• Calories 55   • Sodium 65 mg
  (Calories from Fat 25) • Potassium 50 gm
• Total Fat 3 gm   • Total Carb 7 gm
  (Saturated Fat 0.7 gm, • Dietary Fiber 1 gm
  Trans Fat 0.0 gm, • Sugars 3 gm
  Polyunsat Fat 1.3 gm, • Protein 1 gm
  Monounsat Fat 0.8 gm) • Phosphorus 40 gm
• Cholesterol 5 mg

White Chip
Pumpkin Cookies

Joanna Harrison
Lafayette, CO

*Makes 60 cookies,
1 cookie per serving*

Prep. Time: 15 minutes
Baking Time: 11–14 minutes

2 sticks (1 cup) butter
¼ cup Splenda Brown
  Sugar Blend
¼ cup Splenda Blend for
  Baking
1 egg
2 tsp. vanilla
1 cup cooked, puréed
  pumpkin
2 cups flour
1 tsp. ground cardamom
2 tsp. ground cinnamon
1 tsp. baking soda
1¼ cups white chocolate
  chips
⅔ cup chopped nuts,
  optional

1. Using a mixer, cream
together butter, Splenda, egg,
and vanilla. Beat in pumpkin.
2. Separately, stir together
flour, cardamom, cinnamon,
and baking soda.

3. Stir flour mixture
into butter mixture. Stir in
chocolate chips and optional
nuts.
4. Drop spoonfuls onto
greased cookie sheet.
5. Bake at 350° for 11–14
minutes.

Exchange List Values
• Carbohydrate 0.5 • Fat 1.0

Basic Nutritional Values
• Calories 70   • Sodium 50 mg
  (Calories from Fat 30) • Potassium 30 gm
• Total Fat 4 gm   • Total Carb 8 gm
  (Saturated Fat 1.5 gm, • Dietary Fiber 0 gm
  Trans Fat 0.0 gm, • Sugars 4 gm
  Polyunsat Fat 1.0 gm, • Protein 1 gm
  Monounsat Fat 1.2 gm) • Phosphorus 15 gm
• Cholesterol 5 mg

Forgotten Cookies

Penny Blosser
New Carlisle, OH

*Makes 30 cookies,
1 cookie per serving*

Prep. Time: 20 minutes
***Baking Time: until oven cools or
overnight***

2 egg whites
⅔ cup sugar
pinch salt
1 tsp. vanilla
½ cup chopped nuts
½ cup chocolate chips

1. Preheat oven to 350°.
2. Beat egg whites until
foamy. Gradually add sugar,
beating until stiff. Fold in
remaining ingredients.

3. Drop cookies onto foil-lined cookie sheet. Place in 350° oven.

4. Turn oven *off* immediately. Let cookies in oven until cooled completely or overnight.

Exchange List Values

• Carbohydrate 0.5 • Fat 0.5

Basic Nutritional Values

• Calories 45	• Sodium 0 mg
(Calories from Fat 20)	• Potassium 25 gm
• Total Fat 2 gm	• Total Carb 7 gm
(Saturated Fat 0.6 gm,	• Dietary Fiber 0 gm
Trans Fat 0.0 gm,	• Sugars 6 gm
Polyunsat Fat 1.0 gm,	• Protein 1 gm
Monounsat Fat 0.5 gm)	• Phosphorus 10 gm
• Cholesterol 0 mg	

No-Bake Chocolate Cookies

Penny Blosser
Beavercreek, OH

Makes 3 dozen,
36 servings, 1 cookie per serving

Prep. Time: 20 minutes
Cooking Time: 15 minutes
Cooling Time: 30 minutes

½ **cup trans-fat-free tub margarine**
½ **cup fat-free milk**
1 **cup Splenda Blend for Baking**
1 **cup chocolate chips**
½ **cup peanut butter**
3 **cups quick oats**
1 **tsp. vanilla**

1. Put margarine, milk, Splenda and chocolate chips in a saucepan.

2. Bring to boil, and boil 1 minute. Remove from heat.

3. Stir in peanut butter and vanilla until melted.

4. Add rolled oats. Mix.

5. Drop by heaping tablespoon onto waxed paper lined baking sheet.

6. Let cool until set.

Exchange List Values

• Carbohydrate 1.0 • Fat 1.0

Basic Nutritional Values

• Calories 110	• Sodium 40 mg
(Calories from Fat 55)	• Potassium 70 gm
• Total Fat 6 gm	• Total Carb 14 gm
(Saturated Fat 1.7 gm,	• Dietary Fiber 1 gm
Trans Fat 0.0 gm,	• Sugars 9 gm
Polyunsat Fat 1.5 gm,	• Protein 2 gm
Monounsat Fat 2.1 gm)	• Phosphorus 50 gm
• Cholesterol 0 mg	

Apricot Bars

Shirley Thieszen
Lakin, KS

Virginia Bender
Dover, DE

Makes 20 servings,
2½"×2¼" bar per serving

Prep. Time: 20 minutes
Baking Time: 40–45 minutes

½ **cup egg substitute,** *divided*
½ **cup + 2 Tbsp. trans-fat-free tub margarine,** *divided*
1 **tsp. baking powder**
1 **cup flour**
6 **Tbsp. Splenda Blend for Baking**

1¼ **cups quick oats**
1 **cup sugar-free apricot jam,** *or* **preserves**
½ **cup granular Splenda**
¼ **cup egg substitute**
2 **Tbsp. margarine**
⅔ **cup coconut**

1. Combine ¼ cup egg substitute, ½ cup margarine, baking powder, flour, Splenda and quick oats. Press into greased 9×13 baking pan.

2. Spread batter with apricot jam.

3. Mix together granular Splenda, ¼ cup egg substitute, 2 Tbsp. margarine and coconut. Spread this mixture over apricot jam.

4. Bake at 350° for 40–45 minutes. Cut when cool.

Variation:

Add ⅓ cup pecan or walnut pieces and ½ tsp. vanilla to ingredients in step 3.

Loren J. Zehr
Ft. Myers, FL

Exchange List Values

• Carbohydrate 1.0 • Fat 1.0

Basic Nutritional Values

• Calories 125	• Sodium 80 mg
(Calories from Fat 55)	• Potassium 55 gm
• Total Fat 6 gm	• Total Carb 18 gm
(Saturated Fat 2.0 gm,	• Dietary Fiber 1 gm
Trans Fat 0.0 gm,	• Sugars 6 gm
Polyunsat Fat 1.9 gm,	• Protein 2 gm
Monounsat Fat 1.5 gm)	• Phosphorus 55 gm
• Cholesterol 0 mg	

Date Nut Bars

Anna A. Yoder
Millersburg, OH

Makes 24 servings,
2" square per serving

Prep. Time: 20 minutes
Baking Time: 15–20 minutes

2 eggs
6 Tbsp. Splenda Blend for
  Baking
½ cup trans-fat-free tub
  margarine
¾ cup whole wheat flour
¼ tsp. baking powder
1 cup chopped nuts
1 cup chopped dates

1. Beat eggs and add
Splenda, mixing well. Add
melted margarine.
2. Sift together flour and
baking powder and add to
batter. Beat gently. Fold in
nuts and dates. Pour into
greased 9×13 pan.
3. Bake at 350° for about
15–20 minutes. Cool, cut and
serve.

Exchange List Values
• Carbohydrate 1.0 • Fat 1.0

Basic Nutritional Values
• Calories 105   • Sodium 40 mg
  (Calories from Fat 65) • Potassium 85 gm
• Total Fat 7 gm   • Total Carb 11 gm
  (Saturated Fat 1.1 gm, • Dietary Fiber 1 gm
  Trans Fat 0.0 gm,   • Sugars 7 gm
  Polyunsat Fat 3.6 gm, • Protein 2 gm
  Monounsat Fat 1.5 gm) • Phosphorus 50 gm
• Cholesterol 15 mg

Chocolate Brownies

Sandy Zeiset Richardson
Leavenworth, WA

Makes 16 servings,
2" square per serving

Prep. Time: 20 minutes
Baking Time: 30 minutes

2 eggs
6 Tbsp. Splenda Blend for
  Baking
½ tsp. vanilla
½ cup light (50% less
  calories and sugar)
  chocolate syrup
⅓ cup canola oil
¾ cup flour
½ tsp. salt
½ cup chopped nuts

1. Beat eggs until foamy.
Add Splenda and vanilla.
Beat.
2. Add chocolate syrup and
oil. Beat.
3. Add flour and salt. Mix
thoroughly. Fold in nuts.
4. Spread into 8" square
nonstick pan.
5. Bake at 350° for 30
minutes.

Exchange List Values
• Carbohydrate 1.0 • Fat 1.5

Basic Nutritional Values
• Calories 125   • Sodium 95 mg
  (Calories from Fat 70) • Potassium 50 gm
• Total Fat 8 gm   • Total Carb 13 gm
  (Saturated Fat 0.8 gm, • Dietary Fiber 1 gm
  Trans Fat 0.0 gm,   • Sugars 7 gm
  Polyunsat Fat 3.2 gm, • Protein 2 gm
  Monounsat Fat 3.4 gm) • Phosphorus 35 gm
• Cholesterol 25 mg

Cheesecake

Dot Hess
Willow Street, PA

Makes 15 servings

Prep. Time: 30 minutes
Baking Time: 1 hour 10 minutes
Chilling Time: 3 hours

Crust:
  1½ cups crushed graham
    crackers
  2 Tbsp. Splenda Blend
    for Baking
  ¼ cup trans-fat-free tub
    margarine

Filling:
  3 8-oz. pkgs. fat-free
    cream cheese,
    softened
  5 eggs
  ½ cup Splenda Blend for
    Baking
  1½ tsp. vanilla

Topping:
  1½ pints fat-free sour
    cream
  ⅓ cup granular Splenda
  1½ tsp. vanilla

1. Combine graham crack-
ers, sugar, and margarine.
Press into bottom of 9-inch
spring-form pan.
2. Beat cream cheese well
with mixer. Add eggs, one at
a time, mixing well after each
one.
3. Add Splenda and vanilla.
4. Pour gently over pre-
pared crust.
5. Bake at 300° for 1 hour.
Cool 5 minutes. Do not turn
off oven.
6. As the cake cools, mix

sour cream, Splenda, and vanilla.

7. Spread topping on cake and bake 5 minutes more.

8. Chill for at least 3 hours before serving.

Good Go-Alongs:

Good with canned pie filling on top

Variation:

Omit crust. Bake at 350° for 35 minutes and proceed with topping.

Renée Hankins
Narvon, PA

Exchange List Values

- Fat-Free Milk 0.5 • Fat 1.0
- Carbohydrate 1.5

Basic Nutritional Values

- Calories 200 • Sodium 440 mg
  (Calories from Fat 45) • Potassium 230 gm
- Total Fat 5 gm • Total Carb 26 gm
  (Saturated Fat 1.3 gm, • Dietary Fiber 0 gm
  Trans Fat 0.0 gm, • Sugars 15 gm
  Polyunsat Fat 1.6 gm, • Protein 10 gm
  Monounsat Fat 1.7 gm) • Phosphorus 330 gm
- Cholesterol 75 mg

Date Pudding (an old-fashioned trifle from scratch!)

Clara Byler
Hartville, OH

Makes 12 servings,
2"×2⅔" rectangle per serving

Prep. Time: 30 minutes
Cooking/Baking Time: 45 minutes
Cooling Time: 1 hour

1 cup dates
1 tsp. baking soda
1 Tbsp. butter
1 cup boiling water
½ cup Splenda Blend for Baking
1 egg
1½ cups flour
1 cup chopped nuts
1 tsp. vanilla

Sauce:
  2 cups water
  ½ cup Splenda Brown Sugar Blend
  1 Tbsp. butter
  2 Tbsp. flour
  1 tsp. vanilla
  pinch of salt

whipping cream or whipped topping, *optional*

1. In a heatproof mixing bowl, pour boiling water over the dates, baking soda and butter. Let cool for 30 minutes.

2. Add sugar, flour, egg, and vanilla. Beat well.

3. Stir in nuts.

4. Pour batter into greased 8×8 pan.

5. Bake at 350° for 35 minutes or until toothpick comes out clean. Cool at least 1 hour.

6. To make sauce, bring water to boil in covered saucepan.

7. Add rest of sauce ingredients and bring to a boil again.

8. Remove from heat. Allow to cool for at least 30 minutes.

9. Break the cooled cake (date pudding) into pieces and put in pretty glass serving dish.

10. Drizzle sauce over the pieces.

Tip:

Layer the broken cake pieces and sauce with optional whipped cream.

Exchange List Values

- Carbohydrate 2.5 • Fat 1.5

Basic Nutritional Values

- Calories 245 • Sodium 125 mg
  (Calories from Fat 70) • Potassium 160 gm
- Total Fat 8 gm • Total Carb 39 gm
  (Saturated Fat 1.1 gm, • Dietary Fiber 2 gm
  Trans Fat 0.0 gm, • Sugars 20 gm
  Polyunsat Fat 5.5 gm, • Protein 4 gm
  Monounsat Fat 1.5 gm) • Phosphorus 70 gm
- Cholesterol 15 mg

When a recipe calls for softened cream cheese, remove the cream cheese from the refrigerator at least 2 hours before starting the recipe.
Mamie Christopherson, Rio Rancho, NM

Royal Raspberry Cake

Miriam Christophel
Battle Creek, MI

Makes 20 servings

Prep. Time: 25 minutes
Baking Time: 30–35 minutes

Cake:
2 cups flour
½ tsp. salt
1 Tbsp. baking powder
⅓ cup no-trans-fat tub
   margarine, softened
½ cup Splenda Blend for
   Baking
1 egg, room temperature
1 cup fat-free milk, room
   temperature
1 tsp. vanilla
3½ cups red raspberries

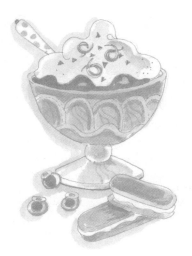

Glaze:
1½ cups granular
   Splenda
¼ cup cornstarch
1⅔ Tbsp. water
½ tsp. vanilla

1. Sift together flour, salt and baking powder. Set aside.
2. Cream margarine with mixer. Add Splenda gradually, beating well after each addition. Stir in egg.
3. Combine milk and vanilla.
4. Add dry ingredients to margarine mixture, alternating with milk and vanilla and beating well after each addition.
5. Spread cake batter into greased 9×13 pan. Spread berries evenly over the top.
6. Bake at 350° for 30–35 minutes or until center of cake springs back when lightly touched. Cool 5 minutes.
7. To make glaze, blend Splenda and cornstarch until a very fine powder. Pour into a small bowl. Add vanilla and water and stir well. Spread over cake.

Tip:
Serve warm with ice cream or frozen yogurt.

Exchange List Values
- Carbohydrate 1.5   • Fat 0.5

Basic Nutritional Values
- Calories 120
  (Calories from Fat 20)
- Total Fat 2.5 gm
  (Saturated Fat 0.6 gm,
  Trans Fat 0.0 gm,
  Polyunsat Fat 1.1 gm,
  Monounsat Fat 0.8 gm)
- Cholesterol 10 mg
- Sodium 145 mg
- Potassium 70 gm
- Total Carb 21 gm
- Dietary Fiber 2 gm
- Sugars 8 gm
- Protein 2 gm
- Phosphorus 105 gm

Blueberry Spice Cake

Rosalle M. Otto
Champaign, IL

Makes 20 servings,
2¼"×2½" rectangle per serving

Prep. Time: 25 minutes
Baking Time: 30 minutes

1 pint blueberries
2 cups flour
2 tsp. baking powder
1 tsp. baking soda
½ tsp. ground cinnamon
½ tsp. ground cloves
½ tsp. ground allspice
½ tsp. salt
⅓ cup trans-fat-free tub
   margarine, softened
½ cup Splenda Blend for
   Baking
1 egg, room temperature
3 Tbsp. molasses
1 cup 1% buttermilk

1. Toss berries in a little flour.
2. Sift flour, measuring 2 cups. Resift flour with baking powder, baking soda, cinnamon, cloves, allspice and salt.
3. Cream butter and white sugar. Beat egg and add to batter.
4. Gradually beat in molasses. Add this mixture alternately with milk to dry ingredients.
5. Fold in blueberries. Spread batter into greased and floured 9×13 pan.
6. Bake at 375° for 30 minutes. Cool on rack.

Desserts

Exchange List Values

- Carbohydrate 1.5
- Fat 0.5

Basic Nutritional Values

- Calories 110
  (Calories from Fat 20)
- Total Fat 2.5 gm
  (Saturated Fat 0.7 gm,
  Trans Fat 0.0 gm,
  Polyunsat Fat 1.1 gm,
  Monounsat Fat 0.9 gm)
- Cholesterol 10 mg
- Sodium 200 mg
- Potassium 95 gm
- Total Carb 20 gm
- Dietary Fiber 1 gm
- Sugars 9 gm
- Protein 2 gm
- Phosphorus 80 gm

German Blueberry Kuchen

Mrs. A. Krueger
Richmond, British Columbia

*Makes 20 servings,
3" square per serving*

*Prep. Time: 30 minutes
Baking Time: 40–45 minutes*

Batter:
3 cups flour
¾ cup Splenda Blend for Baking
4 tsp. baking powder
½ tsp. salt
½ cup no-trans-fat tub margarine
1⅓ cups milk
2 eggs
2 tsp. vanilla
1 tsp. nutmeg
grated rind of 1 lemon
4 cups fresh, *or* frozen blueberries

Crumb Topping:
½ cup granular Splenda
½ cup flour
¼ cup no-trans-fat tub margarine

1. To prepare batter, combine flour, Splenda, baking powder, salt, margarine and milk in large bowl.
2. Beat 2 minutes with electric mixer or 300 strokes by hand. Add eggs, vanilla, nutmeg and lemon rind. Mix thoroughly.
3. Pour batter into greased and floured 12×16 baking pan. (Do not use a smaller pan.) Sprinkle with blueberries.
4. To prepare crumb topping rub together Splenda, flour and margarine until mixture is crumbly. Sprinkle over layer of blueberries.
5. Bake at 350° for 40–45 minutes. Cut into squares.

Exchange List Values
- Carbohydrate 2.0
- Fat 1.0

Basic Nutritional Values
- Calories 190
  (Calories from Fat 55)
- Total Fat 6 gm
  (Saturated Fat 1.3 gm,
  Trans Fat 0.0 gm,
  Polyunsat Fat 2.3 gm,
  Monounsat Fat 1.9 gm)
- Cholesterol 20 mg
- Sodium 200 mg
- Potassium 80 gm
- Total Carb 30 gm
- Dietary Fiber 1 gm
- Sugars 12 gm
- Protein 4 gm
- Phosphorus 145 gm

Dark Apple Cake

Amy Bauer
New Ulm, MN

*Makes 24 servings,
2" square per serving*

*Prep. Time: 30 minutes
Baking Time: 50 minutes*

½ cup trans-fat-free tub margarine
⅓ cup canola oil
4 eggs
1 cup Splenda Blend for baking
1 cup cold coffee
3 cups all-purpose flour
1½ tsp. baking soda
1½ tsp. ground cinnamon
½ tsp. ground nutmeg
½ tsp. ground cloves
½ tsp. salt
1 tsp. vanilla
1 cup chopped nuts
½ cup raisins
2 cups chopped apples

1. Cream sugar, shortening and eggs. Blend in coffee.
2. Add rest of ingredients. Mix well.
3. Pour into greased 9×13 pan. Bake at 350° for 50 minutes.

Exchange List Values
- Carbohydrate 1.5
- Fat 2.0

Basic Nutritional Values
- Calories 200
  (Calories from Fat 90)
- Total Fat 10 gm
  (Saturated Fat 1.4 gm,
  Trans Fat 0.0 gm,
  Polyunsat Fat 4.6 gm,
  Monounsat Fat 3.6 gm)
- Cholesterol 30 mg
- Sodium 170 mg
- Potassium 90 gm
- Total Carb 25 gm
- Dietary Fiber 1 gm
- Sugars 11 gm
- Protein 4 gm
- Phosphorus 55 gm

Raw Apple Cake

Kathryn Yoder
Minot, ND

Makes 20 servings

Prep. Time: 20 minutes
Baking/Cooking Time: 1 hour

Cake:

4 cups diced apples
1 cup Splenda Brown
   Sugar Blend
½ cup canola oil
1 cup nuts, *optional*
2 eggs, beaten
2 tsp. vanilla
2 cups whole wheat
   flour
2 tsp. baking soda
2 tsp. cinnamon
1 tsp. salt

Hard Sauce:

¼ cup margarine
6 Tbsp. Splenda Brown
   Sugar Blend
1⅓ Tbsp. flour
dash salt
1½ cups water
1 tsp. maple flavoring

1. To prepare cake combine apples and brown sugar and mix thoroughly. Add oil, nuts, eggs and vanilla.
2. Mix all dry ingredients and add to batter. Place in greased and floured 9×13 pan.
3. Bake at 350° for 40–50 minutes or until done.
4. To prepare hard sauce, melt margarine in saucepan. Add all other ingredients and cook until mixture thickens.

5. Pour over warm cake. Serve.

Exchange List Values
• Carbohydrate 2.0   • Fat 1.0

Basic Nutritional Values
• Calories 180   • Sodium 275 mg
  (Calories from Fat 70) • Potassium 105 gm
• Total Fat 8 gm   • Total Carb 26 gm
  (Saturated Fat 1.0 gm, • Dietary Fiber 2 gm
  Trans Fat 0.0 gm,   • Sugars 9 gm
  Polyunsat Fat 2.4 gm, • Protein 2 gm
  Monounsat Fat 4.2 gm) • Phosphorus 55 gm
• Cholesterol 20 mg

Carrot Fruitcake

Margaret Wenger Johnson
Keezletown, VA

Makes 2 small loaves,
8 slices per loaf, 1 slice per serving

Prep. Time: 25 minutes
Cooling Time: 30 minutes
Baking/Cooking Time: 1 hour

1 cup grated carrots
1 cup raisins
6 Tbsp. honey
3 Tbsp. Splenda Blend
   for Baking

2 Tbsp. tub no-trans-fat
   margarine
1 tsp. cinnamon
1 tsp. allspice
1 tsp. salt
½ tsp. nutmeg
¼ tsp. cloves
1½ cups water
1½ cups whole wheat flour
1 tsp. baking soda
½ cup wheat germ
½ cup chopped walnuts

1. Cook carrots, raisins, honey, Splenda, margarine and spices in 1½ cups water for 10 minutes. Let cool.
2. Combine flour, baking soda, wheat germ and walnuts. Add dry ingredients to batter and mix well. Pour into 2 small, well-greased loaf pans.
3. Bake at 300° for 45 minutes.

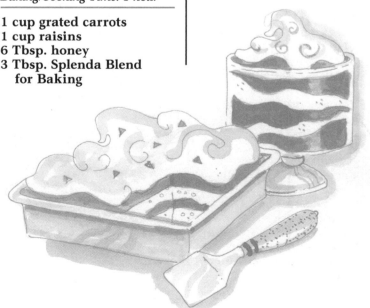

Exchange List Values
- Carbohydrate 2.0 • Fat 0.5

Basic Nutritional Values
- Calories 160
  (Calories from Fat 35)
- Total Fat 4 gm
  (Saturated Fat 0.6 gm,
  Trans Fat 0.0 gm,
  Polyunsat Fat 2.5 gm,
  Monounsat Fat 0.8 gm)
- Cholesterol 0 mg
- Sodium 245 mg
- Potassium 190 gm
- Total Carb 29 gm
- Dietary Fiber 3 gm
- Sugars 17 gm
- Protein 4 gm
- Phosphorus 105 gm

Chocolate Chip Applesauce Cake

Lois Cressman
Plattsville, Ontario
Ruby Lehman
Towson, MD

Makes 20 servings

Prep. Time: 25 minutes
Baking Time: 40 minutes

¾ cup Splenda Blend for
  Baking
½ cup cooking oil
2 eggs
2 cups unsweetened
  applesauce
2 cups flour
1½ tsp. baking soda
½ tsp. cinnamon
2 Tbsp. unsweetened cocoa

Topping:
½ cup chopped nuts
½ cup chocolate chips

1. To prepare cake batter
combine Splenda, oil, eggs
and applesauce. Beat lightly.
2. Add all dry ingredients
and stir to mix.

3. Pour into greased 9×13
pan. Mix topping ingredients
and sprinkle over batter.
4. Bake at 350° for 40
minutes. When cool, cut in 4
rows lengthwise and 5 rows
crosswise to yield 20 pieces.

Exchange List Values
- Carbohydrate 1.5 • Fat 2.0

Basic Nutritional Values
- Calories 185
  (Calories from Fat 80)
- Total Fat 9 gm
  (Saturated Fat 1.6 gm,
  Trans Fat 0.0 gm,
  Polyunsat Fat 3.1 gm,
  Monounsat Fat 4.4 gm)
- Cholesterol 20 mg
- Sodium 105 mg
- Potassium 75 gm
- Total Carb 23 gm
- Dietary Fiber 1 gm
- Sugars 12 gm
- Protein 3 gm
- Phosphorus 45 gm

Chocolate Oatmeal Cake

Dorothy R. Hess
Coolidge, AZ

Makes 20 servings,
2" square per serving

Prep. Time: 20 minutes
Standing Time: 5–10 minutes
Baking Time: 35 minutes

1½ cups boiling water
1 cup rolled oats
⅓ cup canola oil
1 cup Splenda Blend for
  Baking
2 eggs
1 cup flour
½ tsp. salt
1 tsp. baking soda
½ cup cocoa
1 tsp. vanilla
½ cup chopped nuts

3 oz. chocolate chips

1. Pour boiling water over
oatmeal in large mixing
bowl and let stand for 5–10
minutes.
2. Add oil, Splenda, and
eggs. Mix well. Add flour,
salt, baking soda, cocoa and
vanilla. Pour into greased and
floured 9×13 baking pan.
3. Sprinkle nuts and
chocolate chips over batter.
4. Bake at 350° for about
35 minutes.

Exchange List Values
- Carbohydrate 1.0 • Fat 1.5

Basic Nutritional Values
- Calories 135
  (Calories from Fat 65)
- Total Fat 7 gm
  (Saturated Fat 1.3 gm,
  Trans Fat 0.0 gm,
  Polyunsat Fat 2.2 gm,
  Monounsat Fat 2.8 gm)
- Cholesterol 15 mg
- Sodium 110 mg
- Potassium 75 gm
- Total Carb 18 gm
- Dietary Fiber 1 gm
- Sugars 10 gm
- Protein 2 gm
- Phosphorus 55 gm

Gingerbread with Lemon Sauce

Fran Sauder
Mount Joy, PA

Makes 12 servings,
2¼"×3" rectangle per serving

Prep. Time: 20 minutes
Baking Time: 45 minutes
Cooking Time: 20 minutes

2 cups flour
½ cup Splenda Blend for
   Baking
1 tsp. ginger
1 tsp. cinnamon
⅓ cup canola oil
1 egg, beaten
2 Tbsp. molasses
½ tsp. salt
1 tsp. baking soda
1 cup 1%-fat buttermilk
whipped cream, *optional*

1. Sift together flour, sugar, ginger, and cinnamon.
2. Cut shortening into flour mixture to make fine crumbs. Take out ½ cup crumbs and set aside.
3. To remaining, add egg, molasses, salt, baking soda, and buttermilk. Beat well.
4. Pour into 9×9 greased and floured cake pan. Sprinkle with reserved crumbs.
5. Bake at 350° for 45 minutes. Serve with lemon sauce and optional whipped cream.

Lemon Sauce:
2 cups water
4 Tbsp. cornstarch
1½ cups granular
   Splenda
¼ tsp. salt
3 egg yolks
4 tsp. butter
juice of 2 lemons
zest of 1 lemon

1. Bring water to boil in covered saucepan.
2. Combine cornstarch, Splenda, and salt. Mix well. Add to boiling water, stirring constantly. Cook about 5 minutes on low heat. Mixture should be thickened.
3. Stir a small amount of hot sugar mixture into beaten egg yolks, whisking continuously. Return the whole mixture to pan and cook 1 more minute, stirring constantly.
4. Remove from heat; add lemon juice, zest, and butter.

Exchange List Values
• Carbohydrate 2.0 • Fat 2.0

Basic Nutritional Values
• Calories 235
(Calories from Fat 80)
• Total Fat 9 gm
(Saturated Fat 1.9 gm,
Trans Fat 0.1 gm,
Polyunsat Fat 2.1 gm,
Monounsat Fat 4.8 gm)
• Cholesterol 65 mg
• Sodium 295 mg
• Potassium 125 gm
• Total Carb 34 gm
• Dietary Fiber 1 gm
• Sugars 14 gm
• Protein 4 gm
• Phosphorus 70 gm

Apple Cupcakes

24 servings, 1 cupcake per serving

Prep. Time: 20 minutes
Baking Time: 20–25 minutes

1 cup whole wheat flour
1¼ cups white flour
½ cup Splenda Blend for
   Baking
1½ tsp. baking soda
⅜ tsp. baking powder
1 tsp. ground cinnamon
½ tsp. ground cloves
⅔ cup canola oil
2 eggs
⅔ cup fat-free milk
1½ tsp. vanilla
3 cups chopped apples
½ cup raisins, *optional*

Topping:
1 Tbsp. trans-fat-free tub
   margarine, melted
2⅔ Tbsp. Splenda Brown
   Sugar Blend

½ cup chopped nuts
2 tsp. cinnamon
2 tsp. flour
¼ cup quick oats

1. Combine flours, Splenda, baking powder, baking powder, and spices in a bowl.
2. Add margarine, eggs, milk and vanilla and beat well. Fold in apples and raisins.
3. Fill greased and floured muffin cups at least ½ full.
4. Mix all topping ingredients and put 1 tsp. topping on each cupcake.
5. Bake at 350° for 20–25 minutes.

Always check what you are baking a little earlier than stated in the recipe. Ovens do vary.
Mary Jones, Marengo, OH

Exchange List Values
- Carbohydrate 1.0 • Fat 2.0

Basic Nutritional Values
- Calories 160 • Sodium 100 mg
  (Calories from Fat 80) • Potassium 80 gm
- Total Fat 9 gm • Total Carb 18 gm
  (Saturated Fat 0.9 gm, • Dietary Fiber 2 gm
  Trans Fat 0.0 gm, • Sugars 7 gm
  Polyunsat Fat 3.2 gm, • Protein 3 gm
  Monounsat Fat 4.4 gm) • Phosphorus 60 gm
- Cholesterol 15 mg

New England Blueberry Pie

Krista Hershberger
Elverson, PA

*Makes 8 servings,
1 slice per serving*

Prep. Time: 15 minutes
Cooking Time: 12 minutes
Chilling Time: 1 hour

4 cups fresh blueberries, *divided*
½ cup Splenda Blend for Baking
3 Tbsp. cornstarch
¼ tsp. salt
¼ cup water
1 Tbsp. trans-fat-free tub margarine
pre-baked 9"pie shell (see page 203)
whipped cream, *optional*

1. Place 2 cups of blueberries in a baked pie shell.
2. In medium saucepan, cook sugar, cornstarch, salt, water, remaining 2 cups blueberries and butter. Stir continuously until thick.

3. Cool blueberry mixture for ½ hour. Pour cooled mixture over berries in pie crust. Chill.
4. Top with whipped cream before serving if you wish.

Warm Memories:
We have our own blueberry bushes so this is the first recipe to come out when we pick our first batch!

Exchange List Values
- Carbohydrate 2.0 • Fat 0.5

Basic Nutritional Values
- Calories 150 • Sodium 105 mg
  (Calories from Fat 25) • Potassium 65 gm
- Total Fat 3 gm • Total Carb 30 gm
  (Saturated Fat 0.6 gm, • Dietary Fiber 2 gm
  Trans Fat 0.2 gm, • Sugars 19 gm
  Polyunsat Fat 1.0 gm, • Protein 1 gm
  Monounsat Fat 1.2 gm) • Phosphorus 15 gm
- Cholesterol 0 mg

Pumpkin Cupcakes

Shelley Burns
Elverson, PA

*Makes 24 cupcakes,
1 cupcake per serving*

Prep. Time: 20 minutes
Baking Time: 20–25 minutes

1 cup Splenda Blend for Baking
2 cups cooked pumpkin
2 cups flour
1 cup canola oil
¼ cup fat-free milk
4 eggs
1 tsp. salt
2 tsp. baking powder
2 tsp. baking soda
2 tsp. cinnamon
dash of nutmeg
½ cup coconut, *optional*
cinnamon and sugar, *optional*

1. Mix together Splenda, pumpkin, oil, milk and eggs.
2. Add flour, salt, baking powder, baking soda, cinnamon, and nutmeg. Fold in coconut if you wish.
3. Line 24 muffin cups with cupcake papers.
4. Divide batter among them.
5. Sprinkle cinnamon and sugar on tops of cupcakes if you wish.
6. Bake at 350° for 20–25 minutes or until toothpick inserted comes out clean.

Tip:
You can use canned or frozen pumpkin. I use frozen pumpkin. I get it out of the freezer a few hours before I am going to use it. I let it thaw and drain any excess water off before using it in the recipe.

Exchange List Values
- Carbohydrate 1.0 • Fat 2.0

Basic Nutritional Values
- Calories 170 • Sodium 245 mg
  (Calories from Fat 90) • Potassium 70 gm
- Total Fat 10 gm • Total Carb 18 gm
  (Saturated Fat 1.0 gm, • Dietary Fiber 1 gm
  Trans Fat 0.0 gm, • Sugars 9 gm
  Polyunsat Fat 2.8 gm, • Protein 2 gm
  Monounsat Fat 6.1 gm) • Phosphorus 75 gm
- Cholesterol 30 mg

No-Added-Sugar Apple Pie

Faye Pankratz
Inola, OK

Makes 1 9" pie,
8 slices, 1 slice per serving

Prep. Time: 30 minutes
Chilling Time: 1 hours
Baking Time: 45 minutes

Pastry:
½ cup low-fat ricotta
    cheese
5 pkgs. artificial
    sweetener
3 Tbsp. fat-free milk
1 egg white
2 Tbsp. cooking oil
1½ tsp. vanilla
dash salt
2 cups flour
2 tsp. baking powder
2 Tbsp. water

Filling:
6–8 apples
¼ cup flour
½ tsp. cinnamon
10–12 pkgs. artificial
    sweetener

1. Mix pastry ingredients in the order given. Divide pastry into two equal pieces. Chill dough.
2. Roll each piece of dough into a 10" circle. Place 1 piece of pastry in pie pan.
3. Peel and slice apples. Toss with flour, cinnamon and sweetener. Spoon into pie shell.
4. Use remaining pastry for a top crust. Slit in several places.

5. Bake at 375° for 20 minutes. Reduce temperature to 325° and bake 25 minutes longer. (The edges of this pastry tend to get hard.)

Exchange List Values
• Starch 2.0   • Fat 1.0
• Fruit 0.5

Basic Nutritional Values
• Calories 230   • Sodium 140 mg
  (Calories from Fat 40) • Potassium 160 gm
• Total Fat 4.5 gm   • Total Carb 42 gm
  (Saturated Fat 0.8 gm, • Dietary Fiber 2 gm
  Trans Fat 0.0 gm,   • Sugars 12 gm
  Polyunsat Fat 1.3 gm, • Protein 6 gm
  Monounsat Fat 2.4 gm) • Phosphorus 195 gm
• Cholesterol 5 mg

Simple Egg Custard Pie

Peggy Howell
Hinton, WV

Makes 8 servings,
1 slice per serving

Prep. Time: 10 minutes
Baking Time: 25–30 minutes
Cooling Time: 1 hour

4 eggs
¼ cup Splenda Blend for
    Baking
½ tsp. salt
2 cups fat-free milk
1 tsp. vanilla
9" unbaked pie shell (see
    page 203)

nutmeg, *optional*
cinnamon and sugar,
    optional

1. Mix eggs, Splenda, salt, milk, and vanilla together.
2. Pour into unbaked pie shell.
3. Sprinkle with nutmeg or cinnamon and sugar if you wish.
4. Place on lower oven rack. Bake at 425° for 25–30 minutes. Center may still be a little jiggly, but it will firm up as it cools.
5. Allow to cool 1 hour before serving.

Variation:
Spread ½ can prepared pie filling (blueberry or cherry) evenly over bottom of pie crust. Slowly pour custard filling over it so as not to disturb the fruit. Bake as instructed. The fruit under custard makes for a tasty treat!

Exchange List Values
• Carbohydrate 1.0   • Fat 1.0

Basic Nutritional Values
• Calories 120   • Sodium 225 mg
  (Calories from Fat 40) • Potassium 140 gm
• Total Fat 4.5 gm   • Total Carb 14 gm
  (Saturated Fat 1.1 gm, • Dietary Fiber 0 gm
  Trans Fat 0.2 gm,   • Sugars 9 gm
  Polyunsat Fat 0.9 gm, • Protein 6 gm
  Monounsat Fat 1.8 gm) • Phosphorus 115 gm
• Cholesterol 95 mg

Over-ripe bananas can be peeled and frozen in a plastic bag until it's time to bake a bread or a cake.

Deb Kepiro, Strasburg, PA

Basic Pie Crust

Graham Kerr, from his book
Charting a Course to Wellness

Makes 1 9" pie crust
Serving size is ⅛ of a 9" pie

Prep. Time: 10 minutes
Baking Time: 10–12 minutes

¾ cup cake flour
½ tsp. sugar
1⅙ tsp. salt
1 Tbsp. non-aromatic olive oil
2 Tbsp. hard margarine (65% vegetable oil variety), frozen for 15 minutes
½ tsp. vinegar
2 Tbsp. ice water

1. In a mixing bowl, stir together cake flour, sugar, and salt.
2. Cut in olive oil and hard margarine with a pastry cutter or two knives until crumbly.
3. Sprinkle vinegar and ice water over dough. Toss with a fork until the dough is moistened and forms a ball.
4. Roll out on a lightly floured surface.
5. Fold dough gently in half, without creasing. Then fold in half again, also without creasing.
6. Lift folded dough into pie pan with point in center of pan. Unfold dough, patting it into place. Crimp the edge if you wish.
7. If your recipe calls for a baked crust, use a fork to prick the crust in several places over the bottom and sides. Bake at 400° for 10–12 minutes, until lightly browned.

Exchange List Values
- Starch 0.5
- Fat 1.0

Basic Nutritional Values
- Calories 80
  (Calories from Fat 35)
- Total Fat 4 gm
  (Saturated Fat 0.6 gm,
  Trans Fat 0.4 gm,
  Polyunsat Fat 0.9 gm,
  Monounsat Fat 1.7 gm)
- Cholesterol 0 mg
- Sodium 50 mg
- Potassium 15 gm
- Total Carb 10 gm
- Dietary Fiber 0 gm
- Sugars 0 gm
- Protein 1 gm
- Phosphorus 10 gm

Lemon Pie for Beginners

Jean M. Butzer
Batavia, NY

Makes 8 servings

Prep. Time: 10 minutes
Cooking Time: 10–12 minutes
Cooling Time: 15 minutes

9-inch baked pastry shell (see page 203)
½ cup Splenda
4 Tbsp. cornstarch
¼ tsp. salt
1¾ cups water, divided
3 egg yolks, slightly beaten
2 Tbsp. trans-fat-free tub margarine
⅓ cup lemon juice
meringue *or* whipped cream, *optional*

1. Combine Splenda, cornstarch, salt, and ¼ cup water in 1½ quart microwave safe bowl.
2. Microwave remaining ¼ cup water on high until boiling. Stir into sugar mixture.
3. Microwave 4 to 6 minutes until very thick, stirring every 2 minutes.
4. Mix a little hot mixture into egg yolks. Blend yolks into sugar mixture.
5. Microwave 1 minute more.
6. Stir in margarine and lemon juice.
7. Cool for 15 minutes and pour into pie shell.
8. If desired, top with meringue and brown in oven for 10–15 minutes at 350° or serve with whipped cream.

Tips:
1. To make a meringue, beat 3 egg whites adding ¼ tsp. cream of tartar and 3 Tbsp. sugar slowly. Continue beating until stiff peaks form. Cover the lemon filling with meringue to edge of crust. Bake in 350° oven for 10–12 minutes or until meringue is golden.
2. Using the microwave is so much easier than cooking the filling on the top of the stove. You don't have to worry about it sticking or burning to the bottom of the pan.

Exchange List Values
- Carbohydrate 1.5
- Fat 1.0

Basic Nutritional Values
- Calories 140
  (Calories from Fat 55)
- Total Fat 6 gm
  (Saturated Fat 1.4 gm,
  Trans Fat 0.2 gm,
  Polyunsat Fat 1.6 gm,
  Monounsat Fat 2.3 gm)
- Cholesterol 70 mg
- Sodium 125 mg
- Potassium 25 gm
- Total Carb 21 gm
- Dietary Fiber 0 gm
- Sugars 12 gm
- Protein 2 gm
- Phosphorus 30 gm

Creamy Peanut Butter Dessert

Kristine Martin
Newmanstown, PA

Makes 16 servings,
2¼"×3¼" rectangle per serving

Prep. Time: 15 minutes
Chilling Time: 30 minutes + 3 hours

Crust:
 1¾ cups graham cracker crumbs
 ¼ cup trans-fat-free tub margarine
 2 Tbsp. peanut butter

Filling:
 8 oz. fat-free cream cheese, softened
 ½ cup peanut butter
 ½ cup granular Splenda
 2 tsp. vanilla
 16 oz. fat-free frozen whipped topping, thawed
 3 Tbsp. chocolate syrup

1. Combine cracker crumbs, margarine, and peanut butter. Mix well. Set aside ½ cup for topping.
2. Press remaining crumb mixture into greased 9×13 baking dish.
3. Cover and refrigerate 30 minutes.
4. Meanwhile, make the filling. In a mixing bowl, beat cream cheese and peanut butter until smooth.
5. Beat in Splenda and vanilla. Fold in whipped topping.

6. Spoon filling over chilled crust.
7. Drizzle with chocolate syrup. Sprinkle with reserved ½ cup crumbs.
8. Cover. Freeze for at least 3 hours before serving.
9. Remove from freezer 15 minutes before serving.

Warm Memories:
I take this often to hot and cold dish dinners. Everyone always thinks it has ice cream in it, which it doesn't so it's a lot easier to keep from melting than something with ice cream. I always get requests for the recipe.

Tip:
This dessert can be frozen up to three months, so it's convenient to make ahead for many occasions.

Exchange List Values
• Carbohydrate 1.5 • Fat 1.5

Basic Nutritional Values
• Calories 180
 (Calories from Fat 70)
• Total Fat 8 gm
 (Saturated Fat 1.6 gm,
 Trans Fat 0.0 gm,
 Polyunsat Fat 2.6 gm,
 Monounsat Fat 3.4 gm)
• Cholesterol 5 mg
• Sodium 225 mg
• Potassium 145 gm
• Total Carb 21 gm
• Dietary Fiber 1 gm
• Sugars 9 gm
• Protein 5 gm
• Phosphorus 140 gm

Rhubarb Dessert

Ruth Schiefer
Vassar, MI

Makes 20 servings,
2¼" square per serving

Prep. Time: 20 minutes
Cooking Time: 15 minutes
Cooling Time: 30 minutes

 2 cups + 2 Tbsp. granular Splenda, *divided*
 8 cups diced rhubarb
 1 cup water
 3 Tbsp. cornstarch
 0.3-oz. pkg. sugar-free raspberry gelatin
 2 cups graham cracker crumbs
 ½ cup trans-fat-free tub margarine, melted
 8 oz. fat-free frozen whipped topping, thawed
 1½ cups mini marshmallows, melted
 1-oz. pkg. fat-free, sugar-free instant vanilla pudding
 1½ cups fat-free milk

1. Combine 2 cups Splenda, rhubarb, water, and cornstarch in saucepan.
2. Bring to a boil, stirring frequently. Cook until thickened and clear.
3. Remove saucepan from heat. Stir in powdered gelatin.
4. Cool at least 30 minutes.
5. Mix graham cracker crumbs, margarine, and 2 Tbsp. Splenda. Set aside ⅓ cup for topping.
6. Press remaining crumbs in bottom of greased 9×13 pan to form crust.

7. Spread cooled rhubarb over crust.

8. In microwave safe bowl, melt marshmallows in microwave. Check and stir until smooth.

9. Mix together melted marshmallows and whipped topping, stirring vigorously to combine.

10. Spread mixture over rhubarb layer.

11. Mix vanilla pudding with milk for 2 minutes until thickened.

12. Gently spread pudding over marshmallow layer.

13. Sprinkle reserved crumbs on top. Refrigerate.

Tip:
Keep cold. Cut in squares.

Exchange List Values
• Carbohydrate 1.5 • Fat 1.0

Basic Nutritional Values
• Calories 135 • Sodium 175 mg
  (Calories from Fat 40) • Potassium 195 gm
• Total Fat 4.5 gm • Total Carb 21 gm
  (Saturated Fat 0.9 gm, • Dietary Fiber 1 gm
  Trans Fat 0.0 gm, • Sugars 10 gm
  Polyunsat Fat 1.7 gm, • Protein 2 gm
  Monounsat Fat 1.4 gm) • Phosphorus 85 gm
• Cholesterol 0 mg

Fresh Peach Delight

Jan Mast
Lancaster, PA

*Makes 20 servings,
2¼" square per serving*

Prep. Time: 20 minutes
Cooking/Baking Time: 35 minutes
Cooling Time: 1½ hours

½ cup trans-fat-free tub margarine
2 Tbsp. Splenda Brown Sugar Blend
1 cup chopped pecans
1 cup + 2 Tbsp. flour
8 oz. fat-free cream cheese, softened
1 cup confectioners sugar
1 tsp. vanilla
2 cups frozen whipped topping, thawed
2 Tbsp. cornstarch
⅓ cup granular Splenda
1½ cups water
0.3-oz. box sugar-free peach gelatin
4 cups sliced fresh peaches

1. To make a crust, combine margarine, Splenda, pecans, and flour. Press into a 9×13 baking pan.

2. Bake at 350° for 25 minutes. Cool at least 30 minutes.

3. Beat cream cheese until soft and smooth. Beat in vanilla and confectioners sugar.

4. Fold in whipped topping.

5. Spread filling on cooled crust.

6. To make topping, combine cornstarch and granular Splenda in a saucepan. Add water.

7. Cook until boiling. Boil and stir for 2 minutes.

8. Add gelatin and stir well. Allow to cool at least 30 minutes.

9. Combine gelatin mixture with sliced peaches and stir gently.

10. Refrigerate until cool but not gelled – between 15–30 minutes.

11. Pour cooled topping over filling.

12. Chill and cut into squares to serve.

Warm Memories:
Everyone loves this yummy dessert. It works well with fresh strawberries, fresh blueberries, etc. Just change the gelatin flavor and fruit for your own variation!

Exchange List Values
• Carbohydrate 1.5 • Fat 1.5

Basic Nutritional Values
• Calories 165 • Sodium 125 mg
  (Calories from Fat 70) • Potassium 140 gm
• Total Fat 8 gm • Total Carb 21 gm
  (Saturated Fat 1.1 gm, • Dietary Fiber 1 gm
  Trans Fat 0.0 gm, • Sugars 11 gm
  Polyunsat Fat 2.6 gm, • Protein 3 gm
  Monounsat Fat 3.5 gm) • Phosphorus 105 gm
• Cholesterol 0 mg

Beside each dish of food on the buffet, place a stack of cards with its recipe written on them. Then guests can take the recipe if they wish.
Anita Troyer, Fairview, MI

Mom's Baked Rice Pudding

Stacie Skelly
Millersville, PA

*Makes 6 servings,
about ½ cup per serving*

Prep. Time: 5 minutes
Baking Time: 1½ hours
Cooling Time: 30 minutes

1 quart (4 cups) 1% milk
½ cup white rice (not instant)
½ cup granular Splenda
pinch of salt
1 Tbsp. vanilla
cinnamon *or* nutmeg

1. Mix together milk, rice, Splenda, salt, and vanilla.
2. Pour into buttered 1½ quart casserole
3. Bake at 325° for 1½ hours. Stir every 20 minutes.
4. Sprinkle with cinnamon or nutmeg.
5. Cool at least 30 minutes and serve warm, or chill for several hours and serve cold.

Exchange List Values
- Starch 1.0
- Fat-Free Milk 0.5

Basic Nutritional Values
- Calories 140
  (Calories from Fat 15)
- Total Fat 2 gm
  (Saturated Fat 1.1 gm,
  Trans Fat 0.0 gm,
  Polyunsat Fat 0.1 gm,
  Monounsat Fat 0.5 gm)
- Cholesterol 10 mg
- Sodium 100 mg
- Potassium 265 gm
- Total Carb 23 gm
- Dietary Fiber 0 gm
- Sugars 11 gm
- Protein 7 gm
- Phosphorus 170 gm

Cracker Pudding

Anna Musser
Manheim, PA

*Makes 6 servings,
about 7 oz. per serving*

Prep. Time: 15 minutes
Cooking Time: 15 minutes
Chilling Time: 2 hours

1 quart (4 cups) fat-free milk
1 cup coarse saltine cracker crumbs
½ cup egg substitute
¾ cup granular Splenda
⅓ cup flaked coconut
pinch salt
1 Tbsp. vanilla

1. Combine milk and cracker crumbs in saucepan.
2. Heat to steaming.
3. In a mixing bowl, beat egg substitute, Splenda, coconut, and salt.
4. Add egg mixture to hot milk, stirring continuously.
5. Bring to boil, stirring.
6. Add vanilla. Boil 1 minute longer.
7. Pour into a heatproof serving dish. Cover.
8. Refrigerate until chilled, 2 hours.

Variation:
Top the cold pudding with 1½ cups whipped cream and sprinkle with one crushed 5th Avenue candy bar.

Esther S. Martin
Ephrata, PA

Exchange List Values
- Fat-Free Milk 0.5
- Fat 0.5
- Carbohydrate 1.0

Basic Nutritional Values
- Calories 160
  (Calories from Fat 25)
- Total Fat 3 gm
  (Saturated Fat 1.9 gm,
  Trans Fat 0.1 gm,
  Polyunsat Fat 0.5 gm,
  Monounsat Fat 0.4 gm)
- Cholesterol 5 mg
- Sodium 275 mg
- Potassium 320 gm
- Total Carb 23 gm
- Dietary Fiber 1 gm
- Sugars 14 gm
- Protein 9 gm
- Phosphorus 185 gm

Fruit Pudding

Penny Blosser
New Carlisle, OH
Phoebe M. Yoder
Bristol, IN

*Makes 10 servings,
about 5½ oz. per serving*

Prep. Time: 20 minutes

8 oz. can pineapple, undrained
11-oz. can mandarin oranges, undrained
17-oz. can fruit cocktail packed in juice, undrained
⅓ cup coconut
2 Tbsp. lemon juice
1-oz. pkg. sugar-free fat-free lemon instant pudding
1 cup fat-free milk
2 bananas, sliced

1. Combine pineapple, mandarin oranges, fruit cocktail, coconut and lemon juice.
2. Combine pudding and milk and mix well.
3. Combine fruit mixture with pudding mixture and

stir gently to combine all ingredients.

4. Immediately before serving, fold in sliced bananas.

Exchange List Values
- Fruit 1.0
- Carbohydrate 0.5

Basic Nutritional Values
- Calories 105 (Calories from Fat 10)
- Total Fat 1 gm (Saturated Fat 1.0 gm, Trans Fat 0.0 gm, Polyunsat Fat 0.0 gm, Monounsat Fat 0.1 gm)
- Cholesterol 0 mg
- Sodium 145 mg
- Potassium 255 gm
- Total Carb 22 gm
- Dietary Fiber 2 gm
- Sugars 16 gm
- Protein 1 gm
- Phosphorus 115 gm

Easy Baked Apples

Willard and Alice Roth
Elkhart, IN

Makes 12 servings
Prep. Time: 20 minutes
Cooking Time: 6–8 hours

12 medium baking apples, 4 lbs. total
½ cup raisins
½ cup chopped nuts
½ cup Splenda Brown Sugar Blend
½ tsp. nutmeg
1 tsp. cinnamon
3 slices fresh lemon
1¼ cups boiling water

1. Wash and core whole apples. Starting at the stem, peel about ⅓ of the way down.

2. Fill each apple with raisins and nuts. Stack into slow cooker.

3. Combine Splenda, nutmeg and cinnamon in small saucepan. Add lemon slices and pour boiling water over everything. Boil ingredients together for about 5 minutes. Pour over apples in slow cooker.

4. Cover and cook on low 6–8 hours. Serve hot or cold.

Exchange List Values
- Fruit 1.5
- Carbohydrate 0.5
- Fat 0.5

Basic Nutritional Values
- Calories 155 (Calories from Fat 30)
- Total Fat 4 gm (Saturated Fat 0.4 gm, Trans Fat 0.0 gm, Polyunsat Fat 2.4 gm, Monounsat Fat 0.5 gm)
- Cholesterol 0 mg
- Sodium 0 mg
- Potassium 230 gm
- Total Carb 33 gm
- Dietary Fiber 4 gm
- Sugars 22 gm
- Protein 1 gm
- Phosphorus 40 gm

Merry Fruit Compote

A. Catharine Boshart
Lebanon, PA

Makes 20 servings, about ½ cup per serving
Prep. Time: 15 minutes
Cooking Time: 15 minutes
Cooling Time: 30 minutes or more

2 12-oz. pkgs. pitted prunes
12-oz. bottle diet ginger-ale
8-oz. pkg. dried apricots
1 cup raisins
1 cup orange juice
1 tsp. minced, peeled ginger root, *or* ¼ tsp. ground ginger
1 stick cinnamon
20-oz. can pineapple chunks canned in juice
16-oz. can pear halves canned in juice
½ cup granular Splenda

1. In 5-quart saucepan combine prunes, ginger-ale, apricots, raisins, orange juice, ginger and cinnamon. Bring to boiling over high heat. Reduce heat to low; cover and simmer 15 minutes or until fruit is tender.

2. Drain pineapple chunks and pear halves. Cut each pear in half lengthwise.

3. To fruit mixture in saucepan add pineapple, pears, and corn syrup. Stir gently with rubber spatula to mix well.

4. Cool at least 30 minutes before serving or refrigerate and serve chilled.

Exchange List Values
- Fruit 2.5

Basic Nutritional Values
- Calories 145 (Calories from Fat 0)
- Total Fat 0 gm (Saturated Fat 0.0 gm, Trans Fat 0.0 gm, Polyunsat Fat 0.0 gm, Monounsat Fat 0.0 gm)
- Cholesterol 0 mg
- Sodium 0 mg
- Potassium 465 gm
- Total Carb 38 gm
- Dietary Fiber 4 gm
- Sugars 27 gm
- Protein 2 gm
- Phosphorus 40 gm

Lime Poppy Seed Fruit Salad

Diann Dunham
State College, PA

Makes 4½ cups,
½ cup per serving, 9 servings total

Prep. Time: 20 minutes

2 cups pineapple chunks,
    fresh *or* canned, juice
    reserved
1 orange, peeled and
    chopped
1 kiwi fruit, peeled and
    sliced
1 cup red *or* green grapes
1 cup quartered
    strawberries

Dressing:
¼ cup reserved
    pineapple juice
¼ tsp. grated lime peel
2 Tbsp. fresh lime juice
1 Tbsp. honey
1 tsp. poppy seeds

whole strawberries,
    optional

1. Mix pineapple chunks,
orange, kiwi, grapes, and
strawberries in a bowl.
2. In a separate bowl, mix
dressing ingredients. Add
dressing to salad.
3. If desired, garnish with a
few whole strawberries before
serving.

Tips:
1. It looks very pretty in a
clear bowl.
2. The salad is best made
and eaten the same day.
Strawberries get mushy if
stored too long.

Warm Memories:
    People can't tell why it
tastes better than other fruit
salads. The lime juice and
peel with the honey gives
it a refreshing taste. I have
used it for many years. I first
made for a special Mother &
Daughter brunch.

Good Go-Alongs:
    It's lovely for a simple des-
sert with shortbread cookies
or coconut macaroons.

Exchange List Values
• Fruit 1.0

Basic Nutritional Values
• Calories 70
  (Calories from Fat 0)
• Total Fat 0 gm
  (Saturated Fat 0.0 gm,
  Trans Fat 0.0 gm,
  Polyunsat Fat 0.2 gm,
  Monounsat Fat 0.0 gm)
• Cholesterol 0 mg
• Sodium 0 mg
• Potassium 180 gm
• Total Carb 17 gm
• Dietary Fiber 2 gm
• Sugars 14 gm
• Protein 1 gm
• Phosphorus 20 gm

Healthy Fruit Salad

Ida C. Knopp
Salem, OH

Makes 8 servings,
about ½ cup per serving

Prep. Time: 15 minutes

3 tart red apples, chopped
3 oranges, chopped
½ cup chopped celery
⅓ cup raisins
⅓ cup chopped nuts
2 Tbsp. honey
2 Tbsp. lemon juice

1. In a serving bowl toss
apples, oranges, celery, raisins
and nuts.
2. In a small bowl combine
honey and lemon juice.
Drizzle over fruit salad and
serve.

Exchange List Values
• Fruit 1.5   • Fat 0.5

Basic Nutritional Values
• Calories 120
  (Calories from Fat 30)
• Total Fat 4 gm
  (Saturated Fat 0.3 gm,
  Trans Fat 0.0 gm,
  Polyunsat Fat 2.4 gm,
  Monounsat Fat 0.5 gm)
• Cholesterol 0 mg
• Sodium 5 mg
• Potassium 250 gm
• Total Carb 24 gm
• Dietary Fiber 3 gm
• Sugars 19 gm
• Protein 2 gm
• Phosphorus 40 gm

Frozen Fruit

Anna A. Yoder
Millersburg, OH

*Makes 20 servings,
2¼" square per serving*

Prep. Time: 15 minutes
Freezing Time: 3 hours or more
Standing Time: 2 hours

3 cups water
1½ cups granular Splenda
8 medium bananas, sliced
**20-oz. can crushed
    pineapple packed in juice**
**6-oz. can frozen orange
    juice, undiluted**

1. Combine water and sugar and let stand to dissolve.
2. Combine bananas and pineapple. Set aside.
3. Add orange juice to sugar water. Pour mixture over bananas and pineapple, stirring gently until mixed. Pour into 9×13 baking dish with a lid. Cover dish and freeze for at least 3 hours.
4. Remove from freezer 2 hours before serving.

Variation:

Add some sliced fresh peaches and a small bottle of maraschino cherries. Pour ginger-ale over slush immediately before serving.
Veva Zimmerman Mumaw
Hatfield, PA

Exchange List Values
• Fruit 1.5

Basic Nutritional Values

• Calories 85
  (Calories from Fat 0)
• Total Fat 0 gm
  (Saturated Fat 0.1 gm,
  Trans Fat 0.0 gm,
  Polyunsat Fat 0.1 gm,
  Monounsat Fat 0.0 gm)
• Cholesterol 0 mg
• Sodium 0 mg
• Potassium 285 gm
• Total Carb 21 gm
• Dietary Fiber 2 gm
• Sugars 15 gm
• Protein 1 gm
• Phosphorus 20 gm

Fruit Slush

Julette Rush
Harrisonburg, VA

*Makes 16 servings,
about 6 oz. per serving*

Prep. Time: 20 minutes
Freezing Time: 5–12 hours

½ cup granular Splenda
2 cups boiling water
**6-oz. can frozen orange
    juice**
12-oz. can apricot nectar
**6 bananas, firmly ripe,
    mashed**
1 Tbsp. lemon juice
**20-oz. can crushed
    pineapple, undrained**
**16-oz. frozen no-sugar-
    added strawberries**

1. In large bowl, dissolve Splenda in 2 cups boiling water.
2. Add frozen orange juice and 2 cans of water. Add apricot nectar.

3. Mash the bananas with the lemon juice to prevent browning. Add them to the bowl.
4. Add pineapple and strawberries. Stir all gently together.
5. Put bowl in freezer. Stir once an hour for 5 hours until slushy.

Tips:

For a potluck event, make this a day or more in advance. Get it out of the freezer 2–3 hours ahead of time to get to the right slushy consistency. Time to thaw may vary greatly depending on your home's temperature. The slush keeps indefinitely in the freezer.

Exchange List Values
• Fruit 2.0

Basic Nutritional Values

• Calories 105
  (Calories from Fat 0)
• Total Fat 0 gm
  (Saturated Fat 0.1 gm,
  Trans Fat 0.0 gm,
  Polyunsat Fat 0.1 gm,
  Monounsat Fat 0.0 gm)
• Cholesterol 0 mg
• Sodium 0 mg
• Potassium 365 gm
• Total Carb 27 gm
• Dietary Fiber 3 gm
• Sugars 18 gm
• Protein 1 gm
• Phosphorus 25 gm

With a busy life, it is nice to have potluck dishes that can be made a day or two ahead of time.
Sue Hamilton, Benson, AZ

Grandma Moley's Fruit Salad

Elva Evers
North English, IA

*Makes 8 servings,
about 6½ oz. per serving*

Prep Time: 15 minutes
Cooking Time: 8-10 minutes
Standing Time: 20 minutes

20-oz can juice-packed
  pineapple chunks
1 orange
1 lemon
6–8 pkgs. sugar substitute
2 Tbsp. minute tapioca
6 small apples, cored and
  diced
2 bananas, sliced

1. Drain pineapple chunks, reserving juice.

2. Squeeze juice from orange and lemon. Combine all juices, sugar and tapioca. Let stand for about 5 minutes.

3. Heat mixture in microwave for 8–10 minutes, stirring every 2 minutes, until it thickens and tapioca is transparent. Cool.

4. Combine apples and pineapples. Fold in cooled dressing.

5. Immediately before serving, slice in bananas.

Exchange List Values
• Fruit 2.0

Basic Nutritional Values
• Calories 130
  (Calories from Fat 0)
• Total Fat 0 gm
  (Saturated Fat 0.1 gm,
  Trans Fat 0.0 gm,
  Polyunsat Fat 0.1 gm,
  Monounsat Fat 0.0 gm)
• Cholesterol 0 mg
• Sodium 0 mg
• Potassium 310 gm
• Total Carb 33 gm
• Dietary Fiber 3 gm
• Sugars 24 gm
• Protein 1 gm
• Phosphorus 20 gm

Rhubarb Tapioca

Carol Weber
Lancaster, PA
Elaine Gibbel
Lititz, PA

Makes 6 servings

Prep. Time: 10 minutes
Soaking Time: 20 minutes
Cooking Time: 20 minutes
Chilling Time: 1 hour

2 Tbsp. tapioca
⅓ cup cold water
2 cups chopped rhubarb
½ cup granular Splenda
¾ cup water
1 pint frozen strawberries
6 Tbsp. fat-free whipped
  topping, *divided*

1. Soak tapioca in ⅓ cup cold water for 20 minutes.

2. Cook rhubarb, Splenda and ¾ cup water until rhubarb is soft, about 5 minutes. Add tapioca slowly. Cook until mixture is transparent.

3. Fold in strawberries. Cool.

4. Divide among 6 dessert cups and top each cup with a tablespoon of whipped topping.

Exchange List Values
• Carbohydrate 1.0

Basic Nutritional Values
• Calories 55
  (Calories from Fat 0)
• Total Fat 0 gm
  (Saturated Fat 0.0 gm,
  Trans Fat 0.0 gm,
  Polyunsat Fat 0.0 gm,
  Monounsat Fat 0.0 gm)
• Cholesterol 0 mg
• Sodium 5 mg
• Potassium 195 gm
• Total Carb 13 gm
• Dietary Fiber 2 gm
• Sugars 5 gm
• Protein 1 gm
• Phosphorus 15 gm

Prep as much as possible, so that you can enjoy your guests or family during the meal. Sharing food around your table is precious time, don't miss it.

Julie Horst, Lancaster, PA

Orange Tapioca Fruit

Carol Eberly
Harrisonburg, VA

*Makes 15 servings,
about 5 oz. per serving*

Prep. Time: 15 minutes
Cooking Time: 10 minutes
Chilling Time: 2–4 hours

½ cup minute tapioca
1 quart water
½ cup granular Splenda
6-oz. frozen orange juice
    concentrate
2 14-oz. cans mandarin
    oranges, drained
2 15-oz. cans sliced
    peaches, drained
1 banana, sliced

1. In a saucepan, heat water, Splenda, and tapioca, stirring often.
2. Cook until clear.

3. Remove from heat and stir in juice concentrate until dissolved.
4. Mix in fruit. Pour into serving dish.
5. Chill for 2–4 hours.
6. Stir in bananas just before serving.

Variation:
Use 20-oz. pineapple instead of fruit above. Use its juice, plus 6-oz. pineapple juice to make 1 quart liquid. Use same method above, adding 12 oz. frozen orange juice concentrate. Also delicious topped with whipped cream.

Ruth Hershey
Paradise, PA

Exchange List Values
• Carbohydrate 1.0

Basic Nutritional Values
• Calories 75
  (Calories from Fat 0)
• Total Fat 0 gm
  (Saturated Fat 0.0 gm,
  Trans Fat 0.0 gm,
  Polyunsat Fat 0.0 gm,
  Monounsat Fat 0.0 gm)
• Cholesterol 0 mg
• Sodium 5 mg
• Potassium 210 gm
• Total Carb 19 gm
• Dietary Fiber 1 gm
• Sugars 13 gm
• Protein 1 gm
• Phosphorus 20 gm

Fruit Tapioca

Anna Weber
Atmore, AL

Makes 20 servings

Prep. Time: 15 minutes
Cooling Time: 1 hour
Cooking Time: 5 minutes

7 cups water
1 cup minute tapioca
1 cup granular Splenda
12-oz. can frozen orange
    concentrate
2 bananas, sliced
2 oranges, peeled,
    segments diced

1. Bring water to a boil and add tapioca and Splenda. Boil for 1 minute or until tapioca appears clear.
2. Remove from heat and add frozen concentrate. Mix well and cool.
3. Immediately before serving, fold in fruit slices.

Exchange List Values
• Starch 0.5
• Fruit 1.0

Basic Nutritional Values
• Calories 85
  (Calories from Fat 0)
• Total Fat 0 gm
  (Saturated Fat 0.0 gm,
  Trans Fat 0.0 gm,
  Polyunsat Fat 0.0 gm,
  Monounsat Fat 0.0 gm)
• Cholesterol 0 mg
• Sodium 0 mg
• Potassium 230 gm
• Total Carb 21 gm
• Dietary Fiber 1 gm
• Sugars 13 gm
• Protein 1 gm
• Phosphorus 20 gm

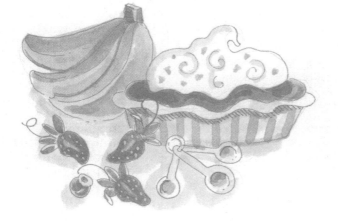

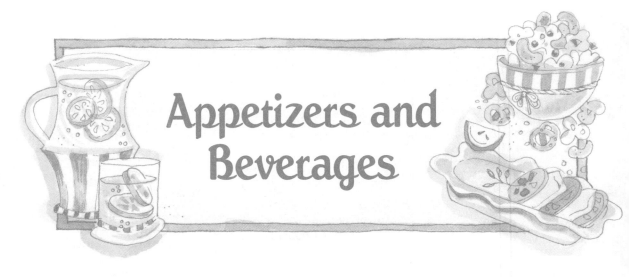

Appetizers and Beverages

Reuben Appetizer Squares

Mary Ann Lefever
Lancaster, PA

*Makes 24 servings,
2" square per serving*

Prep. Time: 20 minutes
Cooking/Baking Time: 12–15 minutes

2 cups baking mix
½ cup fat-free milk
2 Tbsp. vegetable oil
1 cup sauerkraut, well drained
2½-oz. pkg. thinly sliced smoked corned beef, coarsely chopped
⅔ cup light mayonnaise
1 Tbsp. pickle relish
1 Tbsp. ketchup
1½ cups reduced-fat shredded Swiss cheese (about 6 oz.)

1. Mix baking mix, milk, and oil until soft dough forms. Press into ungreased 9×13 baking pan.
2. Top with sauerkraut and corned beef.
3. Mix mayonnaise, relish, and ketchup; spread over corned beef. Sprinkle with cheese.
4. Bake at 450° until cheese is bubbly and crust is golden brown, 12–15 minutes.
5. Cut into 2-inch squares.

Warm Memories:
These squares are very different for church suppers and well received.

Exchange List Values
• Starch 0.5   • Fat 1.0

Basic Nutritional Values
• Calories 90
(Calories from Fat 45)
• Total Fat 5 gm
(Saturated Fat 1.1 gm,
Trans Fat 0.0 gm,
Polyunsat Fat 1.4 gm,
Monounsat Fat 1.9 gm)
• Cholesterol 5 mg
• Sodium 250 mg
• Potassium 45 gm
• Total Carb 8 gm
• Dietary Fiber 1 gm
• Sugars 2 gm
• Protein 4 gm
• Phosphorus 110 gm

Veggie Pizza

Jean Butzer
Batavia, NY
Julette Rush
Harrisonburg, VA

*Makes 18 servings,
2"×3" rectangle per serving*

Prep. Time: 20–30 minutes
Cooking Time: 9–12 minutes
Chilling Time: 30 minutes

2 8-oz. pkgs. refrigerated crescent rolls
8-oz. pkg. fat-free cream cheese, softened
½ cup fat-free mayonnaise
1 tsp. dill weed
½ tsp. onion salt
¾-1 cup broccoli florets
¾-1 cup green pepper *or* mushrooms, chopped fine
¾-1 cup tomato, membranes and seeds removed, chopped fine
½ cup sliced ripe olives
¼ cup sweet onion *or* red onion, chopped fine

¾ **cup cheddar cheese, shredded fine,** *optional*

1. Separate dough into 4 rectangles.
2. Press onto bottom and up sides of 10×13 jelly roll baking pan to form crust.
3. Bake 9–12 minutes at 350° or until golden brown. Cool.
4. Mix cream cheese, dressing, dill, and onion salt until well blended.
5. Spread over cooled crust, but not too thickly. About ¼ cup mixture should be left over.
6. Top with chopped vegetables and optional cheese.
7. Press down lightly into cream cheese mixture.
8. Refrigerate. Cut into squares to serve.

Tips:
1. Add veggies of your preference and availability
2. Do not put the cream cheese mixture on too thick. There may be ¼ cup left after spreading it on the crescent rolls. This can be saved to use as a dip with any leftover vegetables you have.

Exchange List Values
• Starch 1.0   • Fat 1.0

Basic Nutritional Values
• Calories 130   • Sodium 400 mg
  (Calories from Fat 65) • Potassium 110 gm
• Total Fat 7 gm   • Total Carb 12 gm
  (Saturated Fat 1.5 gm, • Dietary Fiber 1 gm
  Trans Fat 0.0 gm,   • Sugars 3 gm
  Polyunsat Fat 0.8 gm, • Protein 3 gm
  Monounsat Fat 4.1 gm) • Phosphorus 150 gm
• Cholesterol 0 mg

Crust from Scratch (for Veggie Pizza)
Mrs. Anna Gingerich
Apple Creek, OH

Makes 12 servings,
2"×5" rectangle per serving

1 cup flour
2 tsp. sugar
2 tsp. baking powder
⅓ tsp. salt
3 Tbsp. tub margarine, no trans fat
½ cup fat-free milk

Mix well. Press dough into 9×13 baking pan. Bake at 350° for 10–15 minutes until golden. Allow to cool and proceed with toppings.

Exchange List Values
• Starch 1.0   • Fat 1.0

Basic Nutritional Values
• Calories 110   • Sodium 460 mg
  (Calories from Fat 40) • Potassium 140 gm
• Total Fat 4.5 gm   • Total Carb 13 gm
  (Saturated Fat 0.7 gm, • Dietary Fiber 1 gm
  Trans Fat 0.0 gm,   • Sugars 3 gm
  Polyunsat Fat 1.1 gm, • Protein 4 gm
  Monounsat Fat 2.2 gm) • Phosphorus 190 gm
• Cholesterol 5 mg

Shrimp Hors d'oeuvres
Barbara A. Hershey, Lititz, PA

Makes 24 servings,
2 pieces per serving

Prep. Time: 20 minutes
Cooking/Baking Time: 20 minutes

½ **cup tub margarine, no trans-fat**
5-oz. **jar Old English cheese spread**
3 Tbsp. **light mayonnaise**
4½-oz. **can shrimp, drained**
6 **English muffins, opened into 12 halves**

1. Melt butter and cheese in heavy saucepan. Add mayonnaise and continue stirring until thick. Add shrimp.
2. Immediately spread on muffin halves.
3. Cut into quarters. Cover with plastic wrap and freeze up to 3 weeks.
4. Bake on cookie sheet at 350° for 10 minutes.

Variation:
Do not freeze assembled muffins. Broil 5–10 minutes – watch carefully!

Exchange List Values
• Starch 0.5   • Fat 1.0

Basic Nutritional Values
• Calories 80   • Sodium 190 mg
  (Calories from Fat 40) • Potassium 40 gm
• Total Fat 4.5 gm   • Total Carb 7 gm
  (Saturated Fat 1.5 gm, • Dietary Fiber 0 gm
  Trans Fat 0.0 gm,   • Sugars 1 gm
  Polyunsat Fat 1.6 gm, • Protein 3 gm
  Monounsat Fat 1.4 gm) • Phosphorus 70 gm
• Cholesterol 15 mg

Shrimp-Stuffed Celery

Lois W. Benner
Lancaster, PA

Makes 25 servings,
1 Tbsp. spread and 1 5" celery stick

Prep. Time: 20 minutes
Cooking Time: 5 minutes
Cooling Time: 20 minutes
Chilling Time: 1 hour

1 lb. fresh unshelled shrimp
3 cups boiling water
1 tsp. salt
¼ cup vinegar
dash pepper
3 oz. ⅓-less-fat cream
    cheese, softened
1 Tbsp. grated onion
½ tsp. Worcestershire sauce
⅓ cup reduced-fat light
    mayonnaise
1 Tbsp. sweet pickle juice
½ tsp. horseradish
dash garlic salt, *optional*
25 celery ribs, each 5" long
cherry tomatoes, olives, *or*
    small radishes, *optional*
    garnishes

1. Rinse shrimp thoroughly. Cook shrimp for 5 minutes in boiling water to which has been added salt, vinegar and pepper. Drain water. Cool shrimp, take off out shells and shred in blender.

2. Combine cream cheese, onion, Worcestershire sauce, mayonnaise, pickle juice, horseradish, garlic salt and shredded shrimp. Mix well and chill at least an hour.

3. Fill celery stalks with shrimp mixture and arrange in an attractive manner on a platter. Add either cherry tomatoes, olives or radishes for additional color.

Exchange List Values
• Fat 0.5

Basic Nutritional Values
• Calories 30
  (Calories from Fat 15)
• Total Fat 2 gm
  (Saturated Fat 0.6 gm,
  Trans Fat 0.0 gm,
  Polyunsat Fat 0.5 gm,
  Monounsat Fat 0.5 gm)
• Cholesterol 25 mg
• Sodium 90 mg
• Potassium 70 gm
• Total Carb 1 gm
• Dietary Fiber 0 gm
• Sugars 1 gm
• Protein 3 gm
• Phosphorus 40 gm

Stuffed Mushrooms

Gloria Lehman, Singers Glen, VA
Melva Baumer, Mifflintown, PA

Makes 10 servings,
2 mushroom caps per serving

Prep. Time: 25 minutes
Cooking/Baking Time: 20–40
    minutes

20 fresh mushrooms, about
    1 lb.
¼ cup tub margarine, no
    trans-fat
2 Tbsp. onion, finely
    chopped
2 Tbsp. mushroom stems,
    finely chopped
½ cup Italian seasoned
    bread crumbs
¼ cup freshly grated
    Parmesan cheese
2 Tbsp. oil

1. Wash mushrooms; remove stems. Place mushrooms in greased baking pan, stem side up.

2. Sauté onion and mushroom stems in margarine. Turn off heat and stir in crumbs.

3. Fill each mushroom cap with mixture. Sprinkle Parmesan cheese over all. Drizzle with oil.

4. Bake at 350° for 20–30 minutes.

Variation:
To plain cracker crumbs, add 1 Tbsp. dried parsley, ½ tsp. garlic salt, 3 Tbsp. minced onion, 2 Tbs. melted butter, pepper to taste, and minced mushroom stems. Do not sauté. Stuff mushroom caps and proceed as listed.
Melva Baumer

Warm Memories:
This is a simple dish to prepare and to shop for. But it is fabulous.

Exchange List Values
• Carbohydrate 0.5   • Fat 1.5

Basic Nutritional Values
• Calories 90
  (Calories from Fat 65)
• Total Fat 7 gm
  (Saturated Fat 1.5 gm,
  Trans Fat 0.0 gm,
  Polyunsat Fat 1.8 gm,
  Monounsat Fat 3.3 gm)
• Cholesterol 0 mg
• Sodium 150 mg
• Potassium 145 gm
• Total Carb 6 gm
• Dietary Fiber 1 gm
• Sugars 1 gm
• Protein 3 gm
• Phosphorus 55 gm

Easy Turkey Roll-Ups

Rhoda Atzeff
Lancaster, PA

Makes 6 servings,
2 roll-ups per serving

Prep. Time: 10 minutes

3 6-inch flour tortillas
3 Tbsp. chive and onion cream cheese
12 slices deli shaved 97%-fat free turkey breast, 6 oz. total
¾ cup shredded lettuce

1. Spread tortillas with cream cheese. Top with turkey. Place lettuce on bottom halves of tortillas; roll up.
2. Cut each into 4 pieces and lay flat to serve.

Tips:
I have also used deli shaved ham and vegetable cream cheese – this is very good! You can use ⅓ less fat cream cheese.

Good Go-Alongs:
A batch of each (turkey and ham) makes a quick lovely dish for a potluck or fellowship meal. Good just as a snack with a few chips or crackers.

Exchange List Values
• Starch 0.5   • Lean Meat 1.0

Basic Nutritional Values
• Calories 90   • Sodium 365 mg
  (Calories from Fat 20)   • Potassium 125 gm
• Total Fat 2.5 gm   • Total Carb 8 gm
  (Saturated Fat 1.1 gm, • Dietary Fiber 1 gm
  Trans Fat 0.0 gm,   • Sugars 1 gm
  Polyunsat Fat 0.5 gm, • Protein 9 gm
  Monounsat Fat 0.8 gm) • Phosphorus 95 gm
• Cholesterol 15 mg

Spinach Roll-ups

Esther Gingerich
Kalona, IA

Makes 23 servings,
3 roll-ups per serving

Prep. Time: 30 minutes
Chilling Time: 12 hours

2 10-oz. boxes frozen spinach, thawed and drained
2-oz. bacon bits (half of a small jar)
¼ cup water chestnuts, chopped
1 pkg. Ranch dressing mix
1 cup fat-free sour cream
6 green onions, chopped
1 cup light mayonnaise
7 10" tortillas
toothpicks

1. Mix together ingredients except tortillas.
2. Spread the mixture on the tortillas. Roll up and secure with toothpicks.
3. Refrigerate overnight. Slice into 1-inch pieces to serve.

Tip:
Arrange on a pretty plate or tray to serve.

Warm Memories:
Our church often has "finger food" potlucks and this works well for that.

Exchange List Values
• Starch 1.0   • Fat 1.0

Basic Nutritional Values
• Calories 120   • Sodium 440 mg
  (Calories from Fat 45)   • Potassium 160 gm
• Total Fat 5 gm   • Total Carb 15 gm
  (Saturated Fat 1.2 gm, • Dietary Fiber 2 gm
  Trans Fat 0.0 gm,   • Sugars 1 gm
  Polyunsat Fat 1.8 gm, • Protein 4 gm
  Monounsat Fat 1.7 gm) • Phosphorus 50 gm
• Cholesterol 5 mg

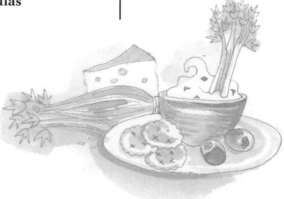

Smoky Barbeque Meatballs

Carla Koslowsky
Hillsboro, KS
Sherry Kreider
Lancaster, PA
Jennie Martin
Richfield, PA

*Makes 10 servings,
1 meatball per serving*

Prep. Time: 30 minutes
Baking Time: 1 hour

1½ lbs. 90%-lean ground beef
½ cup quick oats
½ cup fat-free evaporated milk *or* milk
¼ cup egg substitute
¼-½ cup finely chopped onion, *optional*
¼ tsp. garlic powder
¼ tsp. pepper
¼ tsp. chili powder
1 tsp. salt

Sauce:
 1 cup ketchup
 6 Tbsp. Splenda Brown Sugar Blend
 ¼ cup chopped onion
 ¼ tsp. liquid smoke

1. Mix hamburger, oatmeal, milk, egg, onion, garlic powder, pepper, chili powder, and salt together. Form 10 balls, each weighing about 2 oz. Place in 9×13 baking dish.
2. Bake at 350° for 40 minutes. Mix the sauce ingredients while the meatballs bake. Set aside.
3. Pour off any grease from the meatballs after they baked 40 minutes. Pour sauce over meatballs.
4. Bake meatballs and sauce an additional 10–20 minutes, until bubbling and heated through.

Tips:
 1. It's easy to double the recipe to share, or freeze. You can also make this as a meat loaf.

Carla Koslowsky
Hillsboro, KS

 2. Bring the sauce to a boil and boil 2 minutes. Reserve a little before pouring over the meatballs. Then, at the end of baking and just before serving, brush on the reserved sauce.
 3. You can also bake these meatballs for 2 hours at 300°. Cover with foil the first hour, then uncover.

Sherry Kreider
Lancaster, PA

Good Go-Alongs:
 These meatballs can be served as part of a full cooked meal or luncheon, or just as an appetizer.

Jennie Martin
Richfield, PA

Exchange List Values
• Carbohydrate 1.0   • Fat 0.5
• Lean Meat 2.0

Basic Nutritional Values
• Calories 190   • Sodium 450 mg
 (Calories from Fat 55) • Potassium 375 gm
• Total Fat 6 gm   • Total Carb 18 gm
 (Saturated Fat 2.3 gm, • Dietary Fiber 1 gm
 Trans Fat 0.3 gm,   • Sugars 11 gm
 Polyunsat Fat 0.3 gm, • Protein 16 gm
 Monounsat Fat 2.4 gm) • Phosphorus 170 gm
• Cholesterol 40 mg

Party Kielbasi

Mary C. Wirth
Lancaster, PA

Makes 48 servings, 1 oz. per serving

Prep. Time: 15 minutes
Cooking/Baking Time: 2½ hours

3 lbs. 95%-fat free turkey kielbasa
1 cup ketchup
½ cup chili sauce
½ cup brown sugar, packed
2 Tbsp. Worcestershire sauce
1 Tbsp. lemon juice
¼ tsp. prepared mustard

1. Cut kielbasa or smoked sausage into 6 or 9 large pieces. Lay it in a large pan of water. Simmer 20 minutes. Drain. Cool slightly. Cut into 1-oz. pieces.
2. Mix all other ingredients in 13×9 baking dish. Add kielbasa. Toss to coat with sauce.
3. Bake at 325° for 1½-2 hours, stirring occasionally.

Tip:
 You can keep this warm in a slow cooker or chafing dish.

Warm Memories:
 I first tried this at a house warming party and kept reminding the hostess about the recipe until she remembered to share it.

Exchange List Values
• Carbohydrate 0.5   • Lean Meat 1.0

Basic Nutritional Values
- Calories 65
  (Calories from Fat 15)
- Total Fat 2 gm
  (Saturated Fat 0.8 gm,
  Trans Fat 0.0 gm,
  Polyunsat Fat 0.3 gm,
  Monounsat Fat 0.5 gm)
- Cholesterol 20 mg
- Sodium 380 mg
- Potassium 95 gm
- Total Carb 5 gm
- Dietary Fiber 0 gm
- Sugars 3 gm
- Protein 5 gm
- Phosphorus 55 gm

Jalapeño Popper Dip

Jamie Mowry
Arlington, TX

*Makes 12 servings,
about ¼ cup per serving*

Prep. Time: 15 minutes
Baking Time: 30 minutes

2 8-oz. pkgs. fat-free cream
  cheese, softened
1 cup light mayonnaise
4-oz. can chopped green
  chilies, drained
2-oz. can diced jalapeño
  peppers, drained
½ cup freshly grated
  Parmesan cheese
½ cup panko bread crumbs

1. Mix cream cheese and
mayonnaise in large bowl
until smooth. Stir in chilies
and peppers.
2. Pour pepper mixture in
a greased baking dish.
3. Combine Parmesan and
panko. Put on top of pepper
mixture.
4. Bake at 350° for 30
minutes until golden and
bubbly.

Tip:
  Serve with veggies, pita
chips or regular corn chips,
or whatever "dipper" you like.

Exchange List Values
- Carbohydrate 0.5
- Lean Meat 1.0
- Fat 0.5

Basic Nutritional Values
- Calories 105
  (Calories from Fat 55)
- Total Fat 6 gm
  (Saturated Fat 1.2 gm,
  Trans Fat 0.0 gm,
  Polyunsat Fat 2.7 gm,
  Monounsat Fat 1.6 gm)
- Cholesterol 15 mg
- Sodium 480 mg
- Potassium 130 gm
- Total Carb 6 gm
- Dietary Fiber 0 gm
- Sugars 2 gm
- Protein 6 gm
- Phosphorus 230 gm

Buffalo Chicken Dip

Deb Martin
Gap, PA
Donna Treloar
Muncie, IN

*Makes 26 servings,
¼ cup per serving*

Prep. Time: 15 minutes
Cooking Time: 20–60 minutes

10-oz. can chunk chicken,
  drained
2 8-oz. pkgs. fat-free cream
  cheese, softened
1 cup light Ranch dressing
¾ cup Frank's Red Hot
  sauce
1½ cups shredded cheddar
  jack cheese
tortilla chips

1. Heat chicken and hot
sauce in a large frying pan
over medium heat until
heated through.
2. Stir in cream cheese
and Ranch dressing. Cook,
stirring until well blended
and warm.
3. Mix in half of shredded
cheese.
4. Transfer the mixture to
a small slow cooker. Sprinkle
the remaining cheese over the
top.
5. Cover and cook on low
setting until hot and bubbly.
Serve with tortilla chips.

Variation:
  Replace hot sauce with
1 cup buffalo wing sauce.
Spread cream cheese in bottom of small shallow baking
dish. Layer with shredded
chicken, buffalo wing sauce,
ranch dressing, and shredded
cheese. Bake at 350° for 20
minutes or until cheese is
melted.

Donna Treloar
Muncie, IN

Exchange List Values
- Lean Meat 1.0
- Fat 0.5

Basic Nutritional Values
- Calories 75
  (Calories from Fat 35)
- Total Fat 4 gm
  (Saturated Fat 1.1 gm,
  Trans Fat 0.0 gm,
  Polyunsat Fat 0.8 gm,
  Monounsat Fat 0.9 gm)
- Cholesterol 15 mg
- Sodium 475 mg
- Potassium 90 gm
- Total Carb 2 gm
- Dietary Fiber 0 gm
- Sugars 1 gm
- Protein 6 gm
- Phosphorus 160 gm

Hot Pizza Dip

Linda Abraham
Kimberly, OR
Beverly High
Bradford, PA

Makes 8 servings, 1 slice per serving

Prep. Time: 20 minutes
Cooking/Baking Time: 5–20 minutes

8-oz. pkg. fat-free cream cheese, softened
½ tsp. dried oregano
½ tsp. dried parsley
¼ tsp. dried basil
¾ cup shredded part-skim mozzarella cheese, *divided*
¼ cup freshly grated Parmesan cheese, *divided*
½-1 cup pizza sauce
2 Tbsp. chopped green bell pepper
2 Tbsp. sliced black olives, *optional*
¼ cup chopped onions, *optional*

1. In a small bowl, beat together cream cheese, oregano, parsley, and basil.
2. Spread mixture in bottom of greased 9-inch glass pie plate.
3. Sprinkle 6 Tbsp. mozzarella and 2 Tbsp. Parmesan cheese on top of cream cheese mixture.
4. Spread the pizza sauce over all.
5. Sprinkle with remaining cheese.
6. Top with green pepper, olives, and onions.
7. Cover and microwave 5 minutes or bake at 350° for 20 minutes.
8. Serve hot with sliced French baguette bread, focaccia, tortilla chips, or fresh veggies.

Variations:

1. Use 1 tsp. Italian seasoning in place of the oregano, parsley, and basil.
Beverly High
Bradford, PA

2. Add ½ cup sour cream to the cream cheese and herbs.
Gloria Mumbauer
Singers Glen, VA

3. Add ½ tsp. garlic powder and ⅛ tsp. cayenne pepper to the cream cheese mixture.
Juanita Mellinger
Abbottstown, PA

Tip:

This makes a great Sunday supper or snack for company. You get the pizza flavor without the work of making a crust.
Juanita Mellinger
Abbottstown, PA

Exchange List Values
• Lean Meat 1.0   • Fat 0.5

Basic Nutritional Values
• Calories 70   • Sodium 340 mg
(Calories from Fat 20) • Potassium 155 gm
• Total Fat 2.5 gm   • Total Carb 4 gm
(Saturated Fat 1.5 gm, • Dietary Fiber 0 gm
Trans Fat 0.0 gm,   • Sugars 2 gm
Polyunsat Fat 0.2 gm,   • Protein 7 gm
Monounsat Fat 0.7 gm)   • Phosphorus 220 gm
• Cholesterol 15 mg

Party Starter Bean Dip

Leona M. Slabaugh
Apple Creek, OH

*Makes 16 servings,
¼ cup per serving*

Prep. Time: 20–25 minutes
Baking Time: 20 minutes
Standing Time: 5 minutes

16-oz. can Old El Paso refried beans *or* vegetarian refried beans
8-oz. pkg. fat-free cream cheese, softened
12-oz. jar salsa, *divided*
Nachips Tortilla Chips

1. Spread beans into bottom of a 9" pie pan or a decorative pan, spreading up the sides a bit.
2. In a bowl, beat cream cheese, then add ⅔ cup salsa and beat until smooth.
3. Spread cream cheese mixture over beans. Bake 20 minutes at 350°.
4. Spread remaining salsa over dip which has set for 5 minutes. Serve with Nachips.

Good Go-Alongs:

This is nice with a good dish of fruit and assorted snack crackers when eaten as a snack.

Exchange List Values
• Carbohydrate 0.5

Basic Nutritional Values

- Calories 40
  (Calories from Fat 0)
- Total Fat 0 gm
  (Saturated Fat 0.1 gm,
  Trans Fat 0.0 gm,
  Polyunsat Fat 0.0 gm,
  Monounsat Fat 0.1 gm)
- Cholesterol 0 mg
- Sodium 345 mg
- Potassium 180 gm
- Total Carb 6 gm
- Dietary Fiber 2 gm
- Sugars 1 gm
- Protein 3 gm
- Phosphorus 105 gm

Easy Layered Taco Dip

Lindsey Spencer
Morrow, OH
Jenny R. Unternahrer
Wayland, IA

Makes 10 servings

Prep. Time: 15 minutes

8-oz. fat-free cream cheese,
  softened
8-oz. fat-free sour cream
8-oz. taco sauce *or* salsa
4 cups shredded lettuce
1 cup chopped tomato
chopped green pepper,
  optional
1 cup reduced-fat shredded
  Mexi-blend cheese
tortilla chips

1. Blend cream cheese and sour cream until smooth. Spread in bottom of a 9×13 dish.
2. Layer taco sauce over sour cream mixture, then lettuce, tomato, and cheese.
3. Serve with tortilla chips.

Tips:

1. If you can, add the lettuce, tomato and cheese at the last minute so the lettuce doesn't get soggy.
  Jenny R. Unternahrer
  Wayland, IA

2. Omit salsa and lettuce. Add 3 Tbsp. taco seasoning to the sour cream and cream cheese and add a layer of chopped onion.
  Barbara J. Bey
  Hillsboro, OH

Exchange List Values
- Carbohydrate 0.5
- Lean Meat 1.0

Basic Nutritional Values

- Calories 90
  (Calories from Fat 20)
- Total Fat 2.5 gm
  (Saturated Fat 1.5 gm,
  Trans Fat 0.0 gm,
  Polyunsat Fat 0.1 gm,
  Monounsat Fat 0.6 gm)
- Cholesterol 10 mg
- Sodium 415 mg
- Potassium 175 gm
- Total Carb 9 gm
- Dietary Fiber 1 gm
- Sugars 3 gm
- Protein 7 gm
- Phosphorus 205 gm

Hot Reuben Dip

Leona Miller
Millersburg, OH

*Makes 12 servings,
about ¼ cup per serving*

Prep. Time: 10 minutes
Baking Time: 35 minutes

8-oz. fat-free cream cheese,
  softened
½ cup fat-free sour cream
2 Tbsp. ketchup
½ lb. deli lean corned beef,
  finely chopped
1 cup sauerkraut, chopped,
  rinsed, and drained
1 cup reduced-fat shredded
  Swiss cheese
2 Tbsp. onion, finely
  chopped
Snack rye bread *or* crackers

1. In a mixing bowl, beat cream cheese, sour cream, and ketchup until smooth.
2. Stir in corned beef, sauerkraut, Swiss cheese, and onion until blended.
3. Transfer to a greased 1-quart baking dish.
4. Cover and bake at 375° for 30 minutes. Uncover and bake 5 minutes longer or until bubbly.
5. Serve warm with rye bread or crackers.

Exchange List Values
- Carbohydrate 0.5
- Lean Meat 1.0

Basic Nutritional Values

- Calories 85
  (Calories from Fat 20)
- Total Fat 2.5 gm
  (Saturated Fat 1.2 gm,
  Trans Fat 0.0 gm,
  Polyunsat Fat 0.1 gm,
  Monounsat Fat 0.7 gm)
- Cholesterol 20 mg
- Sodium 415 mg
- Potassium 135 gm
- Total Carb 5 gm
- Dietary Fiber 1 gm
- Sugars 2 gm
- Protein 11 gm
- Phosphorus 190 gm

Basic Deviled Eggs and Variations

*Makes 12 halves,
serving size is 2 egg halves*

Prep. Time: 30 minutes
Cooking Time: 20 minutes

To hardboil eggs:

1. Place eggs in a single layer in a lidded pan.

2. Fill the pan with cold water to just cover the eggs.

3. Bring to a full boil over high heat, covered.

4. As soon as the water begins the full boil, immediately turn the heat down to low for a simmer. Allow to barely simmer for exactly 18 minutes.

5. Pour off hot water. Run cold water and/or ice over the eggs to quickly cool them.

To make deviled eggs:

1. Cut eggs in half lengthwise. Gently remove yolk sections into a bowl.

2. Discard two yolks if using a recipe for 6; discard 4 yolks if using a recipe for 12. Mash remaining yolk sections together with a fork. Stir in remaining ingredients with yolk mixture until smooth.

3. Fill empty egg whites. The filling will make a little mound in the egg white. Garnish, optional.

4. Refrigerate.

Basic Deviled Eggs

6 large eggs, hardboiled
and peeled
¼ cup light mayonnaise
1 tsp. vinegar
1 tsp. prepared mustard
⅛ tsp. salt
sprinkle of pepper
paprika
parsley sprigs for garnish
Joanne Warfel
Lancaster, PA

Exchange List Values
• Med-Fat Meat 1.0

Basic Nutritional Values
• Calories 75   • Sodium 205 mg
  (Calories from Fat 55)   • Potassium 70 gm
• Total Fat 6 gm   • Total Carb 1 gm
  (Saturated Fat 1.4 gm,   • Dietary Fiber 0 gm
  Trans Fat 0.0 gm,   • Sugars 1 gm
  Polyunsat Fat 2.0 gm,   • Protein 6 gm
  Monounsat Fat 1.9 gm)   • Phosphorus 70 gm
• Cholesterol 125 mg

Traditional Eggs

6 large eggs, hardboiled
and peeled
¼ cup plain fat-free yogurt
or light mayonnaise
1 Tbsp. onion, minced
1 tsp. dried parsley
1 tsp. lemon juice
1 tsp. prepared mustard
¼ tsp. salt
¼ tsp. Worcestershire sauce
⅛ tsp. pepper
paprika

olive slices *or* pimento
pieces to garnish
Jan Mast
Lancaster, PA

Exchange List Values
• Med-Fat Meat 1.0

Basic Nutritional Values
• Calories 60   • Sodium 180 mg
  (Calories from Fat 25)   • Potassium 95 gm
• Total Fat 3 gm   • Total Carb 1 gm
  (Saturated Fat 1.1 gm,   • Dietary Fiber 0 gm
  Trans Fat 0.0 gm,   • Sugars 1 gm
  Polyunsat Fat 0.6 gm,   • Protein 6 gm
  Monounsat Fat 1.2 gm)   • Phosphorus 85 gm
• Cholesterol 125 mg

Sweet & Spicy Deviled Eggs

12 large eggs, hardboiled
and peeled
½ cup light mayonnaise
3 Tbsp. sugar-free apricot
preserves
1 tsp. curry powder
½ tsp. salt
⅛ tsp. cayenne pepper
Gwendolyn Chapman
Gwinn, MI

Exchange List Values
• Med-Fat Meat 1.0

Basic Nutritional Values
• Calories 80   • Sodium 245 mg
  (Calories from Fat 55)   • Potassium 75 gm
• Total Fat 6 gm   • Total Carb 2 gm
  (Saturated Fat 1.4 gm,   • Dietary Fiber 0 gm
  Trans Fat 0.0 gm,   • Sugars 1 gm
  Polyunsat Fat 2.0 gm,   • Protein 5 gm
  Monounsat Fat 1.9 gm)   • Phosphorus 70 gm
• Cholesterol 125 mg

Tex Mex Eggs

6 large eggs, hardboiled
  and peeled
¼ cup fat-free plain yogurt
  or light mayonnaise
1 Tbsp. finely diced onion
1 tsp. lemon juice
1 tsp. prepared mustard
1 tsp. taco seasoning
¼ tsp. salt
⅛ tsp. pepper
paprika
black olive slices to garnish

Jan Mast
Lancaster, PA

Exchange List Values
• Med-Fat Meat 1.0

Basic Nutritional Values
• Calories 60
  (Calories from Fat 30)
• Total Fat 4 gm
  (Saturated Fat 1.1 gm,
  Trans Fat 0.0 gm,
  Polyunsat Fat 0.7 gm,
  Monounsat Fat 1.2 gm)
• Cholesterol 125 mg
• Sodium 215 mg
• Potassium 95 gm
• Total Carb 2 gm
• Dietary Fiber 0 gm
• Sugars 1 gm
• Protein 6 gm
• Phosphorus 90 gm

Dill Pickle Eggs

6 large eggs, hardboiled
  and peeled
¼ cup fat-free plain yogurt
  or light mayonnaise
1 Tbsp. pickle relish
1 tsp. dill weed
1 tsp. vinegar
1 tsp. prepared mustard
¼ tsp. salt

¼ tsp. Worcestershire sauce
⅛ tsp. pepper
paprika
pickle slice to garnish

Jan Mast
Lancaster, PA

Exchange List Values
• Med-Fat Meat 1.0

Basic Nutritional Values
• Calories 65
  (Calories from Fat 30)
• Total Fat 4 gm
  (Saturated Fat 1.1 gm,
  Trans Fat 0.0 gm,
  Polyunsat Fat 0.6 gm,
  Monounsat Fat 1.3 gm)
• Cholesterol 125 mg
• Sodium 205 mg
• Potassium 95 gm
• Total Carb 2 gm
• Dietary Fiber 0 gm
• Sugars 2 gm
• Protein 6 gm
• Phosphorus 85 gm

Horseradish Eggs

6 large eggs, hardboiled
  and peeled
¼ cup light mayonnaise
1 or 2 Tbsp. horseradish
½ tsp. dill weed
¼ tsp. ground mustard
⅛ tsp. salt
dash pepper
dash paprika

Anna Marie Albany
Broomall, PA

Exchange List Values
• Med-Fat Meat 1.0

Basic Nutritional Values
• Calories 80
  (Calories from Fat 55)
• Total Fat 6 gm
  (Saturated Fat 1.4 gm,
  Trans Fat 0.0 gm,
  Polyunsat Fat 2.0 gm,
  Monounsat Fat 1.9 gm)
• Cholesterol 125 mg
• Sodium 205 mg
• Potassium 75 gm
• Total Carb 1 gm
• Dietary Fiber 0 gm
• Sugars 1 gm
• Protein 6 gm
• Phosphorus 70 gm

Tuna Eggs

6 large eggs, hardboiled
  and peeled
¼ to ⅓ cup plain fat-free
  yogurt
½ cup tuna, drained and
  flaked
1 tsp. pickle relish
1 tsp. prepared mustard
1 tsp. onion, minced
¼ tsp. salt
⅛ tsp. pepper
paprika, olive slices
  or pimento pieces to
  garnish

Jan Mast
Lancaster, PA

Exchange List Values
• Med-Fat Meat 1.0

Basic Nutritional Values
• Calories 80
  (Calories from Fat 30)
• Total Fat 4 gm
  (Saturated Fat 1.1 gm,
  Trans Fat 0.0 gm,
  Polyunsat Fat 0.7 gm,
  Monounsat Fat 1.3 gm)
• Cholesterol 135 mg
• Sodium 255 mg
• Potassium 135 gm
• Total Carb 1 gm
• Dietary Fiber 0 gm
• Sugars 1 gm
• Protein 10 gm
• Phosphorus 120 gm

Shrimp Appetizer Platter

Tammy Smith
Dorchester, WI

*Makes 5 cups, 20 servings,
¼ cup per serving*

Prep. Time: 15 minutes

8-oz. fat-free cream cheese, softened
½ cup fat-free sour cream
¼ cup reduced-fat mayonnaise
4-oz. can broken shrimp, drained and rinsed
1 cup cocktail sauce
2 cups reduced-fat shredded cheddar cheese
1 bell pepper, chopped
1 tomato, chopped
3 green onions, chopped

1. Beat together cream cheese, sour cream and salad dressing. Put on bottom of a 12-inch platter.
2. Layer rest of ingredients in order given.
3. Cover and chill. Serve with crackers.

Exchange List Values
• Carbohydrate 0.5 • Lean Meat 1.0

Basic Nutritional Values
• Calories 80
  (Calories from Fat 25)
• Total Fat 3 gm
  (Saturated Fat 1.5 gm,
  Trans Fat 0.0 gm,
  Polyunsat Fat 0.3 gm,
  Monounsat Fat 0.8 gm)
• Cholesterol 20 mg
• Sodium 365 mg
• Potassium 155 gm
• Total Carb 8 gm
• Dietary Fiber 1 gm
• Sugars 4 gm
• Protein 6 gm
• Phosphorus 155 gm

Taco Appetizer Platter

Rachel Spicher Hershberger
Sarasota, FL

*Makes 15 servings,
about 3½ oz. per serving*

*Prep. Time: 20 minutes
Cooking/Baking Time: 10 minutes*

1 lb. 90%-lean ground beef
½ cup water
7 tsp. salt-free taco seasoning (see page 271)
2 8-oz. pkgs. cream cheese, softened
¼ cup fat-free milk
4-oz. can chopped green chilies, drained
2 medium tomatoes, seeded and chopped
1 cup chopped green onions
lettuce, *optional*
½ cup honey barbecue sauce
1 cup shredded 75%-less-fat cheddar cheese

1. In a skillet, cook beef over medium heat until no longer pink. Drain. Add water and taco seasoning, simmer for 5 minutes.
2. In a bowl, combine the cream cheese and milk; spread on 14-inch serving platter or pizza pan. Top with meat mixture. Sprinkle with chilies, tomatoes and onions. Add lettuce, if desired.
3. Drizzle with barbecue sauce. Sprinkle with cheddar cheese. Serve with corn chips.

Tip:
I put this on my cake server with a pedestal. It looks great.

Exchange List Values
• Carbohydrate 0.5 • Lean Meat 2.0

Basic Nutritional Values
• Calories 115
  (Calories from Fat 30)
• Total Fat 4 gm
  (Saturated Fat 1.4 gm,
  Trans Fat 0.2 gm,
  Polyunsat Fat 0.2 gm,
  Monounsat Fat 1.2 gm)
• Cholesterol 25 mg
• Sodium 350 mg
• Potassium 285 gm
• Total Carb 7 gm
• Dietary Fiber 1 gm
• Sugars 5 gm
• Protein 12 gm
• Phosphorus 260 gm

Chicken Salad Spread

Lois W. Benner
Lancaster, PA

*Makes 8 servings,
about ¼ cup per serving*

Prep. Time: 20 minutes

2 cups shredded, cooked chicken
½ cup reduced-fat light mayonnaise
½ tsp. cream-style horseradish
½ tsp. prepared mustard
½ tsp. Worcestershire sauce
1 tsp. white sugar
½ tsp. salt
1 Tbsp. finely chopped onion
1 Tbsp. finely chopped celery

1. Prepare cooked chicken by removing all skin, bones and tendons. Save broth and chunks of chicken. Shred chicken chunks in blender. Set aside and cool thoroughly.

2. Combine all other ingredients.

3. Add cooled, shredded chicken to mayonnaise mixture. If consistency is too thick to spread easily, add small amounts of chicken broth until it spreads easily.

4. Spread filling generously between bread or rolls.

Exchange List Values
- Lean Meat 2.0   • Fat 0.5

Basic Nutritional Values
- Calories 105   • Sodium 310 mg
  (Calories from Fat 55)   • Potassium 100 gm
- Total Fat 6 gm   • Total Carb 2 gm
  (Saturated Fat 1.2 gm,   • Dietary Fiber 0 gm
  Trans Fat 0.0 gm,   • Sugars 1 gm
  Polyunsat Fat 2.6 gm,   • Protein 10 gm
  Monounsat Fat 1.9 gm)   • Phosphorus 75 gm
- Cholesterol 35 mg

Molded Crab Spread

Marsha Sabus
Fallbrook, CA

Makes 12 servings

Prep. Time: 10 minutes
Cooking Time: 5–7 minutes
Chilling Time: 4 hours

6-oz. can crab
1 cup celery, chopped
2 green onions, chopped
1 cup light mayonnaise

8-oz. fat-free cream cheese, softened
10¾-oz. can lower-fat, lower-sodium cream of mushroom soup
1-oz. envelope unflavored gelatin
3 Tbsp. cold water

1. In a small microwave safe bowl, sprinkle gelatin over cold water. Let stand 1 minute. Microwave uncovered on high 20 seconds. Stir. Let stand 1 minute or until gelatin is completely dissolved.

2. In a large saucepan, combine soup, cream cheese, mayonnaise, and gelatin. Cook and stir over medium heat for 5–7 minutes or until smooth.

3. Remove from heat and add crab, celery, and onion.

4. Transfer to a 5 cup ring mold, lightly greased. Cover and refrigerate 4 hours or until set.

5. Unmold onto serving platter. Serve with crackers or bread.

Tip:
You can also substitute shrimp for crab.

Exchange List Values
- Carbohydrate 0.5   • Fat 0.5
- Lean Meat 1.0

Basic Nutritional Values
- Calories 95   • Sodium 430 mg
  (Calories from Fat 45)   • Potassium 290 gm
- Total Fat 5 gm   • Total Carb 5 gm
  (Saturated Fat 0.8 gm,   • Dietary Fiber 0 gm
  Trans Fat 0.0 gm,   • Sugars 2 gm
  Polyunsat Fat 2.9 gm,   • Protein 6 gm
  Monounsat Fat 1.5 gm)   • Phosphorus 145 gm
- Cholesterol 20 mg

Tuna Cheese Spread

Elizabeth Yutzy
Wauseon, OH

Makes 15 servings,
about 1½ Tbsp. per serving

Prep. Time: 10 minutes
Chilling Time: 1 hour or more

¼ cup trans-fat-free tub margarine
8-oz. pkg. fat-free cream cheese
6-oz. can tuna, drained
1 onion, minced
½ tsp. Worcestershire sauce
⅛ tsp. dried thyme
⅛ tsp. dried basil
⅛ tsp. dried marjoram
pinch dried parsley

1. Cream together margarine and cream cheese. Add tuna and all other ingredients and mix well.

2. Chill at least an hour and serve with your favorite crackers.

Exchange List Values
- Lean Meat 1.0

Basic Nutritional Values
- Calories 50   • Sodium 160 mg
  (Calories from Fat 20)   • Potassium 85 gm
- Total Fat 2.5 gm   • Total Carb 2 gm
  (Saturated Fat 0.5 gm,   • Dietary Fiber 0 gm
  Trans Fat 0.0 gm,   • Sugars 1 gm
  Polyunsat Fat 1.0 gm,   • Protein 4 gm
  Monounsat Fat 0.7 gm)   • Phosphorus 100 gm
- Cholesterol 5 mg

Shrimp Dip

Joyce Shackelford
Green Bay, WI

*Makes 1½ cups, 9 servings,
2 Tbsp. per serving*

Prep. Time: 15 minutes
Chilling Time: 1 hour

3-oz. pkg. Neufchatel
(⅓-less-fat) cream cheese,
softened
1 cup fat-free sour cream
2 tsp. lemon juice
1-oz. pkg. Italian salad
dressing mix
2 Tbsp. green pepper,
finely chopped
½ cup shrimp, finely
chopped

1. Blend all ingredients
together.
2. Chill at least 1 hour.
3. Serve with chips or
crackers.

Exchange List Values
• Carbohydrate 0.5 • Fat 0.5

Basic Nutritional Values
• Calories 65
  (Calories from Fat 20)
• Total Fat 2.5 gm
  (Saturated Fat 1.4 gm,
  Trans Fat 0.0 gm,
  Polyunsat Fat 0.1 gm,
  Monounsat Fat 0.6 gm)
• Cholesterol 25 mg
• Sodium 385 mg
• Potassium 70 gm
• Total Carb 7 gm
• Dietary Fiber 0 gm
• Sugars 3 gm
• Protein 4 gm
• Phosphorus 65 gm

Mustard Dip

Mary Kay Nolt
Newmanstown, PA
Jessica Stoner
West Liberty, OH

*Makes 18 servings,
2 Tbsp. per serving*

Prep. Time: 10 minutes

1 cup light mayonnaise
1 cup prepared mustard
1 cup fat-free sour cream
or plain yogurt
½ cup granular Splenda
1-oz. pack Hidden Valley
Ranch dressing mix
1 Tbs. horseradish,
optional
½ cup dried minced onion,
optional

1. Stir together and store
covered in refrigerator. Great
as a dip with vegetables,
crackers, or pretzels, or even
as a salad dressing on your
favorite salad.

Warm Memories:
Once you taste it, look out,
you keep coming back for
more.

Exchange List Values
• Carbohydrate 0.5 • Fat 0.5

Basic Nutritional Values
• Calories 60
  (Calories from Fat 30)
• Total Fat 4 gm
  (Saturated Fat 0.5 gm,
  Trans Fat 0.0 gm,
  Polyunsat Fat 1.9 gm,
  Monounsat Fat 1.2 gm)
• Cholesterol 5 mg
• Sodium 395 mg
• Potassium 40 gm
• Total Carb 5 gm
• Dietary Fiber 0 gm
• Sugars 2 gm
• Protein 1 gm
• Phosphorus 30 gm

Mexican Corn Dip

Janie Steele
Moore, OK

*Makes 28 servings,
about ¼ cup per serving*

Prep. Time: 10 minutes

8-oz. fat-free sour cream
1 cup light mayonnaise
2 11-oz. cans Mexican style
corn
4 green onions, chopped
4½-oz. can chopped green
chilies
1¼ cups reduced-fat
shredded cheddar cheese
1–3 jalapeño peppers,
seeds removed, chopped

1. Mix ingredients together.
2. Serve with Fritos Scoops.

Warm Memories:
It's always requested!

Exchange List Values
• Carbohydrate 0.5 • Fat 0.5

Basic Nutritional Values
• Calories 65
  (Calories from Fat 25)
• Total Fat 3 gm
  (Saturated Fat 0.8 gm,
  Trans Fat 0.0 gm,
  Polyunsat Fat 1.3 gm,
  Monounsat Fat 0.8 gm)
• Cholesterol 5 mg
• Sodium 180 mg
• Potassium 70 gm
• Total Carb 7 gm
• Dietary Fiber 1 gm
• Sugars 2 gm
• Protein 2 gm
• Phosphorus 50 gm

Pineapple Salsa

Lorraine Stutzman Amstutz
Akron, PA

*Makes 2½ cups,
10 servings, ¼ cup per serving*

Prep. Time: 30 minutes

1½ cups fresh pineapple
1 cup cucumber
¼ cup red onion
2–4 tsp. jalapeño
1 tsp. garlic
2 Tbsp. fresh cilantro
¼ cup lime juice
1 tsp. grated lime peel
1 tsp. sugar
¼ tsp. salt

1. Pulse ingredients together in food processor until just chopped.

Tips:
1. Serve with your favorite tortilla chips.
2. If you don't have a food processor, simply chop the pineapple, cucumber, onion, jalapeño, garlic and cilantro. Combine with lime, sugar, and salt.

Exchange List Values
• Carbohydrate 0.5

Basic Nutritional Values
• Calories 20
  (Calories from Fat 0)
• Total Fat 0 gm
  (Saturated Fat 0.0 gm,
  Trans Fat 0.0 gm,
  Polyunsat Fat 0.0 gm,
  Monounsat Fat 0.0 gm)
• Cholesterol 0 mg
• Sodium 60 mg
• Potassium 55 gm
• Total Carb 5 gm
• Dietary Fiber 1 gm
• Sugars 3 gm
• Protein 0 gm
• Phosphorus 5 gm

Texas Caviar

Elaine Rineer
Lancaster, PA

*Makes 7½ cups,
30 servings, ¼ cup per serving*

Prep. Time: 15 minutes
Cooking Time: 10 minutes
Chilling Time: 12–24 hours

15½-oz. can black-eyed peas, rinsed
2 11-oz. cans white shoepeg corn
15½-oz. can black beans, rinsed
8-oz. jar chopped pimento
small green bell pepper, finely diced
small red onion, chopped
½ cup sugar
¼ cup oil
salt and pepper, to taste
¾ cup apple cider vinegar
1 Tbsp. water

1. In saucepan, combine sugar, oil, salt, pepper, vinegar and water. Heat until boiling, then cool.
2. Mix together peas, corn, green pepper, beans, pimento and onion. Pour cooked sauce over mixture. Stir. Serve cold.

Tips:
1. Best if refrigerated 24 hours before serving.
2. Serve with scoop Fritos or corn chips.

Variations:
1. Add Rotel, 2 diced Roma tomatoes, and 2 sliced avocados. Omit corn and pimento. As dressing, use 1 cup Zesty Italian dressing with a squeeze of lime juice.
Angie Van Steenvoort
Galloway, OH

2. For dressing, boil together ½ cup olive oil, ½ cup apple cider vinegar, and ½ sugar until sugar is dissolved. Cool.
3. Reduce pimento to 2-oz. and add 1 cup chopped celery.
4. Serve as a salad or dip.
Amy Bauer
New Ulm, MN

Exchange List Values
• Starch 0.5   • Fat 0.5

Basic Nutritional Values
• Calories 70
  (Calories from Fat 20)
• Total Fat 2 gm
  (Saturated Fat 0.2 gm,
  Trans Fat 0.0 gm,
  Polyunsat Fat 0.6 gm,
  Monounsat Fat 1.2 gm)
• Cholesterol 0 mg
• Sodium 85 mg
• Potassium 125 gm
• Total Carb 11 gm
• Dietary Fiber 2 gm
• Sugars 4 gm
• Protein 2 gm
• Phosphorus 40 gm

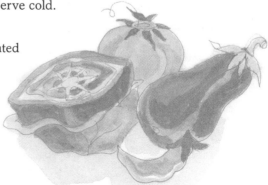

Festive Fruit and Nut Spread

Lucille Hollinger
Richland, PA

*Makes 24 servings,
1 Tbsp. per serving*

***Prep. Time: 15 minutes
Chilling Time: 30 minutes***

**8-oz. Neufchatel (⅓-less-fat)
cream cheese, softened
¼ cup orange juice
½ cup dried cranberries
½ cup pecans, chopped**

1. In a small mixing bowl, beat cream cheese and orange juice until smooth.
2. Fold in cranberries and pecans.
3. Cover and refrigerate 30 minutes.

Good Go-Alongs:

Good with crackers or spread on bagels

Exchange List Values
• Fat 1.0

Basic Nutritional Values
• Calories 50
  (Calories from Fat 35)
• Total Fat 4 gm
  (Saturated Fat 1.4 gm,
  Trans Fat 0.0 gm,
  Polyunsat Fat 0.6 gm,
  Monounsat Fat 1.5 gm)
• Cholesterol 5 mg
• Sodium 40 mg
• Potassium 30 mg
• Total Carb 3 gm
• Dietary Fiber 0 gm
• Sugars 2 gm
• Protein 1 gm
• Phosphorus 20 gm

Cheese and Olive Spread

Suzanne Yoder
Gap, PA

Makes 2 cups, 1 Tbsp. per serving

***Prep. Time: 15 minutes
Chilling Time: 1 hour***

**8-oz. pkg. reduced-fat
shredded mild cheddar
cheese
4 oz. Neufchatel (⅓-less-fat)
cream cheese, softened
4 oz. fat-free cream cheese,
softened
½ cup light mayonnaise
¼ cup stuffed green olives,
chopped
¼ cup green onions,
chopped
2 Tbsp. lemon juice
¼ tsp. ground red pepper
or to taste**

1. Mix ingredients except crackers.
2. Refrigerate at least an hour. Serve with Ritz crackers.

Tips:

I usually have these ingredients on hand so it's simple to have a little something ready for unexpected guests.

It tastes even better after 1–2 days.

Exchange List Values
• Fat 1.0

Basic Nutritional Values
• Calories 45
  (Calories from Fat 30)
• Total Fat 4 gm
  (Saturated Fat 1.5 gm,
  Trans Fat 0.0 gm,
  Polyunsat Fat 0.6 gm,
  Monounsat Fat 0.9 gm)
• Cholesterol 10 mg
• Sodium 145 mg
• Potassium 25 gm
• Total Carb 1 gm
• Dietary Fiber 0 gm
• Sugars 0 gm
• Protein 3 gm
• Phosphorus 65 gm

Father Todd's Favorite Baked Brie

Nanci Keatley
Salem, OR

*Makes 60 servings,
1 Tbsp. per serving*

***Prep. Time: 15 minutes
Baking Time: 20–25 minutes***

**16-oz. round brie
½ cup chopped pecans
¾ cup dried cherries
½ cup Splenda Brown
Sugar Blend
¼ cup amaretto**

1. Place brie in oven-safe round casserole or pie plate.
2. Mix brown sugar and amaretto together; spread on top of cheese.
3. Sprinkle with pecans and cherries.
4. Bake at 375° for 20–25 minutes. Serve with French bread slices.

When choosing high-fat ingredients, such as cheese, pick the most flavorful option and use less.

Tips:
You can use Grand Marnier or a hazelnut liqueur instead. You can also use macadamia nuts or filberts instead of pecans.

Warm Memories:
I've made this for many occasions. The best was when we celebrated our renewing of vows and our priest, Father Todd, came to the small party we had. He loved the baked brie so much that I changed the recipe's name to honor him!

Exchange List Values
• Fat 1.0

Basic Nutritional Values
• Calories 45   • Sodium 55 mg
(Calories from Fat 20) • Potassium 25 gm
• Total Fat 2.5 gm   • Total Carb 4 gm
(Saturated Fat 1.3 gm, • Dietary Fiber 0 gm
Trans Fat 0.0 gm,   • Sugars 2 gm
Polyunsat Fat 0.2 gm, • Protein 1 gm
Monounsat Fat 1.0 gm) • Phosphorus 25 gm
• Cholesterol 5 mg

Pineapple Cheese Dip

Mamie Christopherson
Rio Rancho, NM

*Makes 36 servings,
scant 2 Tbsp. per serving*

Prep. Time: 10 minutes

2 8-oz. pkgs. fat-free cream cheese, softened
8-oz. can no-sugar-added crushed pineapple, drained
2 cups chopped pecans
2 Tbsp. finely chopped onions
1 Tbsp. seasoned salt

1. Soften cream cheese at room temperature. Beat with mixer until fluffy.
2. Add pineapple, pecans, onions, and salt. Serve with crackers.

Variation:
Leave out 1 cup of the pecans. Chill mixture for several hours. Shape into a ball and roll in the reserved pecans.
Joyce Shackelford
Green Bay, WI

Exchange List Values
• Fat 1.0

Basic Nutritional Values
• Calories 55   • Sodium 205 mg
(Calories from Fat 40) • Potassium 65 gm
• Total Fat 4.5 gm   • Total Carb 2 gm
(Saturated Fat 0.4 gm, • Dietary Fiber 1 gm
Trans Fat 0.0 gm,   • Sugars 1 gm
Polyunsat Fat 1.3 gm, • Protein 2 gm
Monounsat Fat 2.7 gm) • Phosphorus 85 gm
• Cholesterol 0 mg

Apple Dippers

Christine Lucke
Aumsville, OR

*Makes 8 servings,
2 Tbsp. per serving*

Prep. Time: 15 minutes

8-oz. fat-free cream cheese
2 tsp. fat-free milk
⅓ cup brown sugar

1. Whip cream cheese, milk, and brown sugar to a smooth, fluffy consistency.
2. Serve with sliced apples for dipping.

Tips:
1. I like Braeburn or Cameo apples.
2. You can use some lemon juice and water to keep the apples from browning, but I just slice right before serving and the Braeburns don't turn brown before they are eaten.

Warm Memories:
We make this as a VBS snack and we have adults lingering in the kitchen hoping for handouts!

Exchange List Values
• Carbohydrate 0.5

Basic Nutritional Values
• Calories 50   • Sodium 185 mg
(Calories from Fat 0) • Potassium 90 gm
• Total Fat 0 gm   • Total Carb 8 gm
(Saturated Fat 0.0 gm, • Dietary Fiber 0 gm
Trans Fat 0.0 gm,   • Sugars 7 gm
Polyunsat Fat 0.0 gm, • Protein 3 gm
Monounsat Fat 0.0 gm) • Phosphorus 150 gm
• Cholesterol 5 mg

Pretty Fruit Kabobs with Dip

Anya Kauffman
Sheldon, WI

Makes 40 servings,
1 kabob and 2 Tbsp. dip per serving

Prep. Time: 30 minutes

8-oz. Neufchatel (⅓-less-fat) cream cheese, softened
9-oz. fat-free frozen whipped topping, thawed
6 oz. marshmallow cream
¼ cup fat-free milk
1 tsp. vanilla

1 honeydew, cut in 80 pieces
1 pineapple, cut in 80 pieces
2 lbs. strawberries, cut in 40 pieces
1 lb. red grapes
1 lb. green grapes
40 8-inch skewers

1. Beat cream cheese until fluffy.
2. Fold in whipped topping and marshmallow cream. Add vanilla and milk.
3. Refrigerate until ready to serve.
4. For kabobs, thread green grape, pineapple, red grape, honeydew, strawberry, honeydew, red grape, pineapple, green grape on skewers. Serve.

Tips:
1. A bright delicious combination!
2. Fresh fruit is always a big hit, especially if there are guests with diet restrictions.

3. Tester stuck the kabobs in a foam block placed in a low pan and covered with lettuce, making a "fruit bouquet."

Exchange List Values
- Fruit 0.5
- Carbohydrate 0.5

Basic Nutritional Values
- Calories 80
  (Calories from Fat 15)
- Total Fat 2 gm
  (Saturated Fat 0.8 gm,
  Trans Fat 0.0 gm,
  Polyunsat Fat 0.1 gm,
  Monounsat Fat 0.3 gm)
- Cholesterol 5 mg
- Sodium 40 mg
- Potassium 175 gm
- Total Carb 16 gm
- Dietary Fiber 1 gm
- Sugars 12 gm
- Protein 1 gm
- Phosphorus 30 gm

Fruit Salsa with Cinnamon Chips

Jackie Halladay
Lancaster, PA

Makes 12 servings, 6 chips and
about ⅓ cup salsa per serving

Prep. Time: 45 minutes
Baking Time: 12 minutes

Cinnamon Chips:
6 6" flour tortillas
2 Tbsp. sugar
¾ tsp. cinnamon
Butter Flavor cooking spray

Salsa:
1 orange, peeled and chopped
1 apple, chopped
1 kiwi, peeled and chopped
1 cup chopped strawberries
½ cup blueberries

2 Tbsp. honey
2 Tbsp. sugar-free jam (any flavor)
¼ cup orange juice
¼-½ tsp. cinnamon
¼ tsp. nutmeg
pinch salt

1. To make cinnamon chips, cut tortillas into 12 wedges and arrange on a baking sheet. Lightly mist with cooking spray.
2. Mix cinnamon and sugar together.
3. Sprinkle tortilla wedges with the cinnamon sugar.
4. Bake 10 minutes at 350°; broil 2 minutes. Remove from pan until cool.
5. To make salsa, toss all prepared fruit together in a large bowl.
6. In a smaller bowl, mix honey, orange juice, jam, cinnamon, nutmeg, and salt.
7. Stir honey mixture into fruit. Tastes best when allowed to marinate in the refrigerator for several hours.

Tips:
1. A food processor helps with all the chopping.
2. You can really use any combination of fruit.
3. Whole wheat tortillas make it even healthier.

Exchange List Values
- Starch 0.5
- Carbohydrate 0.5
- Fruit 0.5

Basic Nutritional Values
- Calories 95
  (Calories from Fat 15)
- Total Fat 2 gm
  (Saturated Fat 0.3 gm,
  Trans Fat 0.0 gm,
  Polyunsat Fat 0.3 gm,
  Monounsat Fat 0.7 gm)
- Cholesterol 0 mg
- Sodium 95 mg
- Potassium 125 gm
- Total Carb 21 gm
- Dietary Fiber 2 gm
- Sugars 10 gm
- Protein 2 gm
- Phosphorus 30 gm

Dressed-Up Fruit Salad

Michelle D. Hostetler
Indianapolis, IN

Makes 10 servings,
2 Tbsp. per serving

Prep. Time: 10 minutes

1 cup fat-free sour cream
2 Tbsp. brown sugar
½ tsp. cinnamon
¼ tsp. vanilla

1. Mix together.
2. Serve with cut-up apples, grapes and bananas.

Warm Memories:

People always take seconds and rave over it.

Exchange List Values
• Carbohydrate 0.5

Basic Nutritional Values
• Calories 30
  (Calories from Fat 0)
• Total Fat 0 gm
  (Saturated Fat 0.1 gm,
  Trans Fat 0.0 gm,
  Polyunsat Fat 0.0 gm,
  Monounsat Fat 0.0 gm)
• Cholesterol 0 mg
• Sodium 30 mg
• Potassium 35 gm
• Total Carb 7 gm
• Dietary Fiber 0 gm
• Sugars 4 gm
• Protein 1 gm
• Phosphorus 25 gm

Strawberry Yogurt Dip

Teresa Koenig
Leola, PA

Makes 5½ cups,
22 servings, ¼ cup per serving

Prep. Time: 20 minutes

8-oz. frozen lite whipped
  topping, thawed
2 6-oz. cartons light
  strawberry yogurt
1–1½ cups mashed
  strawberries, fresh *or*
  thawed frozen

1. Combine whipped topping, yogurt, and mashed berries.
2. Serve with variety of sliced fresh fruit.

Tips:

Also tastes good with pretzels or as a topping for scones.

Exchange List Values
• Carbohydrate 0.5

Basic Nutritional Values
• Calories 35
  (Calories from Fat 15)
• Total Fat 2 gm
  (Saturated Fat 1.2 gm,
  Trans Fat 0.0 gm,
  Polyunsat Fat 0.0 gm,
  Monounsat Fat 0.1 gm)
• Cholesterol 0 mg
• Sodium 15 mg
• Potassium 45 gm
• Total Carb 6 gm
• Dietary Fiber 0 gm
• Sugars 5 gm
• Protein 1 gm
• Phosphorus 25 gm

Creamy Caramel Dip

Mary Kay Nolt
Newmanstown, PA

Makes 40 servings,
1 Tbsp. per serving

Prep. Time: 20 minutes
Chilling Time: 1 hour

8-oz. fat-free cream cheese,
  softened
¾ cup brown sugar
1 cup fat-free sour cream
2 tsp. vanilla
1 cup fat-free milk
3.4-oz. instant vanilla
  pudding mix

1. Beat cream cheese and brown sugar.
2. Add sour cream, vanilla, milk, and pudding and mix.
3. Chill at least 1 hour. Serve as a dip for pineapples, apples, grapes, strawberries, etc.

Exchange List Values
• Carbohydrate 0.5

Basic Nutritional Values
• Calories 30
  (Calories from Fat 0)
• Total Fat 0 gm
  (Saturated Fat 0.0 gm,
  Trans Fat 0.0 gm,
  Polyunsat Fat 0.0 gm,
  Monounsat Fat 0.0 gm)
• Cholesterol 0 mg
• Sodium 80 mg
• Potassium 40 gm
• Total Carb 7 gm
• Dietary Fiber 0 gm
• Sugars 5 gm
• Protein 1 gm
• Phosphorus 60 gm

Use low-fat ingredients, such as low-fat yogurt or milk, in recipes whenever possible.

Sweet Cheese Ball

Mary Ann Lefever
Lancaster, PA

Makes 35 servings,
2 Tbsp. per serving

Prep. Time: 10 minutes
Chilling Time: 4 hours

2 8-oz. pkgs. fat-free cream
   cheese, softened
3-oz. French vanilla
   instant pudding mix
15-oz. can fruit cocktail,
   well drained
4 Tbsp. orange juice
1 cup sliced almonds

1. Mix cream cheese,
pudding, fruit, and juice.
2. Refrigerate to set up,
approximately 4 hours.
3. Shape into a ball and roll
in almonds.
4. Store in refrigerator.
Serve with buttery crackers
such as Town House, graham
crackers, or apple slices.

Warm Memories:
A friend always brought
this to get-togethers or served
at her home and would not
"give out" the recipe. Finally
she got tired of me asking and
gave me the recipe. Always a
hit at get-togethers.

Exchange List Values
• Carbohydrate 0.5

Basic Nutritional Values
• Calories 40
  (Calories from Fat 15)
• Total Fat 2 gm
  (Saturated Fat 0.1 gm,
  Trans Fat 0.0 gm,
  Polyunsat Fat 0.3 gm,
  Monounsat Fat 0.8 gm)
• Cholesterol 0 mg
• Sodium 120 mg
• Potassium 65 gm
• Total Carb 5 gm
• Dietary Fiber 0 gm
• Sugars 3 gm
• Protein 2 gm
• Phosphorus 100 gm

Orange Pecans

Janice Muller
Derwood, MD

Makes 44 servings,
2 Tbsp. per serving, 5½ cups total

Prep. Time: 3 minutes
Cooking Time: 10 minutes
Cooling Time: 30 minutes

¼ cup orange juice
1 Tbsp. grated orange rind
½ tsp. cinnamon
¼ tsp. allspice
¼ tsp. ginger
pinch salt
1 cup sugar
1 lb. pecan halves, whole

1. Combine orange juice,
orange rind, cinnamon,
allspice, ginger, salt, and
sugar in a large flat pot so
that it will be easy to coat
pecans with the hot mixture.
2. Cook on medium heat
until mix comes to a full boil.
3. Stir in pecans. Keep
stirring until the pecans are
well coated and the syrup is
absorbed.
4. Remove from heat; stir
until pecans separate. Spread
onto waxed paper to cool.

Tip:
I always double this recipe
because I buy the pecans in a
2 lb. bag at a club/warehouse,
and once you assemble your
ingredients, why not – they go
fast when you serve them.

Warm Memories:
I can't keep enough of
these in the house during the
holidays, and they're fun to
take to gatherings. People can
take as few or as many as
they want. The orange flavor
and pecan crunch make them
addictive. I've also packaged
these in pretty bags as gifts for
neighbors during the holidays.

Good Go-Alongs:
The sugared pecans are
good by themselves, or you
can sprinkle them over a
dish of vanilla ice cream, or a
green salad.

Exchange List Values
• Carbohydrate 0.5   • Fat 1.5

Basic Nutritional Values
• Calories 90
  (Calories from Fat 70)
• Total Fat 8 gm
  (Saturated Fat 0.6 gm,
  Trans Fat 0.0 gm,
  Polyunsat Fat 2.1 gm,
  Monounsat Fat 4.5 gm)
• Cholesterol 0 mg
• Sodium 0 mg
• Potassium 45 gm
• Total Carb 6 gm
• Dietary Fiber 1 gm
• Sugars 5 gm
• Protein 1 gm
• Phosphorus 30 gm

When a recipe calls for softened cream cheese,
remove the cream cheese from the refrigerator at least
2 hours before starting the recipe.
Mamie Christopherson, Rio Rancho, NM

Popcorn

Rosetta Martin
Columbiana, OH

*Makes 17 servings,
about 2 cups per serving*

Prep. Time: 15 minutes

2 tsp. salt
2 tsp. garlic powder
2 Tbsp. cheese powder
½ cup no-trans-fat tub
  margarine, melted
8 quarts air-popped
  popcorn with no salt or
  butter
1 cup small cheese crackers

1. Mix together salt, garlic powder and cheese powder.

2. Pour melted margarine over popcorn, mixing so it's spread evenly. Pour seasonings over popcorn and mix well.

3. Add cheese crackers and serve.

Exchange List Values
• Starch 1.0   • Fat 1.0

Basic Nutritional Values
• Calories 115   • Sodium 385 mg
  (Calories from Fat 55) • Potassium 60 gm
• Total Fat 6 gm   • Total Carb 14 gm
  (Saturated Fat 1.4 gm, • Dietary Fiber 2 gm
  Trans Fat 0.0 gm,   • Sugars 0 gm
  Polyunsat Fat 2.0 gm, • Protein 3 gm
  Monounsat Fat 1.9 gm) • Phosphorus 70 gm
• Cholesterol 0 mg

Crisp Snack Bars

Norma Saltzman
Shickley, NE

Makes 16 servings, 1 bar per serving

**Prep. Time: 30 minutes
Cooking Time: 10 minutes**

¼ cup honey
½ cup chunky peanut
  butter
½ cup non-fat dry milk
⅓ cup fat-free milk
4 cups crisp rice cereal

1. In a large saucepan, combine honey, peanut butter, and milk powder.

2. Cook and stir over low heat until peanut butter is melted and mixture is warm. Remove from heat. If the mixture is too thick to stir easily, thin with a little milk.

3. Stir in cereal.

4. Press into an 8-inch square dish coated with non-stick cooking spray. Let stand until set.

5. Cut into 16 square bars.

Variations:
Melt chocolate chips along with the peanut butter mixture. Reduce the cereal to 2 cups.

Karen Burkholder
Narvon, PA

Exchange List Values
• Carbohydrate 1.0   • Fat 1.0

Basic Nutritional Values
• Calories 100   • Sodium 120 mg
  (Calories from Fat 40) • Potassium 100 gm
• Total Fat 4.5 gm   • Total Carb 13 gm
  (Saturated Fat 0.8 gm, • Dietary Fiber 1 gm
  Trans Fat 0.0 gm,   • Sugars 7 gm
  Polyunsat Fat 1.2 gm, • Protein 3 gm
  Monounsat Fat 2.0 gm) • Phosphorus 60 gm
• Cholesterol 0 mg

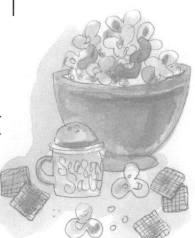

Soft Pretzels

Lydia K. Stoltzfus
Gordonville, PA

*Makes 24 pretzels,
1 pretzel per serving*

**Prep. Time: 15 minutes
Rising Time: 30 minutes
Cooking/Baking Time: 15
minutes**

**4 tsp. active dry yeast
3 cups lukewarm water
pinch of salt
⅓ cup brown sugar
7½ cups flour
3 Tbsp. baking soda
2 cups water
pretzel salt**

1. Dissolve yeast in water.
2. Add brown sugar and pinch salt.
3. Stir in flour slowly. Knead well.
4. Cover and let rise 30 minutes.
5. Divide dough into small pieces and form into pretzel shapes.
6. Meanwhile mix baking soda and 2 cups water in a saucepan and heat until hot.
7. Dip each twisted pretzel in hot solution and rub back side on paper towels, so it will not stick to pan.
8. Lay dipped pretzels on greased baking sheets.
9. Sprinkle salt on pretzels.
10. Bake at 500° for 7–10 minutes.

Exchange List Values
• Starch 2.0

Basic Nutritional Values

• Calories 150 (Calories from Fat 0)	• Sodium 175 mg
	• Potassium 55 gm
• Total Fat 0 gm (Saturated Fat 0.1 gm, Trans Fat 0.0 gm, Polyunsat Fat 0.2 gm, Monounsat Fat 0.0 gm)	• Total Carb 32 gm
	• Dietary Fiber 1 gm
	• Sugars 3 gm
	• Protein 4 gm
	• Phosphorus 50 gm
• Cholesterol 0 mg	

Raspberry Punch

Gloria Martin
Ephrata, PA

*Makes 4 quarts, 32 servings, ½ cup
per serving*

Prep. Time: 20 minutes

**3 3-oz. pkgs. sugar-free raspberry gelatin
4 cups boiling water
¾ cup granular Splenda
4 cups cold water
2¼ cups orange juice concentrate
1¼ cups lemonade concentrate
1 quart diet ginger-ale
10-oz. pkg. frozen raspberries**

1. Dissolve gelatin in boiling water.
2. Add Splenda and cold water and stir to dissolve.
3. In a punch bowl, mix orange juice concentrate, lemon juice concentrate, ginger-ale, and raspberries.
4. Pour gelatin mixture into punch bowl. Stir. Serve with ice.

Variation:
Float scoops of raspberry sherbet on top of the punch.

Exchange List Values
• Carbohydrate 1.0

Basic Nutritional Values

• Calories 70 (Calories from Fat 0)	• Sodium 30 mg
	• Potassium 155 gm
• Total Fat 0 gm (Saturated Fat 0.0 gm, Trans Fat 0.0 gm, Polyunsat Fat 0.0 gm, Monounsat Fat 0.0 gm)	• Total Carb 17 gm
	• Dietary Fiber 1 gm
	• Sugars 16 gm
	• Protein 1 gm
	• Phosphorus 25 gm
• Cholesterol 0 mg	

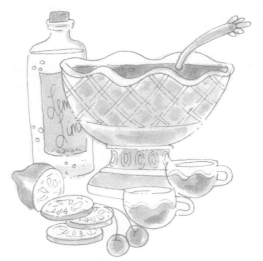

Orange Lemon Drink

Rhonda Freed
Croghan, NY

*Makes 1 gallon,
16 servings of 1 cup each*

Prep. Time: 10 minutes

12-oz. can frozen orange juice concentrate
1 cup granular Splenda
½ cup lemon juice
1 gallon water, *divided*

1. Mix juice concentrate, Splenda, lemon juice, and ½ gallon water.
2. Add water to make a full gallon. Serve cold.

Exchange List Values
• Fruit 1.0

Basic Nutritional Values
• Calories 50
  (Calories from Fat 0)
• Total Fat 0 gm
  (Saturated Fat 0.0 gm,
  Trans Fat 0.0 gm,
  Polyunsat Fat 0.0 gm,
  Monounsat Fat 0.0 gm)
• Cholesterol 0 mg
• Sodium 10 mg
• Potassium 185 gm
• Total Carb 12 gm
• Dietary Fiber 0 gm
• Sugars 12 gm
• Protein 1 gm
• Phosphorus 15 gm

Lemonade

Ruth R. Nissley
Mount Joy, PA

*Makes 60 servings,
about ¾ cup per serving*

Prep. Time: 10 minutes

3 cups Realemon
6 oz. frozen orange juice
4 cups granulated Splenda
water to fill 3 gallons

1. Mix Realemon, orange juice and Splenda.
2. Add water and ice to make an ice-cold drink.

Exchange List Values
• Free food

Basic Nutritional Values
• Calories 15
  (Calories from Fat 0)
• Total Fat 0 gm
  (Saturated Fat 0.0 gm,
  Trans Fat 0.0 gm,
  Polyunsat Fat 0.0 gm,
  Monounsat Fat 0.0 gm)
• Cholesterol 0 mg
• Sodium 10 mg
• Potassium 35 gm
• Total Carb 4 gm
• Dietary Fiber 0 gm
• Sugars 3 gm
• Protein 0 gm
• Phosphorus 0 gm

Very Simple Punch

Mrs. Lewis L. Beachy
Sarasota, FL

*Makes 60 servings,
a scant ½ cup per serving*

Prep. Time: 10 minutes

46-oz. can pineapple juice
46-oz. can grapefruit juice
46-oz. can orange juice
2 quarts diet ginger-ale
1 quart orange sherbet

1. Mix all liquids together.
2. Immediately before serving, cut sherbet into chunks and add to punch.

Exchange List Values
• Carbohydrate 0.5

Basic Nutritional Values
• Calories 45
  (Calories from Fat 0)
• Total Fat 0 gm
  (Saturated Fat 0.1 gm,
  Trans Fat 0.0 gm,
  Polyunsat Fat 0.0 gm,
  Monounsat Fat 0.1 gm)
• Cholesterol 0 mg
• Sodium 10 mg
• Potassium 110 gm
• Total Carb 10 gm
• Dietary Fiber 0 gm
• Sugars 8 gm
• Protein 0 gm
• Phosphorus 10 gm

Wash and dry whole lettuce leaves. Put a scoop of tuna or egg salad in each one. Enjoy your lettuce boats! You can also slip these into wraps or pitas.
Donna Conta, Saylorsburg, PA

My Mother's Holiday Punch

Geraldine A. Ebersole
Hershey, PA

*Makes 32 servings,
½ cup per serving*

***Prep Time: 15 minutes
Cooking time: 10 minutes***

2 cups granular Splenda
3 cups water
4 cups diet cranberry juice
    drink
6-oz. can frozen lemon juice
6-oz. can frozen orange juice
3 cups pineapple juice
ice
1 quart diet ginger-ale
springs of mint, *optional*

1. Make a sugar syrup with sugar and water. Place sugar and water in a saucepan and bring to a boil. Boil 1 minute and take off heat. Cool.

2. Add all fruit juices to cooled sugar syrup. When ready to serve, pour mixture over ice in punch bowl and add ginger-ale.

3. If desired, garnish with sprigs of mint.

Exchange List Values
• Fruit 0.5

Basic Nutritional Values
• Calories 30
  (Calories from Fat 0)
• Total Fat 0 gm
  (Saturated Fat 0.0 gm,
  Trans Fat 0.0 gm,
  Polyunsat Fat 0.0 gm,
  Monounsat Fat 0.0 gm)
• Cholesterol 0 mg
• Sodium 10 mg
• Potassium 80 gm
• Total Carb 8 gm
• Dietary Fiber 0 gm
• Sugars 7 gm
• Protein 0 gm
• Phosphorus 5 gm

Cocoa for a Crowd

Joy Reiff
Mt. Joy, PA

Makes 65 1-cup servings

***Prep. Time: 5 minutes
Cooking Time: 20–30 minutes***

5 cups baking cocoa
4 cups granular Splenda
2 tsp. salt
5 quarts (20 cups) water,
    divided
10 quarts (2½ gallons)
    fat-free milk
1 quart fat-free half-and-
    half
2 Tbsp. vanilla
whipped cream and
    additional baking cocoa
    for garnish, *optional*

1. In each of two large stockpots, combine 2½ cups cocoa, 2 cups Splenda and 1 teaspoon salt.

2. Gradually stir 5 cups water into each pot.

3. Bring to a boil, covered. Turn heat to low.

4. Whisk in milk, half-and-half, remaining 10 cups water; heat through, but do not boil.

5. Turn off heat. Stir in vanilla. Taste, and add sugar to your taste.

6. Garnish with whipped topping and additional cocoa.

Warm Memories:
I like to serve this at my open house in the winter.

Exchange List Values
• Fat-Free Milk 1.0

Basic Nutritional Values
• Calories 80
  (Calories from Fat 10)
• Total Fat 1 gm
  (Saturated Fat 0.7 gm,
  Trans Fat 0.0 gm,
  Polyunsat Fat 0.0 gm,
  Monounsat Fat 0.4 gm)
• Cholesterol 5 mg
• Sodium 150 mg
• Potassium 365 gm
• Total Carb 14 gm
• Dietary Fiber 2 gm
• Sugars 10 gm
• Protein 7 gm
• Phosphorus 225 gm

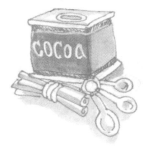

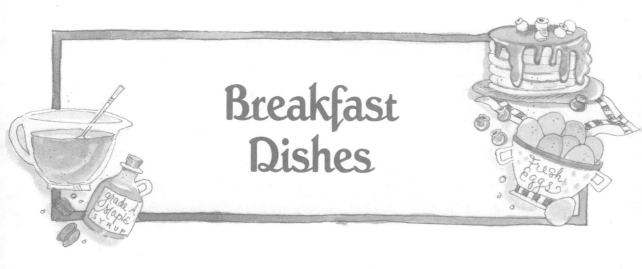

Breakfast Dishes

4. Bake at 350° for 25–30 minutes, or until a knife inserted in center comes out clean.

Exchange List Values
- Carbohydrate 0.5
- Lean Meat 2.0

Basic Nutritional Values
- Calories 125
  (Calories from Fat 30)
- Total Fat 4 gm
  (Saturated Fat 1.9 gm,
  Trans Fat 0.0 gm,
  Polyunsat Fat 0.2 gm,
  Monounsat Fat 0.7 gm)
- Cholesterol 10 mg
- Sodium 480 mg
- Potassium 350 gm
- Total Carb 10 gm
- Dietary Fiber 1 gm
- Sugars 4 gm
- Protein 14 gm
- Phosphorus 140 gm

California Egg Bake

Leona M. Slabaugh
Apple Creek, OH

Makes 2 servings

Prep. Time: 10–15 minutes
Baking Time: 25–30 minutes

¾ cup egg substitute
¼ cup fat-free sour cream
⅛ tsp. salt
1 medium tomato, chopped
1 green onion, sliced
¼ cup reduced-fat
  shredded cheddar cheese

1. In a small bowl, beat eggs, sour cream, and salt.
2. Stir in tomato, onion, and cheese.
3. Pour into greased 2-cup baking dish.

We occasionally plan a breakfast meal, asking persons whose last names begin with A–K to bring fruits and persons whose last names begin with L–Z to bring breads or coffee cakes. The food committee provides coffee and tea. Joy Kauffman, Goshen, IN

Eggs a la Shrimp

Willard E. Roth
Elkhart, IN

Makes 6 servings

Prep. Time: 15 minutes
Cooking Time: 15 minutes

1 Tbsp. canola oil
3 green onions with tops,
   sliced, *or* 1 small onion,
   chopped fine
¼ cup finely chopped
   celery with leaves
4 oz. shrimp, frozen, *or*
   canned
3 Tbsp., plus ¼ cup white
   wine, *divided*
4 large eggs
1 cup egg substitute
4 oz. frozen peas, *or* fresh
¼ tsp. salt
¼ tsp. pepper
3 Tbsp., plus ¼ cup white
   wine
fresh parsley

1. Preheat electric skillet
to 375°, or cast iron skillet to
medium high.
2. Heat oil in skillet. Sauté
onions, until limp.
3. Add celery and sauté
until softened.
4. Add shrimp and 3 Tbsp.
white wine. Cover and steam
over low heat for 3 minutes.
5. In a medium-sized mix-
ing bowl, toss eggs and egg
substitute with ¼ cup white
wine. Pour into skillet.
6. Stir in peas and seasonings.
7. Turn skillet to 300°, or
medium low. Stir gently as
mixture cooks. Cook just

until mixture sets according
to your liking.
8. Serve on warm platter
surrounded with fresh
parsley.

Good Go-Alongs:
   Freshly baked muffins
   Fresh fruit in season

Note:
   A simple but special
brunch—or supper—entrée.

Exchange List Values
• Lean Meat 2.0   • Fat 1.0

Basic Nutritional Values
• Calories 135   • Sodium 415 mg
(Calories from Fat 55)   • Potassium 195 gm
• Total Fat 6 gm   • Total Carb 4.5 gm
(Saturated Fat 1.3 gm,   • Dietary Fiber 1 gm
Trans Fat 0.0 gm,   • Sugars 2 gm
Polyunsat Fat 1.4 gm,   • Protein 14 gm
Monounsat Fat 2.8 gm)   • Phosphorus 145 gm
• Cholesterol 165 mg

Baked Eggs

Esther J. Mast
Lancaster, PA

Make 8 servings,
2¾"×3½" rectangle per serving

Prep. Time: 15 minutes
Baking Time: 40–45 minutes

2 Tbsp. no trans-fat tub
   margarine
1 cup reduced-fat
   buttermilk baking mix
1½ cups fat-free cottage
   cheese
2 tsp. chopped onion
1 tsp. dried parsley

½ cup grated reduced-fat
   cheddar cheese
1 egg, slightly beaten
1¼ cups egg substitute
1 cup fat-free milk

1. Cut butter into chunks
and place in 7×11 baking
dish. Turn oven to 350°
and put dish in oven to melt
butter.
2. Meanwhile, mix
together buttermilk baking
mix, cottage cheese, onion,
parsley, salt, cheese, egg,
egg substitute, and milk in
large mixing bowl.
3. Pour mixture over
melted butter. Stir slightly to
distribute butter.
4. Bake 40–45 minutes
until firm but not drying out.
5. Allow to stand 10
minutes. Cut in squares and
serve.

Tip:
   Serve with muffins and
fresh fruit cup.

Exchange List Values
• Carbohydrate 1.0   • Lean Meat 2.0

Basic Nutritional Values
• Calories 155   • Sodium 460 mg
(Calories from Fat 45)   • Potassium 195 gm
• Total Fat 5 gm   • Total Carb 15 gm
(Saturated Fat 1.5 gm,   • Dietary Fiber 0 gm
Trans Fat 0.0 gm,   • Sugars 4 gm
Polyunsat Fat 1.2 gm,   • Protein 12 gm
Monounsat Fat 1.8 gm)   • Phosphorus 250 gm
• Cholesterol 30 mg

Breakfast Soufflé

Freda Friesen
Hillsboro, KS

Makes 12 servings,
3" square per serving

Prep. Time: 20 minutes
Standing Time: 12 hours or
overnight
Baking Time: 1 hour

½ lb. reduced-fat pork
   sausage
2¼ cups egg substitute
3 cups fat-free milk
1½ tsp. dry mustard
¾ tsp. salt
3 slices bread, cubed
¾ cup grated 75%-less-fat
   cheddar cheese

1. Brown pork sausage and
drain excess fat. Set aside.
2. Combine egg substitute,
milk, mustard and salt. Add
sausage, bread and cheese.
3. Spoon into greased 9 × 13
pan. Cover and refrigerate
overnight.
4. Bake, uncovered, at 350°
for 1 hour.

Exchange List Values
• Carbohydrate 0.5   • Lean Meat 2.0

Basic Nutritional Values
• Calories 115
  (Calories from Fat 35)
• Total Fat 4 gm
  (Saturated Fat 1.4 gm,
  Trans Fat 0.0 gm,
  Polyunsat Fat 0.5 gm,
  Monounsat Fat 1.5 gm)
• Cholesterol 15 mg
• Sodium 440 mg
• Potassium 220 gm
• Total Carb 7 gm
• Dietary Fiber 0 gm
• Sugars 4 gm
• Protein 12 gm
• Phosphorus 135 gm

Egg Scramble

Elva Bare, Lancaster, PA

Makes 6 servings,
4½ to 5½ oz. per serving

Prep. Time: 30–45 minutes
Cooking Time: 10 minutes

1 medium-large potato,
   enough to make ¾ cup
   grated potatoes
1 Tbsp. canola oil
½ cup chopped red bell
   pepper
¼ cup chopped green bell
   pepper
½ cup chopped onion
4 eggs
1 cup egg substitute
⅓ cup fat-free sour cream
¼ cup fat-free milk
½ tsp. onion salt
¼ tsp. garlic salt
⅛ tsp. pepper
½ cup real bacon bits
½ cup shredded 75%-less-
   fat cheddar, *or* Cooper
   sharp, cheese

1. Place a whole potato with
skin on in a small pan. Add
about ½" water, cover, and cook
over low heat until fork-tender.
2. Remove and allow to
reach room temperature.
3. Chill thoroughly. Grate.
4. Sauté peppers and onion
in canola oil 3–5 minutes.
5. In a blender, combine
eggs, egg substitute, sour
cream, milk, onion salt, garlic
salt, and pepper. Cover and
process until smooth.
6. Stir grated potato and
bacon into vegetables in
skillet.

7. Pour egg mixture over
vegetables.
8. Cook and stir over medium
heat until eggs are set.
9. Sprinkle with cheese.
Cover skillet with lid until
cheese melts.
10. Cut in wedges in skillet
and serve on heated dinner
plates.

Tips:
1. You can do a lot of the
prep for this dish the day or
evening before serving it.
Cook the potato in advance
and chill it. Chop the
vegetables ahead of time and
refrigerate them. You can
even blend the eggs, sour
cream, milk, salts, and pepper the day before and then
refrigerate the mixture. The
morning of your breakfast
you're ready to go.
2. I heat the dinner plates
in my oven, turned on Low,
for 5–10 minutes.

Good Go-Alongs:
Serve toasted bagels and
fresh fruit. Add a broiled
tomato, which you've cut
in half and sprinkled with
Parmesan cheese before
running under the broiler.

Exchange List Values
• Carbohydrate 1.0   • Fat 0.5
• Lean Meat 2.0

Basic Nutritional Values
• Calories 180
  (Calories from Fat 70)
• Total Fat 8 gm
  (Saturated Fat 2.5 gm,
  Trans Fat 0.0 gm,
  Polyunsat Fat 1.3 gm,
  Monounsat Fat 3.2 gm)
• Cholesterol 130 mg
• Sodium 485 mg
• Potassium 385 gm
• Total Carb 12 gm
• Dietary Fiber 1 gm
• Sugars 3 gm
• Protein 15 gm
• Phosphorus 175 gm

Egg Casserole

Marie Davis
Mineral Ridge, OH

Makes 6 servings

Prep. Time: 15 minutes
Baking Time: 35–40 minutes

4- or 6½-oz. jar marinated artichoke hearts
½ cup chopped green onions
2–3 garlic cloves
1 Tbsp. vegetable oil
2 cups egg substitute
4½-oz. can sliced mushrooms, drained
1 cup 75%-less-fat shredded sharp cheddar cheese
⅔ cup butter-flavored cracker crumbs (about 16 crackers, crushed)

1. Drain. Cut artichokes into small pieces.
2. In small skillet, sauté green onions and garlic in oil until tender.
3. In large bowl, beat egg substitute.
4. Stir in artichokes, onion mixture, mushrooms, cheese, and cracker crumbs.
5. Bake at 350° for 35–40 minutes.

Tip:
You can use ¼ lb. fresh mushrooms, sliced, instead of canned mushrooms in this dish. If you use fresh ones, sauté with onion and garlic in Step 2.

Exchange List Values
- Carbohydrate 1.0   • Fat 0.5
- Lean Meat 2.0

Basic Nutritional Values
- Calories 165
  (Calories from Fat 55)
- Total Fat 6 gm
  (Saturated Fat 1.3 gm,
  Trans Fat 0.0 gm,
  Polyunsat Fat 2.2 gm,
  Monounsat Fat 2.0 gm)
- Cholesterol 5 mg
- Sodium 480 mg
- Potassium 230 gm
- Total Carb 11 gm
- Dietary Fiber 1 gm
- Sugars 2 gm
- Protein 16 gm
- Phosphorus 150 gm

Southwestern Egg Casserole

Eileen Eash
Lafayette, CO

Makes 12 servings, approximately 3"×3" square per serving

Prep. Time: 20–30 minutes
Baking Time: 35–45 minutes
Standing Time: 5–10 minutes

2½ cups egg substitute
½ cup flour
1 tsp. baking powder
⅛ tsp. salt
⅛ tsp. pepper
1½ cups shredded 75%-less-fat sharp cheddar cheese
2 cups fat-free cottage cheese
¼ cup no-trans-fat tub margarine
2 4-oz. cans chopped green chilies

1. Beat egg substitute in a large mixing bowl.
2. In a smaller bowl, combine flour, baking powder, salt, and pepper. Stir into egg substitute. Batter will be lumpy.
3. Add cheeses, butter, and chilies to batter.
4. Pour into greased 9×13 baking dish.
5. Bake at 350° for 35–45 minutes, or until knife inserted near center comes out clean.
6. Let stand 5–10 minutes before cutting.

Tips:
1. This is a great recipe for brunch. I usually put it together the night before and then refrigerate it.
2. To take to a potluck after baking it, I transport it in an insulated carrier which I wrap in an old mattress pad. It stays hot for at least an hour.

Exchange List Values
- Carbohydrate 0.5   • Lean Meat 2.0

Basic Nutritional Values
- Calories 130
  (Calories from Fat 35)
- Total Fat 4 gm
  (Saturated Fat 1.4 gm,
  Trans Fat 0.0 gm,
  Polyunsat Fat 1.2 gm,
  Monounsat Fat 1.2 gm)
- Cholesterol 10 mg
- Sodium 450 mg
- Potassium 180 gm
- Total Carb 9 gm
- Dietary Fiber 1 gm
- Sugars 1 gm
- Protein 14 gm
- Phosphorus 190 gm

Easy Quiche

Becky Bontrager Horst
Goshen, IN

Makes 6 servings, 1 slice per serving
Prep. Time: 15 minutes
Baking Time: 55 minutes

¼ cup chopped onion
¼ cup chopped mushroom, *optional*
1 tsp. canola oil
3 oz. 75%-less-fat cheddar cheese, shredded
2 Tbsp. bacon bits, chopped ham *or* browned sausage
4 eggs
¼ tsp. salt
1½ cups fat-free milk
½ cup whole wheat flour
1 Tbsp. trans-fat-free tub margarine

1. Sauté onion and mushroom in oil. Combine cheese, meat and vegetables in greased 9" pie pan.
2. Combine remaining ingredients in medium bowl. Pour over meat and vegetables mixture.
3. Bake at 350° for 45 minutes. This quiche will make its own crust.

Exchange List Values
• Carbohydrate 1.0   • Lean Meat 2.0

Basic Nutritional Values
• Calories 135   • Sodium 400 mg
  (Calories from Fat 35) • Potassium 255 mg
• Total Fat 4 gm   • Total Carb 12 gm
  (Saturated Fat 1.5 gm, • Dietary Fiber 1 gm
  Trans Fat 0.0 gm,   • Sugars 4 gm
  Polyunsat Fat 0.9 gm, • Protein 13 gm
  Monounsat Fat 1.4 gm) • Phosphorus 170 gm
• Cholesterol 10 mg

Breakfast Pie

Darlene Bloom
San Antonio, TX

Makes 6 servings
Prep. Time: 20 minutes
Baking Time: 30 minutes

8 oz. lower-sodium ham
1 cup chopped onions
1 cup chopped bell pepper, red *or* green
1 cup 75%-less-fat shredded cheddar cheese
½ cup reduced-fat buttermilk baking mix
1 cup fat-free milk
2 eggs

1. Brown meat, onion, and bell pepper in skillet on stove until done. Drain off drippings.
2. Place cooked ingredients in a greased 9" pie plate.
3. Top with layer of shredded cheese.
4. In a mixing bowl, whisk baking mix, milk, and eggs together. Pour over ingredients in pie plate.
5. Bake at 400° for 30 minutes.
6. Allow to stand 5–10 minutes before cutting and serving.

Tips:
1. Double this recipe and prepare in a 9×13 baking pan. I take this to potlucks all the time (warm) out of the oven.
2. You can use ground turkey or beef as your choice of meats and add 1 envelope taco seasoning mix to the skillet as you cook. I call this version Taco Bake and often make it for dinner.

Exchange List Values
• Carbohydrate 1.0   • Lean Meat 2.0

Basic Nutritional Values
• Calories 170   • Sodium 595 mg
  (Calories from Fat 40) • Potassium 295 gm
• Total Fat 4.5 gm   • Total Carb 15 gm
  (Saturated Fat 1.8 gm, • Dietary Fiber 1 gm
  Trans Fat 0.0 gm,   • Sugars 6 gm
  Polyunsat Fat 0.6 gm, • Protein 17 gm
  Monounsat Fat 1.7 gm) • Phosphorus 310 gm
• Cholesterol 85 mg

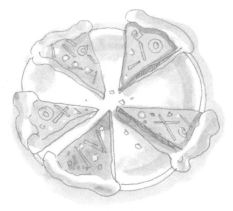

Southwest Brunch Casserole

Janita Mellinger
Abbottstown, PA

Makes 4 servings,
½ an English muffin per serving

Prep. Time: 20–30 minutes
Chilling Time: 3–8 hours
Baking Time: 25 minutes

1 Tbsp. no-trans-fat tub
  margarine
2 English muffins, split
1 oz. cooked reduced-fat
  bulk pork sausage
1 cup egg substitute
¼ cup fat-free sour cream
¼ cup grated 75%-less-fat
  cheddar cheese
¼ cup chopped chilies,
  optional

1. Spread margarine over
cut sides of each muffin half.
Place margarine-side up in
8" square baking pan coated
with non-stick cooking spray.

2. In a small skillet, cook
sausage. Drain off drippings.

3. Spoon sausage over
muffin halves.

4. In a small mixing bowl,
whisk egg substitute and sour
cream together.

5. Pour over sausage.

6. Sprinkle with cheese and
chilies if you wish.

7. Cover and refrigerate 3
hours or overnight.

8. Remove from refrigerator
30 minutes before baking.

9. Bake uncovered at 350°
for 20–25 minutes, or until
knife inserted near center
comes out clean.

Tip:
    This is great for sleep-in
mornings or overnight guests.
You can avoid the morning
rush.

Exchange List Values
- Starch 1.0   • Fat 0.5
- Lean Meat 1.0

Basic Nutritional Values
- Calories 160
  (Calories from Fat 40)
- Total Fat 4.5 gm
  (Saturated Fat 1.5 gm,
  Trans Fat 0.0 gm,
  Polyunsat Fat 1.2 gm,
  Monounsat Fat 1.5 gm)
- Cholesterol 10 mg
- Sodium 365 mg
- Potassium 170 gm
- Total Carb 16 gm
- Dietary Fiber 1 gm
- Sugars 2 gm
- Protein 13 gm
- Phosphorus 95 gm

Potato-Bacon Gratin

Valerie Drobel
Carlisle, PA

Makes 8 servings,
about 5 oz. per serving

Prep. Time: 15 minutes
Baking Time: 1 hour

6-oz. bag fresh spinach
1 clove garlic, minced
1 Tbsp. olive oil
4 large potatoes, peeled or
  unpeeled, *divided*
6-oz. Canadian bacon
  slices, *divided*
5-oz. reduced-fat grated
  Swiss cheddar, *divided*
1 cup lower-sodium, lower-
  fat chicken broth

1. In large skillet, sauté
spinach and garlic in olive oil
just until spinach is wilted.

2. Cut potatoes into thin
slices.

3. In 2-quart baking dish,
layer ⅓ the potatoes, half the
bacon, ⅓ the cheese, and half
the wilted spinach.

4. Repeat layers ending
with potatoes. Reserve ⅓
cheese for later.

5. Pour chicken broth over
all.

6. Cover and bake at 350°
for 45 minutes.

7. Uncover and bake 15
more minutes. During last 5
minutes, top with cheese.

8. Allow to stand 10
minutes before serving.

Tip:
    Leftovers are delicious.
Make two of these Bakes at a
time and freeze one.

Good Go-Alongs:
    Baked apples or applesauce

Exchange List Values
- Carbohydrate 2.0   • Lean Meat 2.0

Basic Nutritional Values
- Calories 220
  (Calories from Fat 65)
- Total Fat 7 gm
  (Saturated Fat 2.4 gm,
  Trans Fat 0.0 gm,
  Polyunsat Fat 0.5 gm,
  Monounsat Fat 2.7 gm)
- Cholesterol 25 mg
- Sodium 415 mg
- Potassium 710 gm
- Total Carb 28 gm
- Dietary Fiber 3 gm
- Sugars 2 gm
- Protein 14 gm
- Phosphorus 285 gm

Shredded Potato Omelet

Mary H. Nolt
East Earl, PA

Makes 6 servings

Prep. Time: 15 minutes
Cooking Time: 20 minutes

3 slices bacon
cooking spray
2 cups shredded cooked
  potatoes
¼ cup minced onion
¼ cup minced green bell
  pepper
1 cup egg substitute
¼ cup fat-free milk
¼ tsp. salt
⅛ tsp. black pepper
1 cup 75%-less-fat
  shredded cheddar cheese

1. In large skillet, fry bacon until crisp. Remove bacon and crumble. Wipe skillet, and spray lightly with cooking spray.
2. Mix potatoes, onion, and green peppers in bowl. Spoon into skillet. Cook over low heat—without stirring—until underside is crisp and brown.
3. Blend egg substitute, milk, salt, and pepper in mixing bowl. Pour over potato mixture.
4. Top with cheese and bacon.
5. Cover. Cook over low heat approximately 10 minutes, or until set. Loosen omelet and serve.

Warm Memories:
The first time I remember eating this Omelet was when we were helping to pick raspberries before breakfast at our son's place in New York. We were so hungry when we went to the house, and our daughter-in-law served this omelet. I have made it a lot since, often serving it to overnight guests for breakfast.

Exchange List Values
- Starch 1.0
- Lean Meat 1.0

Basic Nutritional Values
- Calories 130
  (Calories from Fat 25)
- Total Fat 3 gm
  (Saturated Fat 1.4 gm,
  Trans Fat 0.0 gm,
  Polyunsat Fat 0.2 gm,
  Monounsat Fat 0.9 gm)
- Cholesterol 10 mg
- Sodium 415 mg
- Potassium 280 gm
- Total Carb 13 gm
- Dietary Fiber 2 gm
- Sugars 2 gm
- Protein 12 gm
- Phosphorus 150 gm

Grits New-Mexico Style

Karen Bryant
Corrales, NM

Makes 24 servings

Prep. Time: 20 minutes
Baking Time: 1 hour and 20 minutes

6 cups boiling water
1½ cups uncooked grits
¼ cup no trans-fat tub
  margarine, at room
  temperature
4-oz. can chopped green
  chilies, drained
1 lb. 75%-less-fat shredded
  cheddar cheese
3 eggs, separated
2 tsp. salt
dash of Tabasco sauce
¼ tsp. garlic powder

1. Cook grits in large pan according to package directions until thick.
2. Stir in margarine cut into chunks, chilies, cheese, beaten egg yolks, salt, Tabasco sauce, and garlic powder. Continue stirring until margarine is completely melted.
3. Beat egg whites until soft peaks form. Fold into hot ingredients.
4. Pour into well-greased 4-quart baking dish.
5. Bake at 350° for 1 hour and 20 minutes.

Tip:
This dish is like a soufflé and makes a great brunch or light supper dish.

Exchange List Values
- Starch 0.5
- Lean Meat 1.0
- Fat 0.5

Basic Nutritional Values
- Calories 100
  (Calories from Fat 35)
- Total Fat 4 gm
  (Saturated Fat 1.5 gm,
  Trans Fat 0.0 gm,
  Polyunsat Fat 0.8 gm,
  Monounsat Fat 1.0 gm)
- Cholesterol 30 mg
- Sodium 360 mg
- Potassium 50 gm
- Total Carb 9 gm
- Dietary Fiber 0 gm
- Sugars 0 gm
- Protein 8 gm
- Phosphorus 110 gm

Brunch Delight

Jean Butzer
Batavia, NY

Makes 12 servings,
3" square per serving

Prep. Time: 15 minutes
Baking Time: 35–45 minutes

½ cup chopped onion
½ cup chopped green bell
   pepper
4 eggs
2 cups egg substitute
1 cup milk
½ lb. extra-lean 95%-fat-
   free cooked ham, cut
   into small cubes
16 oz. frozen shredded
   hash brown potatoes,
   thawed
1 cup shredded 75%-less-
   fat cheddar cheese
¼ tsp. salt
½ tsp. pepper
½ tsp. dill weed

1. Sauté onion and green
pepper in small nonstick
skillet. Or cook just until soft
in microwave.
2. In large bowl whisk
together eggs, egg substitute,
and milk.
3. Stir in cooked vegetables,
ham, potatoes, cheese, salt,
pepper, and dill weed.
4. Spoon into well-greased
9×13 baking pan.
5. Bake at 350° for 35–45
minutes, or until knife blade
inserted in center comes out
clean.
6. Allow to stand 10
minutes before cutting into
squares to serve.

Variation:
   Add ½ cup diced green
chilies to Step 3.
       Mamie Christopherson
           Rio Rancho, NM

Tips:
   1. This is a flexible recipe,
so vary the ingredients as
you wish. For example, you
can use ½ lb. cooked bacon
or sausage, turkey ham, or no
meat.
   2. Frozen cubed potatoes
work well, too. Or you can
make your own from-scratch
potatoes, cooking, cooling,
and cubing them.
   3. When we make this
for a breakfast at church,
we prepare all the pans
the afternoon before, and
then cover and refrigerate
them until the morning of
the event. We remove the
pans from the refrigerator
and let them stand at room
temperature for 30 minutes
before baking, or we bake the
dish 15–20 minutes longer
than called for.

Exchange List Values
- Starch 0.5   • Lean Meat 2.0

Basic Nutritional Values
- Calories 135   • Sodium 460 mg
  (Calories from Fat 30) • Potassium 335 gm
- Total Fat 4 gm   • Total Carb 10 gm
  (Saturated Fat 1.4 gm, • Dietary Fiber 1 gm
  Trans Fat 0.0 gm,   • Sugars 2 gm
  Polyunsat Fat 0.5 gm,   • Protein 15 gm
  Monounsat Fat 1.3 gm)   • Phosphorus 160 gm
- Cholesterol 75 mg

Brunch Enchiladas

Ann Good
Perry, NY

Makes 16 servings,
1 filled tortilla per serving

Prep. Time: 20–35 minutes
Chilling Time: 8 hours, or
overnight
Baking Time: 45–60 minutes

¾ cup chopped onion
¾ cup chopped bell
   peppers
1 Tbsp. canola oil
2 cups extra-lean chopped
   cooked ham
8-oz. container fat-free
   sour cream, *divided*

8 eggs
2 cups egg substitute
1½ cups fat-free milk
2 Tbsp. flour
½ tsp. pepper
16 6" flour tortillas
1½ cups shredded
   75%-less-fat cheese,
   divided
3 medium tomatoes, sliced

1. In saucepan, sauté peppers
and onion in oil until soft.
2. Stir in meat and cook
until heated through.
3. Spread 1 Tbsp. of sour
cream in a strip through the
center of each tortilla.
4. Spoon 2 Tbsp. meat
mixture on top of sour cream
on each tortilla.
5. Top with 1½ Tbsp.
cheese on each tortilla.
(Reserve 1 cup cheese for
topping enchiladas after
baking.)

6. Roll up and place seams down in two well-greased 9×13 baking pans.

7. In a large mixing bowl, beat together egg substitute, eggs, milk, flour, salt, and pepper.

8. Pour over tortillas. Cover and refrigerate overnight.

9. Remove from refrigerator for 30 minutes before baking.

10. Bake uncovered at 350° for 45–60 minutes, or until heated through.

11. Remove from oven. Top with tomato slices.

12. Let stand 5–10 minutes before serving.

Tips:

1. Serve with salsa and sour cream.

2. This dish freezes well.

Exchange List Values
- Starch 1.0
- Lean Meat 2.0
- Carbohydrate 0.5
- Fat 0.5

Basic Nutritional Values
- Calories 230
  (Calories from Fat 70)
- Total Fat 8 gm
  (Saturated Fat 2.4 gm,
  Trans Fat 0.0 gm,
  Polyunsat Fat 1.3 gm,
  Monounsat Fat 3.3 gm)
- Cholesterol 110 mg
- Sodium 595 mg
- Potassium 330 gm
- Total Carb 23 gm
- Dietary Fiber 2 gm
- Sugars 4 gm
- Protein 17 gm
- Phosphorus 225 gm

Brunch Pizza
Rachel King
Castile, NY

*Makes 8 servings,
3¼"×4½" rectangle per serving*

Prep. Time: 1 hour
Baking Time: 15–18 minutes

8-oz. pkg. reduced-fat crescent rolls
2 Tbsp. chopped bacon
½ lb. fresh mushrooms, sliced
1 small onion, finely chopped
1 small green bell pepper, finely chopped
1 Tbsp. canola oil, *divided*
2 cups egg substitute
3 oz. fat-free cream cheese, softened to room temperature
⅓ cup fat-free sour cream
1 garlic clove, minced
¼ tsp. Italian seasoning
2 plum tomatoes, sliced thin
¾ cup shredded 75%-reduced fat cheddar cheese
salsa and additional sour cream, *optional*

1. Open crescent dough tube and unroll. Press crescent dough over bottom and partway up sides of 9×13 baking pan.

2. Bake at 375° for 6–8 minutes.

3. Meanwhile, cook bacon in large skillet until crispy. Remove bacon and allow to drain on a paper towel.

4. Sauté mushrooms, onions, and peppers in ½ Tbsp. oil until just tender.

5. Remove vegetables from pan and set aside.

6. Heat other ½ Tbsp. oil in skillet. Add egg substitute and cook, stirring until almost set.

7. In a mixing bowl, beat together cream cheese, sour cream, garlic, and Italian seasoning. Spread over crescent-dough crust in baking pan.

8. Top with egg mixture, and then meat, and then sautéed vegetables.

9. Top with tomato slices and then cheese.

10. Bake at 375° for 15–18 minutes, or until cheese is melted.

11. Serve with salsa and additional sour cream for each person to add as they wish.

Exchange List Values
- Starch 1.0
- Lean Meat 2.0
- Vegetable 1.0
- Fat 0.5

Basic Nutritional Values
- Calories 200
  (Calories from Fat 70)
- Total Fat 8 gm
  (Saturated Fat 2.5 gm,
  Trans Fat 0.0 gm,
  Polyunsat Fat 1.6 gm,
  Monounsat Fat 1.9 gm)
- Cholesterol 5 mg
- Sodium 555 mg
- Potassium 380 gm
- Total Carb 19 gm
- Dietary Fiber 1 gm
- Sugars 6 gm
- Protein 15 gm
- Phosphorus 270 gm

Because of the Sunday morning hassle, I have simplified my own preparations for potluck meals by taking plain, raw vegetables and fruits which children enjoy but will not eat if they are concealed in a fruit salad or other concoction.

Melodie Davis, Harrisonburg, VA

Country Breakfast Pizza

Zoë Rohrer
Lancaster, PA

Makes 10 servings

Prep. Time: 25–30 minutes
Baking Time: 27 minutes

1½ Tbsp. olive oil
1 cup whole wheat pastry
   flour
⅔ cup, plus 2 Tbsp., all-
   purpose flour
1 Tbsp. flax meal, *optional*
2 tsp. baking powder
½ tsp. salt
¼ cup real maple syrup
scant ½ cup fat-free milk
half a green pepper, diced
¼ lb. lower-fat bulk pork
   sausage
2¼ cups egg substitute
1 cup shredded
   75%-reduced-fat cheddar
   cheese, *divided*

maple syrup, *or* ketchup,
   for serving

1. Place oil in a 9×13
baking dish.
2. In a good-sized bowl,
mix together flours, flax if
you wish, baking powder, and
salt.
3. Add maple syrup and
milk. Stir to combine.
4. Knead a few minutes
in bowl, or on countertop, to
make a ball.
5. Press dough into oiled
pan.
6. Bake 12 minutes at 425°.
Remove from the oven.

7. While crust is baking,
brown sausage and peppers
in skillet until pink is gone
from meat and peppers are
just tender. Stir frequently to
break up meat. Place cooked
meat and peppers on platter
and keep warm. Discard
drippings.
8. Beat egg substitute
in mixing bowl. Pour into
skillet used for sausage. Stir
frequently. Add ⅔ cup cheese
while eggs are cooking.
9. When crust is done, top
with sausage, then eggs, and
then remaining cheese.
10. Bake 10 more minutes
or until cheese is melted.
11. Serve immediately with
maple syrup or ketchup.

Exchange List Values

- Starch 1.0   • Lean Meat 2.0
- Carbohydrate 0.5

Basic Nutritional Values

- Calories 200   • Sodium 435 mg
  (Calories from Fat 45)   • Potassium 225 gm
- Total Fat 5 gm   • Total Carb 25 gm
  (Saturated Fat 1.5 gm, • Dietary Fiber 2 gm
  Trans Fat 0.0 gm,   • Sugars 6 gm
  Polyunsat Fat 0.6 gm, • Protein 13 gm
  Monounsat Fat 2.5 gm) • Phosphorus 235 gm
- Cholesterol 10 mg

Bacon Cheese Squares

Katie Ebersol
Ronks, PA

Makes 12 servings,
3" square per serving

Prep. Time: 30 minutes
Baking Time: 18–20 minutes

2 cups reduced-fat
   buttermilk baking mix
½ cup cold water
4 oz. 75%-reduced-fat
   cheese, sliced
½ lb. 50–70% reduced-fat
   turkey bacon, sliced,
   cooked crisp, and
   crumbled
3 eggs
¾ cup egg substitute
½ cup fat-free milk
½ tsp. onion powder

1. In a bowl, combine the
baking mix and water. Stir 20
strokes.
2. Turn onto a floured
surface. Knead 10 times.
3. Roll into a 10×14
rectangle. Fold into quarters
(without pressing down on the
folds) and place on the bottom
and half-way up the sides of a
greased 9×13 baking dish.
4. Lay cheese evenly over
dough. Sprinkle with bacon.
5. In the mixing bowl, beat
together egg substitute, eggs,
milk, and onion powder.
6. Pour egg-milk mixture
over bacon.
7. Bake at 425° for 18–20
minutes, or until a knife
blade inserted in center

comes out clean. If it doesn't, continue baking another 4 minutes. Test again. Continue baking if needed, or remove from oven.

8. Allow to stand 10 minutes before cutting into squares and serving.

Exchange List Values

- Starch 1.0
- Fat 0.5
- Lean Meat 1.0

Basic Nutritional Values

- Calories 140
  (Calories from Fat 45)
- Total Fat 5 gm
  (Saturated Fat 1.5 gm,
  Trans Fat 0.0 gm,
  Polyunsat Fat 0.9 gm,
  Monounsat Fat 2.0 gm)
- Cholesterol 60 mg
- Sodium 440 mg
- Potassium 110 gm
- Total Carb 15 gm
- Dietary Fiber 1 gm
- Sugars 2 gm
- Protein 9 gm
- Phosphorus 215 gm

Sausage and Eggs Baked in Mugs

Peggy C. Forsythe
Memphis, TN

Makes 10 servings

Prep. Time: 30 minutes
Baking Time: 25–30 minutes for mugs & ramekins; 1 hour for 9×13 baking dish

12 oz. sourdough bread, sliced and cut into ½" cubes
6 oz. 50%-reduced-fat pork bulk sausage
2½ cups fat-free milk
4 large eggs
1 Tbsp. Dijon mustard
½ cup fat-free buttermilk
10¾-oz. can cream of mushroom soup

¾ cup shredded 75%-less-fat sharp cheddar cheese

1. Spray insides of 10 oven-proof coffee mugs with non-stick cooking spray.
2. Divide bread cubes evenly among mugs.
3. Brown bulk sausage in skillet, breaking up with wooden spoon and stirring until all pink is gone. Drain off drippings.
4. Top bread cubes in each mug with crumbled sausage.
5. In a mixing bowl, whisk together milk, eggs, and Dijon mustard. Pour evenly over bread and sausage.
6. In same bowl, whisk together buttermilk and cream of mushroom soup. Spoon over bread mixture.
7. Sprinkle each mug with cheddar cheese.
8. Place coffee mugs on baking sheet.
9. Bake at 350° for 25–30 minutes, or until individual casseroles are set and puffed. Serve immediately.

Tips:
1. You can prepare the mugs through Step 7 in advance of serving. Cover mugs with plastic wrap and then foil. Freeze up to one month. When ready to use, thaw overnight in refrigerator. Bake as directed.
2. You may omit the mugs and use ramekins. Or use a 9×13 baking dish instead, and then increase baking time to 1 hour, or until casserole is set. Insert a knife blade in center of baking dish. If blade comes out clean, the dish is

done. If it doesn't, continue baking another 5 minutes. Test again. Repeat if needed.

3. To make the dish spicier, add Tabasco to milk/egg/mustard mixture in Step 5. Or use hot sausage.
4. If you don't have buttermilk, make your own substitute. Mix 1 Tbsp. white vinegar and ⅞ cup milk. Let sit 15 minutes; do not stir.

Exchange List Values

- Starch 1.0
- Lean Meat 2.0
- Carbohydrate 0.5
- Fat 0.5

Basic Nutritional Values

- Calories 225
  (Calories from Fat 55)
- Total Fat 6 gm
  (Saturated Fat 2.3 gm,
  Trans Fat 0.0 gm,
  Polyunsat Fat 1.3 gm,
  Monounsat Fat 2.4 gm)
- Cholesterol 90 mg
- Sodium 525 mg
- Potassium 435 gm
- Total Carb 26 gm
- Dietary Fiber 1 gm
- Sugars 5 gm
- Protein 15 gm
- Phosphorus 225 gm

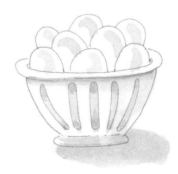

Blueberry French Toast

Stacie Skelly
Millersville, PA

Makes 12 servings

***Prep. Time:** 30 minutes*
***Chilling Time:** 6–8 hours or
overnight*
***Baking Time:** 1 hour*

12 slices day-old bread
4 oz. cream cheese
4 oz. Neufchatel (⅓-less-fat)
cream cheese
1 cup frozen blueberries
6 eggs
1½ cups egg substitute
2 cups fat-free milk
⅓ cup honey

Sauce:
¼ cup Splenda Blend for
Baking
2 Tbsp. cornstarch
1 cup water
1 cup blueberries

1. Grease 9×13 baking pan.
2. Cube bread and spread
in pan.

3. Cube cream cheese.
Distribute evenly over bread.
4. Sprinkle blueberries on
top.
5. In a mixing bowl, blend
eggs, egg substitute, milk, and
honey.
6. Pour over baking-pan
contents.
7. Cover. Refrigerate 6–8
hours, or overnight.
8. Remove from refrigerator
30 minutes before baking.
9. Bake, covered, at 350°
for 30 minutes.
10. Uncover. Bake 30 more
minutes. Serve with sauce.

To make Sauce:
1. Mix Splenda, cornstarch,
and water in a saucepan.
Bring to a boil.
2. Stir in blueberries.
3. Reduce heat, cooking
until blueberries burst.
4. Serve warm over French
Toast.

Warm Memories:
Every summer 5 good
friends and I have "Breakfast
Club" each Wednesday
morning. When it's my turn
to host, this is always at the
top of the request list.

Exchange List Values
- Starch 1.0   • Lean Meat 1.0
- Carbohydrate 1.0 • Fat 0.5

Basic Nutritional Values
- Calories 225   • Sodium 380 mg
  (Calories from Fat 55) • Potassium 230 gm
- Total Fat 6 gm   • Total Carb 32 gm
  (Saturated Fat 2.2 gm, • Dietary Fiber 1 gm
  Trans Fat 0.0 gm,   • Sugars 18 gm
  Polyunsat Fat 1.0 gm, • Protein 12 gm
  Monounsat Fat 1.7 gm) • Phosphorus 185 gm
- Cholesterol 100 mg

Fast, Friendly French Toast

Donna Barnitz
Rio Rancho, NM

Makes 8 servings

***Prep. Time:** 15 minutes*
***Soaking Time:** 1–24 hours*
***Baking Time:** 15 minutes*

1 lb. loaf French bread, cut
1" thick slices
1½ cups fat-free milk
4 eggs
½ cup orange juice
¼ cup sugar
1 Tbsp. vanilla
cinnamon, *optional*

1. Arrange bread slices in a
9×13 baking pan.
2. In a mixing bowl, beat
milk, eggs, orange juice,
sugar, and vanilla together
until well blended.
3. Pour over bread.
4. Cover and refrigerate
1–24 hours, according to your
schedule and how much time
you have.

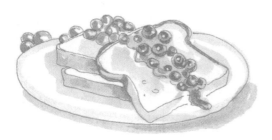

5. Heat oven to 400°. Grease jelly-roll pan.

6. Transfer bread to pan, making sure slices don't touch. Dust with cinnamon, if you wish.

7. Bake 15 minutes, or until puffy and lightly browned.

Exchange List Values

- Starch 2.0
- Lean Meat 1.0
- Carbohydrate 1.0

Basic Nutritional Values

- Calories 250
  (Calories from Fat 30)
- Total Fat 4 gm
  (Saturated Fat 1.1 gm,
  Trans Fat 0.0 gm,
  Polyunsat Fat 0.9 gm,
  Monounsat Fat 1.1 gm)
- Cholesterol 95 mg
- Sodium 345 mg
- Potassium 210 gm
- Total Carb 43 gm
- Dietary Fiber 1 gm
- Sugars 12 gm
- Protein 11 gm
- Phosphorus 165 gm

Baked French Toast with Cream Cheese

Blanche Nyce
Hatfield, PA

Makes 10 servings

Prep. Time: 15–20 minutes
Cooking/Baking Time: 40–45 minutes

1-lb. loaf firm bread, *divided*
8-oz. pkg. fat-free cream cheese
10 eggs
½ cup fat-free half-and-half
¼ cup maple syrup, *or* **pancake syrup**
¼ cup tub margarine, no trans-fat
2 cup berries of your choice—strawberries, blueberries, *or* **raspberries**

1. Cube bread and layer half in well-greased 9×13 baking pan.

2. Cut cream cheese into small pieces and scatter across bread.

3. Sprinkle with berries.

4. Cover berries with remaining half of bread.

5. In mixing bowl, beat together eggs, half-and-half, syrup, and melted butter.

6. Pour over bread contents of baking pan.

7. Press down until bread is submerged as much as possible.

8. Cover and refrigerate for 8 hours, or overnight.

9. Bake uncovered at 375° for 40–45 minutes, or until lightly browned and puffy.

Tip:
Day-old bread works best for this toast.

Exchange List Values

- Starch 1.5
- Lean Meat 2.0
- Carbohydrate 0.5
- Fat 0.5

Basic Nutritional Values

- Calories 270
  (Calories from Fat 70)
- Total Fat 8 gm
  (Saturated Fat 2.4 gm,
  Trans Fat 0.0 gm,
  Polyunsat Fat 2.4 gm,
  Monounsat Fat 3.0 gm)
- Cholesterol 190 mg
- Sodium 485 mg
- Potassium 245 gm
- Total Carb 33 gm
- Dietary Fiber 1 gm
- Sugars 9 gm
- Protein 13 gm
- Phosphorus 285 gm

Choose whole grains — barley, bulgur, quinoa, and whole-wheat couscous — as healthier alternatives to traditional starches such as potatoes, white rice, white bread, grits, and pasta.

Overnight Apple French Toast

Eileen Eash
Lafayette, CO
Peggy C. Forsythe
Memphis, TN

Makes 9 servings,
1 slice per serving

Prep. Time: 40–45 minutes
Soaking Time: 8 hours, or
* overnight*
Baking Time: 35–40 minutes

6 Tbsp. Splenda Brown
  Sugar Blend
3 Tbsp. no trans-fat tub
  margarine
3–4 large tart apples,
  peeled and sliced ¼-inch
  thick
3 eggs
1 cup fat-free milk
1 tsp. vanilla
9 slices day old French
  bread, ¾" thick, about 1
  oz. each

Syrup:
  ½ cup unsweetened
    applesauce
  ¼ tsp. cinnamon
  ¼ cup apple jelly
  ¹⁄₁₆ tsp. ground cloves
  sprinkle of nutmeg,
    optional
  maple syrup for serving,
    optional
  whipped cream, *optional*

1. In a small saucepan,
melt Splenda and margarine
together about 3–4 minutes,
stirring constantly, until
slightly thick.

2. Pour into ungreased
9 × 13 baking pan.
  3. Top with apple slices.
  4. In a medium-sized
mixing bowl, beat together
eggs, milk, and vanilla.
  5. Dip bread slices in egg
mixture, one by one, and then
lay over top of apples.
  6. Cover and refrigerate
overnight.
  7. Remove from refrigerator
30 minutes before baking.
Sprinkle with nutmeg if you
wish.
  8. Bake uncovered at 350°
for 35–40 minutes.
  9. Meanwhile, prepare
syrup by cooking applesauce,
cinnamon, apple jelly, and
ground cloves in small
saucepan until hot.
  10. Serve over toast.
  11. Offer maple syrup and
whipped cream as toppings,
too.

Variation:
  Crab apple jelly, instead
of apple jelly, in the syrup is
also delicious.

Exchange List Values
- Starch 1.0
- Fruit 1.0
- Carbohydrate 1.0
- Fat 1.0

Basic Nutritional Values
- Calories 245
  (Calories from Fat 45)
- Total Fat 5 gm
  (Saturated Fat 1.3 gm,
  Trans Fat 0.0 gm,
  Polyunsat Fat 1.8 gm,
  Monounsat Fat 1.6 gm)
- Cholesterol 65 mg
- Sodium 220 mg
- Potassium 195 gm
- Total Carb 43 gm
- Dietary Fiber 2 gm
- Sugars 19 gm
- Protein 7 gm
- Phosphorus 105 gm

Waffles with Cinnamon Apple Syrup

Betty L. Moore
Plano, IL

Makes 12 5" waffles and
1¾ cups syrup, 1 waffle and
2⅓ Tbsp. syrup per serving

Prep. Time: 15 minutes
Cooking Time: about 3 minutes
* per waffle*

Waffles:
  2 cups flour
  2 Tbsp. sugar
  3 tsp. baking powder
  ½ tsp. salt
  2 eggs
  1½ cups fat-free milk
  4 Tbsp. canola oil

Cinnamon Apple Syrup:
  2 Tbsp. cornstarch
  ½ tsp. cinnamon
  ⅛ tsp. salt
  1 cup water
  ¾ cup unsweetened
    apple juice concentrate
  ½ tsp. vanilla

1. To make waffles, mix
flour, sugar, baking powder,
and salt together in large
bowl.
  2. In a separate bowl, beat
eggs, milk, and oil together.
  3. Add wet ingredients to
dry ingredients. Beat just
until mixed.
  4. Pour scant ½ cup batter
onto hot waffle iron. Cook
according to your waffle
iron's instructions.
  5. To make syrup, combine

cornstarch, cinnamon, and salt in saucepan.

6. Gradually stir in water and apple juice concentrate until smooth.

7. Over medium heat, and stirring continually, bring to boil.

8. Cook, stirring continually, for 2 minutes, or until thickened.

9. Remove from heat. Stir in vanilla.

10. Serve warm over waffles.

Tips:

1. You can refrigerate any leftover syrup, covered, until the next time you make waffles.

2. We have friends over quite frequently for waffles for breakfast. I serve them with sausage, strawberries, assorted syrups, and orange juice. This recipe works in both my regular waffle iron and my Belgian waffle-maker. We sometimes have waffles for supper if we have leftover batter.

Exchange List Values
- Starch 1.0
- Fat 1.0
- Carbohydrate 1.0

Basic Nutritional Values
- Calories 180
  (Calories from Fat 55)
- Total Fat 6 gm
  (Saturated Fat 0.6 gm,
  Trans Fat 0.0 gm,
  Polyunsat Fat 1.6 gm,
  Monounsat Fat 3.3 gm)
- Cholesterol 30 mg
- Sodium 240 mg
- Potassium 145 gm
- Total Carb 28 gm
- Dietary Fiber 1 gm
- Sugars 11 gm
- Protein 4 gm
- Phosphorus 185 gm

Oatmeal Pancakes

Barbara J. Bey
Hillsboro, OH

*Makes 6 servings,
1 pancake per serving*

Prep. Time: 5 minutes
Cooking Time: 10 minutes

½ cup flour
½ cup dry oats, rolled *or* quick-cooking
1 Tbsp. Splenda
1 tsp. baking powder
½ tsp. baking soda
¾ cup fat-free buttermilk
¼ cup fat-free milk
2 Tbsp. canola oil
1 egg, beaten

1. Stir together flour, oats, Splenda, baking powder, and baking soda in a large mixing bowl.

2. In a separate bowl, blend buttermilk, milk, oil, and egg until smooth.

3. Stir wet ingredients into dry ingredients, just until moistened.

4. Drop by scant half-cupfuls into skillet or onto griddle.

5. Cook until small bubbles form on top.

6. Flip and cook until lightly browned.

Exchange List Values
- Starch 1.0
- Fat 1.0

Basic Nutritional Values
- Calories 140
  (Calories from Fat 55)
- Total Fat 6 gm
  (Saturated Fat 0.7 gm,
  Trans Fat 0.0 gm,
  Polyunsat Fat 1.7 gm,
  Monounsat Fat 3.4 gm)
- Cholesterol 30 mg
- Sodium 215 mg
- Potassium 110 gm
- Total Carb 17 gm
- Dietary Fiber 1 gm
- Sugars 4 gm
- Protein 4 gm
- Phosphorus 170 gm

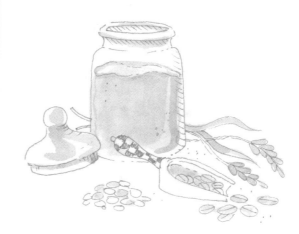

Baked Oatmeal

Esther Porter
Minneapolis, MN

*Makes 12 servings,
3" square per serving*

**Prep. Time: 10 minutes
Cooking/Baking Time: 20–25
minutes**

3 Tbsp. Splenda Brown
  Sugar Blend
2 Tbsp. tub margarine, no
  trans-fat, melted
2 eggs, slightly beaten
3 cups quick oatmeal
2 tsp. baking powder
1 cup fat-free milk
1 tsp. salt
½ cup raisins *or* dried
  cranberries

1. Combine brown sugar
blend, margarine, and eggs
in mixing bowl.
2. Mix and add
oatmeal, baking powder,
milk, and salt. Stir in
raisins or cranberries.
3. Pour into 9×13
baking pan.
4. Bake at
350° for 20–25
minutes.

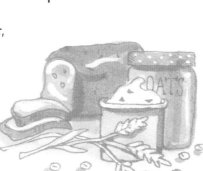

Try to use healthy oils instead of solid fats when cooking: scramble an egg in olive oil instead of margarine.

Tips:
Serve with hot milk,
cinnamon, baked apple slices,
etc. You may cut leftover
baked oatmeal in pieces to
freeze and microwave for
later. Great for brunch.

Exchange List Values
• Starch 1.0   • Fat 0.5
• Fruit 0.5

Basic Nutritional Values
• Calories 140
  (Calories from Fat 30)
• Total Fat 4 gm
  (Saturated Fat 0.8 gm,
  Trans Fat 0.0 gm,
  Polyunsat Fat 1.2 gm,
  Monounsat Fat 1.2 gm)
• Cholesterol 30 mg
• Sodium 290 mg
• Potassium 165 gm
• Total Carb 23 gm
• Dietary Fiber 2 gm
• Sugars 6 gm
• Protein 5 gm
• Phosphorus 205 gm

B&B Blueberry Coffee Cake

Kim Rapp
Longmont, CO

*Makes 18 servings,
2"×3" rectangle per serving*

**Prep. Time: 15–20 minutes
Baking Time: 55–65 minutes**

4 cups flour
¾ cup Splenda Blend for
  Baking
5 tsp. baking powder
1 tsp. salt
6 Tbsp. tub margarine,
  no trans-fat
1½ cups fat-free milk
2 eggs
4 cups fresh, *or* frozen,
  blueberries

Topping:
  2 Tbsp. Splenda Blend
    for Baking
  ⅔ cup flour
  1 tsp. cinnamon
  ½ tsp. nutmeg
  6 Tbsp. tub margarine,
    no trans-fat

1. In an electric-mixer
bowl, mix together flour,
sweetener, baking powder,
salt, margarine, milk, and
eggs. Using mixer, beat
vigorously for 30 seconds.
2. If using frozen blueberries, place in large bowl and
stir in 3 Tbsp. flour until each
blueberry is well coated. (If
using fresh berries, no need
to add flour.)
3. Carefully fold blueberries into batter.

4. Pour into lightly greased 9×13 baking pan.

5. For topping, combine sweetener, flour, cinnamon, and nutmeg in a bowl.

6. Using a pastry cutter, or two forks, cut in margarine until small crumbs form.

7. Sprinkle crumbs evenly over batter.

8. Bake at 350° for 55–65 minutes, or until toothpick inserted in center of cake comes out clean.

Exchange List Values

- Starch 1.5
- Fat 1.0
- Carbohydrate 1.0

Basic Nutritional Values

- Calories 240
  (Calories from Fat 55)
- Total Fat 6 gm
  (Saturated Fat 1.5 gm,
  Trans Fat 0.0 gm,
  Polyunsat Fat 2.6 gm,
  Monounsat Fat 2.1 gm)
- Cholesterol 20 mg
- Sodium 305 mg
- Potassium 105 gm
- Total Carb 40 gm
- Dietary Fiber 2 gm
- Sugars 14 gm
- Protein 5 gm
- Phosphorus 200 gm

Finnish Coffee Cake

Sharon Shank
Bridgewater, VA
Martha Ann Auker
Landisburg, PA

Makes 24 servings,
2" square bar per serving

Prep. Time: 10–20 minutes
Baking Time: 30–35 minutes

10 Tbsp. Splenda Blend for Baking
1 cup canola oil
2 eggs, beaten
1 cup fat-free buttermilk
1 tsp. vanilla
2 cups flour
¾ tsp. baking powder
½ tsp. salt
½ tsp. baking soda
2 Tbsp. Splenda Brown Sugar Blend
1–3 tsp. cinnamon, according to your taste preference

Glaze, *optional*
  2 cups confectioners sugar, *optional*
  1–2 tsp. vanilla, according to your taste preference, *optional*
  1–2 Tbsp. hot water, or a bit more, *optional*

1. In good-sized mixing bowl, beat together sugar, oil, eggs, buttermilk, and 1 tsp. vanilla.

2. In a separate bowl, sift together flour, baking powder, salt, and baking soda.

3. Stir dry ingredients into buttermilk mixture.

4. Pour half of batter into greased 9×13 baking dish.

5. Mix together brown sugar and cinnamon in bowl. Sprinkle half of mixture over batter.

6. Repeat layers.

7. Bake at 350° for 30–35 minutes, or until toothpick inserted in center comes out clean.

8. If you're using glaze, poke holes in cake with fork while cake is still warm. In a medium-sized bowl, mix together confectioners sugar, vanilla, and just enough water to make a thin glaze. Drizzle glaze over cake while still warm.

Variation:

Add ¾ cup chopped walnuts to brown sugar-cinnamon mixture in Step 5.
Carrie Darby
Moreno Valley, CA

Exchange List Values

- Starch 0.5
- Fat 2.0
- Carbohydrate 0.5

Basic Nutritional Values

- Calories 155
  (Calories from Fat 90)
- Total Fat 10 gm
  (Saturated Fat 0.8 gm,
  Trans Fat 0.0 gm,
  Polyunsat Fat 2.7 gm,
  Monounsat Fat 5.9 gm)
- Cholesterol 15 mg
- Sodium 105 mg
- Potassium 35 gm
- Total Carb 15 gm
- Dietary Fiber 0 gm
- Sugars 6 gm
- Protein 2 gm
- Phosphorus 45 gm

Healthy Blueberry Muffins

Gloria Lehman
Singers Glen, VA

*Makes 18 servings,
1 muffin per serving*

Prep. Time: 20 minutes
Baking Time: 20 minutes

1 cup flour
½ cup whole wheat flour
6 Tbsp. Splenda Blend for
   Baking
¼ cup oat bran
¼ cup wheat germ
¼ cup quick, *or* old-
   fashioned, oats
1 tsp. baking powder
1 tsp. baking soda
½ tsp. cinnamon
¼ tsp. nutmeg
¼ tsp. allspice
¼ tsp. salt
1 cup blueberries, fresh
   or frozen and partially
   thawed
½ cup chopped walnuts
1 banana, mashed
1 cup buttermilk
1 egg
1 Tbsp. vegetable oil
1 tsp. vanilla

1. In large bowl, stir together all dry ingredients (through salt) until well blended.

2. Gently stir in blueberries and walnuts. (Adding the blueberries to dry ingredients first helps to prevent turning the batter blue from any juice.)

3. In a separate container, mix together mashed banana, buttermilk, egg, oil, and vanilla.

4. Make a well in dry ingredients. Pour wet ingredients into well. Mix just until blended.

5. Fill greased muffin cups almost to the top.

6. Bake at 350° for approximately 20 minutes, or until toothpick inserted in centers of muffins comes out clean.

Tip:

This moist muffin is made better and healthier by using a banana instead of more oil.

Exchange List Values
• Carbohydrate 1.0 • Fat 1.0

Basic Nutritional Values
• Calories 115 • Sodium 140 mg
  (Calories from Fat 30) • Potassium 120 gm
• Total Fat 4 gm • Total Carb 18 gm
  (Saturated Fat 0.4 gm, • Dietary Fiber 2 gm
  Trans Fat 0.0 gm, • Sugars 7 gm
  Polyunsat Fat 2.1 gm, • Protein 3 gm
  Monounsat Fat 1.0 gm) • Phosphorus 110 gm
• Cholesterol 10 mg

All-Bran Date Muffins

Mrs. Lewis L. Beachy
Sarasota, FL

*Makes 16 servings,
1 muffin per serving*

Prep. Time: 20 minutes
Standing Time: 20 minutes
Baking Time: 20–25 minutes

1 cup chopped dates
1 cup chopped nuts
1 tsp. baking soda
1 Tbsp. vegetable
   shortening
1 cup boiling water
¾ cup brown sugar
1 egg, well beaten
1 cup flour
1 cup All-Bran
1 tsp. baking powder

1. Combine dates, nuts, baking soda and shortening. Pour boiling water over mixture and let cool.

2. Add sugar, egg, flour, All-Bran and baking powder. Fold together until blended. Do not use mixer.

3. Spoon batter into well-greased muffin tins.

4. Bake at 350° for 20–25 minutes.

Exchange List Values
• Carbohydrate 1.5 • Fat 1.0

Basic Nutritional Values
• Calories 150 • Sodium 120 mg
  (Calories from Fat 55) • Potassium 160 gm
• Total Fat 6 gm • Total Carb 24 gm
  (Saturated Fat 0.8 gm, • Dietary Fiber 3 gm
  Trans Fat 0.0 gm, • Sugars 14 gm
  Polyunsat Fat 4.0 gm, • Protein 3 gm
  Monounsat Fat 1.1 gm) • Phosphorus 120 gm
• Cholesterol 10 mg

Strawberry Muffins

Janessa Hochstedler
East Earl, PA

*Makes 14 muffins,
1 muffin per serving*

Prep. Time: 10–15 minutes
Standing Time: 30 minutes
Baking Time: 10–12 minutes

1½ cups mashed
  strawberries
6 Tbsp. Splenda Blend for
  Baking, *divided*
1¾ cups flour
¼ tsp. nutmeg
¼ tsp. salt
½ tsp. baking soda
2 eggs, beaten
¼ cup tub margarine, no
  trans-fat
1 tsp. vanilla

1. In a small mixing bowl, combine strawberries and 2 Tbsp. sweetener. Set aside for 30 minutes. Drain strawberries, reserving liquid.

2. In a large mixing bowl, combine flour, nutmeg, salt, and baking soda. Set aside.

3. In yet another bowl, mix together eggs, melted margarine, vanilla, 4 Tbsp. sweetener, and juice from berries.

4. Add to flour mixture, stirring just until combined.

5. Fold in berries.

6. Spoon batter into greased muffin tins.

7. Bake at 425° for 10–12 minutes, or until toothpick inserted in centers of muffins comes out clean.

Zucchini Oatmeal Muffins

Donna Lantgen
Arvada, CO

*Makes 30 muffins,
1 muffin per serving*

Prep. Time: 15 minutes
Baking Time: 20–25 minutes

2½ cups flour
¾ cup Splenda Blend for
  Baking
½ cup dry oatmeal, quick
  or old-fashioned
1 Tbsp. baking powder
1 tsp. salt
1 tsp. cinnamon
1 cup chopped walnuts
4 eggs
10 oz. zucchini (1¼ cups
  shredded), peeled *or*
  unpeeled
¾ cup canola oil

1. Mix flour, sweetener, dry oatmeal, baking powder, salt, cinnamon, and walnuts together in large mixing bowl.

2. In a separate bowl, combine eggs, zucchini, and oil.

3. Stir wet ingredients into dry ingredients, until just mixed. Do not over-stir.

4. Fill greased baking tins half-full. (Or use paper liners instead of greasing tins.)

5. Bake at 400° for 25 minutes, or until toothpick inserted in centers of muffins comes out clean.

Tip:
  Shredding zucchini in your food processor makes things easier.

Replace some of the all-purpose flour in a recipe with whole-wheat flour to increase fiber.

Banana Chocolate Chip Muffins

Jen Hoover
Akron, PA

Jane Steiner
Orrville, OH

Makes 24 servings,
1 muffin per serving

Prep. Time: 15 minutes
Baking Time: 12–20 minutes

4 large ripe bananas,
 mashed
6 Tbsp. Splenda Blend for
 Baking
1 egg
1½ cups flour
1 tsp. baking soda
1 tsp. baking powder
5⅓ Tbsp. no-trans-fat tub
 margarine, melted
½ cup chocolate chips

1. In a good-sized mixing bowl, blend together bananas, Splenda, egg, and flour.

2. Mix in baking soda, baking powder, and melted margarine.

3. Stir in chocolate chips.

4. Bake in lined muffin tins at 375° for 12–18 minutes, or until toothpick inserted in center comes out clean. Check after 12 minutes to prevent muffins from over-baking.

Tips:

1. I freeze overly ripe bananas with these muffins in mind. Microwave frozen bananas until soft; then follow recipe.

2. Tip from tester: You can use ¾ cup whole wheat flour and ¾ cup white flour for these. You can also add 1 Tbsp. wheat germ or flax seed to Step 1.

3. Another tip from tester: Before baking these, I placed a pecan half on top of each muffin. I served them at breakfast with softened cream cheese and with peanut butter for the kids.

Warm Memories:

My boys love these! I make them to take along every time we go on a trip.

Exchange List Values
- Carbohydrate 1.0 • Fat 0.5

Basic Nutritional Values
- Calories 100
 (Calories from Fat 25)
- Total Fat 3 gm
 (Saturated Fat 1.2 gm,
 Trans Fat 0.0 gm,
 Polyunsat Fat 0.9 gm,
 Monounsat Fat 1.1 gm)
- Cholesterol 10 mg
- Sodium 90 mg
- Potassium 105 gm
- Total Carb 17 gm
- Dietary Fiber 1 gm
- Sugars 8 gm
- Protein 1 gm
- Phosphorus 40 gm

Morning Maple Muffins

Connie Lynn Miller
Shipshewana, IN

Makes 18 muffins,
1 muffin per serving

Prep. Time: 15 minutes
Baking Time: 15–20 minutes

Muffins:
 2 cups flour
 ¼ cup Splenda Brown
  Sugar Blend
 2 tsp. baking powder
 ½ tsp. salt
 ¾ cup fat-free milk
 ½ cup no trans-fat tub
  margarine, melted
 ¼ cup maple syrup
 ¼ cup fat-free sour cream
 1 egg
 ½ tsp. vanilla

Topping:

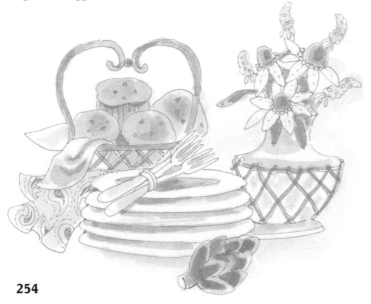

Topping:
- 3 Tbsp. flour
- 3 Tbsp. sugar
- 2 Tbsp. chopped pecans
- ½ tsp. cinnamon
- 2 Tbsp. no trans-fat tub margarine

1. To make muffins, combine flour, brown sugar blend, baking powder, and salt in a large bowl.

2. In another bowl, combine milk, melted margarine, maple syrup, sour cream, egg, and vanilla.

3. Stir wet ingredients into dry ingredients just until moistened.

4. Fill greased or paper-lined muffin cups ⅔ full.

5. For topping, combine flour, sugar, nuts, and cinnamon.

6. Cut in margarine, using a pastry cutter or two knives, until crumbly.

7. Sprinkle over batter in muffin cups.

8. Bake at 400° for 15–20 minutes, or until a toothpick inserted near the center comes out clean.

9. Cool 5 minutes before removing from pans to wire racks. Serve warm.

Tip:
The maple syrup gives these muffins the hint of a hearty pancake breakfast without all the fuss.

Exchange List Values
- Starch 1.0
- Fat 1.0
- Carbohydrate 0.5

Basic Nutritional Values
- Calories 140 (Calories from Fat 55)
- Total Fat 6 gm (Saturated Fat 1.2 gm, Trans Fat 0.0 gm, Polyunsat Fat 2.2 gm, Monounsat Fat 2.0 gm)
- Cholesterol 10 mg
- Sodium 165 mg
- Potassium 60 gm
- Total Carb 20 gm
- Dietary Fiber 1 gm
- Sugars 6 gm
- Protein 3 gm
- Phosphorus 90 gm

Cranberry Buttermilk Scones

Edwina Stoltzfus
Narvon, PA

Makes 16 servings,
1 scone per serving

Prep. Time: 20 minutes
Baking Time: 15–20 minutes

- 3 cups flour
- 2⅔ Tbsp. Splenda Blend for Baking
- 2½ tsp. baking powder
- ¾ tsp. salt
- ½ tsp. baking soda
- 12 Tbsp. cold no trans-fat tub margarine
- 1 cup fat-free buttermilk
- 1 cup dried cranberries
- 1 tsp. grated orange peel
- 1 Tbsp. fat-free milk
- 2 Tbsp. sugar
- ¼ tsp. ground cinnamon

1. In a bowl, combine flour, Splenda, baking powder, salt, and baking soda.

2. Cut in margarine, using a pastry cutter or two knives, until mixture resembles small peas.

3. Stir in buttermilk, just until combined.

4. Fold in cranberries and orange peel.

5. Turn dough onto floured surface. Divide dough in half.

6. Shape each portion into a ball. Pat each into a 6" circle.

7. Cut each circle into six wedges.

8. Place on lightly greased baking sheet.

9. Brush tops with milk.

10. In a small bowl, combine 2 Tbsp. sugar with cinnamon. Sprinkle on top of wedges.

11. Bake at 400° for 15–20 minutes, or until golden brown.

Tips:
1. These freeze well after baking.

2. They're best served warm.

3. I make smaller scones than called for here – at least 8 from a 6" circle.

4. I make my own orange peel by grating the peel of 1 whole orange and then freezing it. It's handy for whenever I need it.

Exchange List Values
- Starch 1.5
- Fat 1.0
- Fruit 0.5

Basic Nutritional Values
- Calories 185 (Calories from Fat 65)
- Total Fat 7 gm (Saturated Fat 1.4 gm, Trans Fat 0.0 gm, Polyunsat Fat 2.8 gm, Monounsat Fat 2.1 gm)
- Cholesterol 0 mg
- Sodium 290 mg
- Potassium 55 gm
- Total Carb 29 gm
- Dietary Fiber 1 gm
- Sugars 10 gm
- Protein 3 gm
- Phosphorus 115 gm

Glazed Cinnamon Biscuits

Virginia Graybill
Hershey, PA

Makes 12 servings,
1 biscuit per serving

Prep. Time: 30 minutes
Baking Time: 18–20 minutes

2 cups flour
4 tsp. baking powder
½ tsp. salt
2 Tbsp. Splenda Blend for Baking
1 tsp. cinnamon
6 Tbsp. no trans-fat tub margarine, *divided*
¾ cup fat-free milk

Glaze:
1 cup Splenda granular
2⅔ Tbsp. cornstarch
¼ tsp. vanilla
1⅓ Tbsp. water

1. In a large bowl, combine flour, baking powder, salt, sugar, and cinnamon.
2. Using a pastry cutter or two knives, cut in 4 Tbsp. margarine until mixture resembles coarse crumbs.
3. Stir in milk just until moistened.
4. Turn onto a lightly floured surface. Rub a bit of vegetable oil on your hands to keep dough from sticking to your fingers while kneading.
5. Knead gently 8–10 times.
6. Roll dough into an 8×11 rectangle, ½" thick.
7. Melt remaining 2 Tbs.

margarine and brush 1 Tbsp. over dough.
8. Roll up jelly-roll style, starting with long end.
9. Cut roll into 12 equal slices.
10. Place slices cut-side down in greased 7×11 baking pan. Make 3 rows with 4 slices in each row.
11. Brush slices with remaining margarine.
12. Bake at 375° for 18–20 minutes, or until golden brown.
13. While biscuits bake, make glaze. Blend Splenda and cornstarch in blender until a very fine powder.
14. In a small bowl, stir water and vanilla together and add Splenda mixture.
15. When biscuits finish baking, allow them to cool 5 minutes.
16. Spread with glaze. Serve immediately.

Exchange List Values

- Starch 1.0
- Fat 0.5
- Carbohydrate 0.5

Basic Nutritional Values

- Calories 140
  (Calories from Fat 40)
- Total Fat 4.5 gm
  (Saturated Fat 0.9 gm,
  Trans Fat 0.0 gm,
  Polyunsat Fat 1.8 gm,
  Monounsat Fat 1.4 gm)
- Cholesterol 0 mg
- Sodium 270 mg
- Potassium 50 gm
- Total Carb 23 gm
- Dietary Fiber 1 gm
- Sugars 5 gm
- Protein 3 gm
- Phosphorus 190 gm

Sticky Buns

Dorothy Schrock
Arthur, IL

Makes 15 buns, 1 bun per serving

Prep. Time: 35 minutes
Rising Time: 30 minutes
Baking Time: 15 minutes

Dough:
½ cup warm water
1 Tbsp. yeast
¾ cup milk
2 Tbsp. no-trans-fat tub margarine
2 Tbsp. canola oil
1 tsp. salt
¼ cup sugar
1 egg, beaten
3 cups flour

Sauce:
6 Tbsp. no-trans-fat tub margarine
¾ tsp. cinnamon
½ cup Splenda Brown Sugar Blend
1 Tbsp. water
⅓ cup pecans

1. In a small bowl, stir yeast into warm water until dissolved. Set aside.
2. Heat milk, margarine, and oil in medium-sized saucepan over low heat until margarine melts. Remove pan from heat.
3. Stir salt and sugar into milk mixture until dissolved.
4. Stir yeast water, egg, and flour into other ingredients.
5. Set in warm place and let rise for 30 minutes.
6. Meanwhile, prepare sauce. In a medium-sized

saucepan, heat margarine, cinnamon, Splenda, and water together. Make good and hot, but do not allow to boil.

7. Stir in pecans.

8. Pour sauce into well-greased 9×13 baking pan. Spread over bottom of pan.

9. Stir down batter. Drop by tablespoons over sauce. You should be able to make 12–15 batter "buns."

10. Bake at 350° for 15 minutes.

11. Cool for 1 minute.

12. Cover baking pan with rimmed cookie sheet. Turn upside down carefully to release sticky buns onto cookie sheet.

Exchange List Values
- Starch 1.5
- Fat 1.5
- Carbohydrate 0.5

Basic Nutritional Values
- Calories 210
  (Calories from Fat 70)
- Total Fat 8 gm
  (Saturated Fat 1.3 gm,
  Trans Fat 0.0 gm,
  Polyunsat Fat 2.9 gm,
  Monounsat Fat 3.8 gm)
- Cholesterol 15 mg
- Sodium 210 mg
- Potassium 85 gm
- Total Carb 30 gm
- Dietary Fiber 1 gm
- Sugars 7 gm
- Protein 4 gm
- Phosphorus 65 gm

Cinnamon Rolls— Easy Method

Betty L. Moore
Plano, IL

Makes 12 rolls, 1 roll per serving

Thawing Time: 8 hours or overnight
Prep. Time: 15–20 minutes
Rising Time: 4–5 hour, or overnight
Baking Time: 20–25 minutes

1 lb. loaf frozen bread dough
8 Tbsp. no trans-fat tub margarine
2 tsp. cinnamon
1½ cups granular Splenda, *divided*
2⅔ Tbsp. cornstarch
1½ Tbsp. fat-free milk

1. Thaw dough at room temperature.

2. Grease a 9×13 baking pan.

3. In a long, flat dish, mix together cinnamon and ½ cup sugar substitute.

4. Melt margarine.

5. Cut thawed bread dough diagonally into 12 pieces.

6. Roll each piece of dough between your hands until it forms a rope.

7. Brush each piece of dough with melted margarine, and then dip in cinnamon-sugar. Use a spoon to cover rope well with mixture.

8. Tie each buttered-sugared piece in a loose knot. Lay in greased 9×13 baking pan, keeping as much space as possible between knots to allow for rising.

9. Cover loosely and let set until knots double in size, or refrigerate overnight.

10. Set out in morning and allow to rise until doubled, if knots haven't risen fully.

11. Bake at 350° for 20–25 minutes.

12. Meanwhile, prepare glaze. Blend 1 cup Splenda in blender with cornstarch until a fine powder.

13. Mix the blended sugar and milk together in a bowl until smooth.

14. Drizzle glaze over cooled buns.

Tips:

These are messy to make, but they taste wonderful. We make these at camp to serve 300–400 people.

Exchange List Values
- Starch 1.5
- Fat 1.0

Basic Nutritional Values
- Calories 170
  (Calories from Fat 65)
- Total Fat 7 gm
  (Saturated Fat 1.5 gm,
  Trans Fat 0.0 gm,
  Polyunsat Fat 2.9 gm,
  Monounsat Fat 2.1 gm)
- Cholesterol 0 mg
- Sodium 280 mg
- Potassium 50 gm
- Total Carb 24 gm
- Dietary Fiber 1 gm
- Sugars 4 gm
- Protein 3 gm
- Phosphorus 45 gm

Eat breakfast every day. People who eat breakfast are less likely to overeat later in the day.

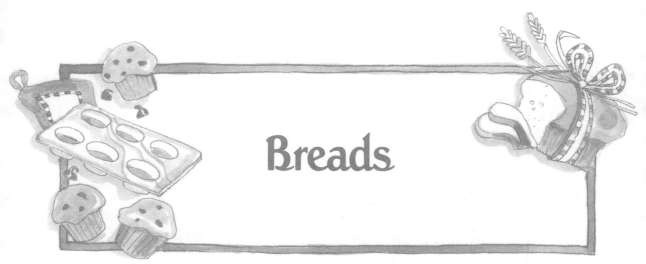

Breads

Oatmeal Herb Bread

Stacy Stoltzfus
Grantham, PA

*Makes 1 loaf, 16 slices in the loaf,
1 slice per serving*

Prep. Time: 20 minutes
Rising Time: 65–85 minutes
**Cooking/Baking Time: 30–35
minutes**
Standing Time: 30–45 minutes

1 cup warm water (110–115°)
2 Tbsp. brown sugar
1 Tbsp. yeast
1 egg, lightly beaten
3 Tbsp. olive oil
1 tsp. salt
½ cup dry quick oats
1 tsp. dried parsley
1 tsp. dried sage
1 tsp. dried oregano
1 tsp. dried basil
1 tsp. dried thyme
3½–4 cups unbleached
   bread flour, also called
   occident flour

1. Dissolve sugar in warm water in a large mixing bowl.
2. Sprinkle yeast over top.
3. Let rest 5–10 minutes until yeast begins to foam.
4. Stir in egg, olive oil, salt, oats, and herbs.
5. Gradually add in flour, one cup at a time, mixing until a ball forms that is not too dense. Dough should be soft but not sticky.
6. Knead about 5 minutes on floured surface.
7. Grease a large bowl. Place dough in bowl and cover with a tea towel.
8. Place in warm spot. Let rise until doubled, about 30–45 minutes.
9. Punch down. Form into a loaf.
10. Place in greased loaf pan. Let rise until dough comes to top of pan, about 35–40 minutes.
11. Meanwhile, preheat oven to 350°. Place risen loaf in oven. Bake approximately 30–35 minutes. Loaf should be golden brown and should sound hollow when tapped.
12. Cool 10 minutes before removing from pan.
13. Let cool until lukewarm before slicing to keep moisture in the loaf. Slice the loaf just before serving.

Tips:
1. I always use an instant-read thermometer to ensure the bread is completely baked through. It should register 190–200° when done.
2. You can use fresh herbs instead of dried herbs. The formula? 1 tsp. dried herbs for 3 tsp. fresh herbs.

Exchange List Values
• Starch 2.0   • Fat 0.5

Basic Nutritional Values
• Calories 175   • Sodium 175 mg
  (Calories from Fat 45)   • Potassium 85 gm
• Total Fat 5 gm   • Total Carb 26 gm
  (Saturated Fat 1.0 gm,   • Dietary Fiber 1 gm
  Trans Fat 0.0 gm,   • Sugars 2 gm
  Polyunsat Fat 0.9 gm,   • Protein 7 gm
  Monounsat Fat 2.7 gm) • Phosphorus 85 gm
• Cholesterol 70 mg

Pumpernickel Bread

Helene Funk
Laird, Saskatchewan

*Makes 4 loaves, 16 slices per loaf,
1 slice per serving*

Prep. Time: 35 minutes
Rising Time: about 3 hours
Cooking/Baking Time: 1 hour

3 Tbsp. yeast
2 tsp. sugar
1 cup warm water
3¼ cups water
½ cup dark molasses
1 Tbsp. no-trans-fat tub
  margarine
1 tsp. salt
3½ cups whole wheat flour
4½ cups white flour
3½ cups rye flour
1 Tbsp. unsweetened
  cocoa, *optional*
1 cup bran
¾ cup yellow cornmeal
½ cup millet, *optional*
2 cups mashed potatoes
2 tsp. caraway seeds
½ cup flax

1. Dissolve yeast with sugar in 1 cup warm water. Let stand 10 minutes until bubbly. Stir well.

2. Combine 3¼ cups water, molasses and margarine in saucepan. Heat over low heat until margarine is dissolved. When room temperature, add salt and yeast mixture.

3. Combine all flours and cocoa in large bowl.

4. Add bran, cornmeal, millet and mashed potatoes.

Add to liquid yeast mixture and beat until thoroughly mixed. Stir in caraway seeds and flax and mix well.

5. Let dough rest 15 minutes. Knead until smooth.

6. Let rise until double in bulk, about 1 hour.

7. Punch down. Let rise again for 30 minutes.

8. Divide into 4 pieces and shape into loaves or balls and place in greased tins.

9. Cover and let rise in warm place, about 45 minutes.

10. Bake at 325° for 45–50 minutes or until done.

Bran Rolls

Johanna Badertscher
Apple Creek, OH

Makes 32 rolls, 1 roll per serving

Prep. Time: 30 minutes
Rising Time: 2 hours
Baking Time: 20 minutes

1 cup wheat bran
1 cup boiling water
½ cup honey, *or* brown sugar
1½ tsp. salt

1 cup canola oil
2 pkgs. yeast
1 cup warm water
2 eggs
6½ cups flour

1. Combine bran, boiling water, honey or brown sugar, salt and oil. Cool to lukewarm.

2. Dissolve yeast in warm water and add to bran mixture.

3. Beat in eggs and 3½ cups flour. Knead in remaining 3 cups flour to make a smooth, soft dough.

4. Place in greased bowl and let rise until double in size, about an hour. Alternatively, cover with plastic wrap with space for dough to expand and place in refrigerator until ready to use.

5. Shape into rolls. Place rolls in greased pans and let rise until double in size.

6. Bake at 375° for 20 minutes.

Variation:

This dough makes wonderful hamburger rolls. After shaping, place on greased cookie sheets at least 1" apart.

French Bread— No-knead

Naomi Ressler
Harrisonburg, VA

*Makes 2 loaves, 19 slices per loaf,
1 slice per serving*

Prep. Time: 1½ hours
**Cooking/Baking Time: 20
minutes**

2 Tbsp. all-vegetable
 shortening
2 Tbsp. sugar
2 tsp. salt
1 cup boiling water
1 cup cold water
2¼-oz. pkgs. yeast
1 scant Tbsp. sugar
6 cups flour
½ cup warm water

1. Dissolve shortening,
sugar and salt in boiling
water.
2. Add cold water to
shortening mixture.
3. Dissolve yeast and sugar
in warm water. Add to the
shortening mixture.
4. Add flour. Do NOT beat.
Stir with big spoon every
10 minutes, 4 or 5 times, for
approximately an hour.
5. Divide dough in half.
Flour dough board or
counter and hands and pat
each section into rectangle
shape about ½-inch thick.

Roll lengthwise in jelly roll
fashion and tuck in ends. Cut
slits diagonally 2–3" apart
(shallow) on top of loaves.
6. Put on lightly greased
baking sheet. Let rise until
double, about 20–30 minutes
depending on temperature of
room.
7. Bake at 375–400° for
approximately 20 minutes.

Tips:
1. May wish to brush
butter or margarine on top of
loaf after baking.
2. Delicious with any meal
but especially with pasta.
3. Dough will be stiff/thick
so difficult to stir but do the
best you can!

Warm Memories:
Good friend shared this
bread with us. I've made
<u>many</u> loaves to donate to our
Mennonite Relief Sale. It's
so quick and easy as well as
delicious and makes large
loaves.

Exchange List Values
• Starch 1.0

Basic Nutritional Values
• Calories 85	• Sodium 125 mg
(Calories from Fat 10)	• Potassium 30 gm
• Total Fat 1 gm	• Total Carb 16 gm
(Saturated Fat 0.2 gm,	• Dietary Fiber 1 gm
Trans Fat 0.0 gm,	• Sugars 1 gm
Polyunsat Fat 0.3 gm,	• Protein 2 gm
Monounsat Fat 0.3 gm)	• Phosphorus 25 gm
• Cholesterol 0 mg	

Use slices of avocado on a sandwich instead of mayonnaise.

Whole Wheat Rolls

Faye Pankratz
Inola, OK

*Makes 2 dozen rolls,
1 roll per serving*

Prep. Time: 25 minutes
Cooling Time: 20 minutes
Rising Time: about 2 hours
Baking Time: 20 minutes

2 pkgs. dry yeast
½ cup warm water
1 tsp. sugar
1¾ cups fat-free milk,
 scalded
¼ cup sugar
1 Tbsp. salt
3 Tbsp. all-vegetable
 shortening
2 cups whole wheat flour
3 egg whites
3 cups white flour, *or more*

1. Combine yeast and
warm water in small bowl.
Sprinkle 1 tsp. sugar over
yeast and water. Set aside.
2. Pour scalded milk
over ¼ cup sugar, salt and
shortening in large bowl.
Cool until lukewarm. Add
yeast mixture and stir well.
3. Add whole wheat flour
and egg whites. Beat well and
gradually add white flour
until you have soft dough.
4. Turn onto floured surface
and knead until dough is
elastic, about 5–7 minutes.
Place in greased bowl, turning
dough to grease top. Cover
with clean cloth and let rise
until doubled in bulk.
5. Punch down and shape
into rolls. Place on greased

cookie sheets and let rise until double.

6. Bake at 350° for 20 minutes or until lightly browned.

Exchange List Values
- Starch 1.5

Basic Nutritional Values
- Calories 125
  (Calories from Fat 20)
- Total Fat 2 gm
  (Saturated Fat 0.4 gm,
  Trans Fat 0.0 gm,
  Polyunsat Fat 0.6 gm,
  Monounsat Fat 0.7 gm)
- Cholesterol 0 mg
- Sodium 305 mg
- Potassium 105 gm
- Total Carb 23 gm
- Dietary Fiber 2 gm
- Sugars 3 gm
- Protein 4 gm
- Phosphorus 80 gm

Homemade Rolls

Ruth S. Weaver
Reinholds, PA

*Makes 20 servings,
1 roll per serving*

Prep. Time: 25 minutes
Rising Time: 2 hours
Baking Time: 14–20 minutes

5¾–6¾ cups bread flour, *divided*
⅓ cup instant non-fat dry milk solids
¼ cup sugar
1 Tbsp. salt
2 pkgs. dry yeast
5 Tbsp. (⅓ cup) margarine, softened
2 cups warm tap water, 120–130°

1. In large bowl mix 2 cups flour, milk, sugar, salt, and yeast. Add margarine.

2. Gradually add water to dry ingredients and beat 2 minutes at medium speed with a mixer. Add 1 more cup flour and beat 2 minutes on high speed. Stir in enough flour to make a stiff dough.

3. Turn out onto a lightly floured board and knead about 8–10 minutes. Place in greased bowl, turning to grease top of dough.

4. Cover with a kitchen towel and let rise in warm place until doubled in bulk (about 45 minutes). Punch down and allow to rise again for 20 minutes.

5. Divide dough in half and cut each half into 10 equal pieces. Form into rolls and place on greased baking sheet about 2" apart. Cover and let rise again about 1 hour.

6. Bake at 375° for 15–20 minutes. Remove from baking sheet and brush with melted margarine.

Tip:

Not many other people bring homemade bread or rolls to a church potluck, and I always bake them several days before the fellowship meal so I have no last minute rush.

Exchange List Values
- Starch 2.0
- Fat 0.5

Basic Nutritional Values
- Calories 190
  (Calories from Fat 25)
- Total Fat 3 gm
  (Saturated Fat 0.5 gm,
  Trans Fat 0.0 gm,
  Polyunsat Fat 1.2 gm,
  Monounsat Fat 0.8 gm)
- Cholesterol 0 mg
- Sodium 380 mg
- Potassium 75 gm
- Total Carb 34 gm
- Dietary Fiber 1 gm
- Sugars 4 gm
- Protein 6 gm
- Phosphorus 60 gm

Herb Toast

Hazel N. Hassan
Goshen, IN

*Makes 25 servings,
1 slice per serving with 1 tsp. spread*

Prep. Time: 20 minutes
Standing Time: a few hours or a day
Baking Time: 30–40 minutes

½ cup no-trans-fat tub margarine, melted
1½ tsp. curry powder
1¼ tsp. paprika
1 tsp. dried savory
¼ tsp. dried thyme
1 loaf Roman meal bread or other thinly sliced bread, 25 slices of ¾ oz. each

1. Mix margarine and seasonings together a few hours or a day ahead.

2. Spread mixture on thin slices of bread.

3. Toast at 300° for 30–40 minutes.

4. Serve in basket lined with a cloth napkin.

Exchange List Values
- Starch 1.0
- Fat 0.5

Basic Nutritional Values
- Calories 95
  (Calories from Fat 30)
- Total Fat 4 gm
  (Saturated Fat 0.8 gm,
  Trans Fat 0.0 gm,
  Polyunsat Fat 1.5 gm,
  Monounsat Fat 1.1 gm)
- Cholesterol 0 mg
- Sodium 165 mg
- Potassium 55 gm
- Total Carb 12 gm
- Dietary Fiber 1 gm
- Sugars 1 gm
- Protein 3 gm
- Phosphorus 45 gm

Icebox Butterhorns

Jolyn Nolt
Leola, PA

Makes 36 rolls, 1 roll per serving

Prep. Time: 15 minutes
Chilling Time: 8 hours or
* overnight*
Rising Time: 1 hour
Baking Time: 15–20 minutes

2 cups fat-free milk
1 Tbsp. yeast
2 Tbsp. warm water,
  110–115°
½ cup sugar
1 egg
1 tsp. salt
6 cups flour
¾ cup butter-oil blend,
  such as Land O Lakes
  tub butter with canola,
  at room temperature

1. Heat milk in small
saucepan just until steaming.
2. Remove from heat and
allow to cool to 110–115°.
3. Meanwhile, in a large
mixing bowl, dissolve yeast in
warm water.
4. When milk has cooled,
add it, plus sugar, egg, salt,
and 3 cups flour to yeast
mixture.
5. Beat until smooth.
6. Beat in butter spread and
remaining flour. The dough
will be sticky.
7. Cover bowl. Refrigerate
8 hours or overnight.
8. Then divide dough into
three balls.
9. Roll each piece into a
12" circle on lightly floured
surface.

10. Cut each circle into 12
wedges each.
11. Roll up each wedge
crescent-style, starting with
the wide end. Place rolls
point-side down, 2" apart on
waxed paper-lined baking
sheets. Curve ends, if you
wish, to shape into crescents.
12. Cover and set in warm
place. Let rise 1 hour.
13. Bake at 350° for 15–20
minutes.

Exchange List Values

• Starch 1.5   • Fat 0.5

Basic Nutritional Values

• Calories 125   • Sodium 100 mg
  (Calories from Fat 35) • Potassium 50 gm
• Total Fat 4 gm   • Total Carb 19 gm
  (Saturated Fat 1.4 gm, • Dietary Fiber 1 gm
  Trans Fat 0.0 gm,   • Sugars 4 gm
  Polyunsat Fat 0.8 gm,   • Protein 3 gm
  Monounsat Fat 1.8 gm) • Phosphorus 45 gm
• Cholesterol 10 mg

Garlic Breadsticks

Sadie Mae Stoltzfus
Gordonville, PA

Makes 26 servings,
1"×9" breadstick per serving

Prep. Time: 10 minutes
Rising Time: 20 minutes
Baking Time: 20 minutes

1½ cups warm water,
  110–115°
1 Tbsp. yeast
1 Tbsp. oil
1 Tbsp. sugar
1¼ tsp. salt
4 cups bread flour, also
  called unbleached
  occident flour

Topping:
3 Tbsp. olive oil, *divided*
½ cup tub margarine, no
  trans-fat, melted
1 tsp. coarsely ground
  salt
3 Tbsp. Parmesan cheese
1½ tsp. garlic powder
3 Tbsp. dried parsley
  flakes

1. Stir yeast into water
in large bowl, stirring until
dissolved.
2. Add 1 Tbsp. oil, sugar, salt
and flour. Knead a little in the
bowl to make sure ingredients
are fully incorporated.
3. Cover with tea towel. Let
rise 5–8 minutes in warm spot.
4. Place 1 tsp. olive oil in
each of two 9×13 baking
pans. Grease pan.
5. Divide dough between
baking pans. Spread to cover
bottom of each pan. Set aside.
6. Prepare topping by
placing melted margarine in
bowl.
7. Stir in remaining ingredients.
8. Pour topping mixture
evenly over 2 pans of dough.
9. Bake at 350° for 20
minutes, or until golden brown.
10. Allow to cool slightly.
Then using a pizza cutter, start
on the 13" side of the pan and
cut dough into 1" sticks.

Tips:
1. For lighter breadsticks
let dough, topped with butter
mixture, rise 15–20 minutes.
2. You can use half whole
wheat flour and half white
bread flour.
3. Sometimes I serve these
with salsa as an appetizer.

Grilled Pizza Crusts

Tammy Smith
Dorchester, WI

*Makes 2 large pizza crusts,
each cut into 8 servings*

Prep. Time: 10–15 minutes
Rising Time: 1 hour, or so
Grilling Time: 2–3 minutes

1¼ cups warm water
3½ cups flour, plus more if
  necessary
1 envelope active dry yeast
1 tsp. sugar
1½ tsp. coarse salt
1¼ cups warm water
¼ cup olive oil

1. Put water in bowl of mixer with a dough hook.

2. Add flour, yeast, sugar, and salt.

3. Add oil. Mix well.

4. If too sticky, add more flour, a tablespoon at a time, until dough pulls away from sides of bowl.

5. Place ball of dough on lightly floured surface. Knead by hand a few minutes.

6. Cover with plastic wrap. Set in warm place.

7. Let rise until double in bulk, an hour or so.

8. Generously oil 2 baking sheets. Divide dough in half, and place one half on each pan.

9. Stretch each ball of dough to form a 9×13 rectangle, about ⅛-¼" thick.

10. Slide crust off baking sheet and right onto grill grate after grill is hot.

11. Grill 1–2 minutes until first side is lightly browned.

12. Flip over. Grill 1–2 minutes on that side until lightly browned.

13. When crust is done, cover with your favorite toppings. Put back on grill on LOW heat until heated through.

14. Cut into wedges and serve.

Cheesy Garlic Bread

Loretta Krahn
Mountain Lake, MN

*Makes 12 servings,
1 slice per serving*

Prep. Time: 15 minutes
Baking Time: 10 minutes

4 Tbsp. trans-fat-free tub
  margarine
4 Tbsp. freshly grated
  Parmesan cheese
1 Tbsp. Italian seasoning
  (see page 270)
½ Tbsp. finely chopped
  onion
½ tsp. garlic powder
½ tsp. salt
16-oz. loaf French bread

1. Warm margarine until softened. Stir in all remaining ingredients except bread.

2. Slice bread and spread mixture thinly on each slice.

3. Warm in microwave or slow oven (200–300°) until margarine melts immediately before serving.

Bagels

Bob Litt
London, OH

*Makes 32 servings,
1 bagel per serving*

Prep. Time: 30 minutes
Rising Time: 2–2½ hours
Baking/Cooking Time: 45 minutes

2 Tbsp. active dry yeast
1 tsp. sugar
1½ cups warm water
¼ cup sugar
4–4½ cups flour, *divided*
2 eggs
cornmeal
egg whites, *optional*
chopped onion or poppy
　seeds, *optional*

1. Dissolve yeast and 1 tsp. sugar in warm water. Let stand until foamy.

2. Add ¼ cup sugar, 2 cups flour and eggs. Beat until well mixed, approximately 200 strokes.

3. Slowly add remaining flour to make soft dough. Turn out onto lightly floured surface. Knead dough until smooth and elastic, approximately 8–10 minutes.

4. Place dough in greased bowl, turning to coat top of dough. Cover and let stand in warm place until doubled in size, approximately 1½ hours.

5. Punch down and divide into 32 pieces (cut in half, then in half again, and so on).

6. Shape each piece into a ball and punch finger through each piece to make a bagel shape. Let rise until double in size.

7. Bring a large pot of water to boil. Boil each bagel for 2 minutes, turning after first minute.

8. Grease baking pan and coat with cornmeal. Bake at 375° for 25–30 minutes.

9. Top each bagel with egg white and either onion or poppy seeds if you wish.

Exchange List Values
• Starch 1.0

Basic Nutritional Values

• Calories 75	• Sodium 0 mg
(Calories from Fat 0)	• Potassium 35 mg
• Total Fat 0 gm	• Total Carb 15 gm
(Saturated Fat 0.1 gm,	• Dietary Fiber 1 gm
Trans Fat 0.0 gm,	• Sugars 2 gm
Polyunsat Fat 0.1 gm,	• Protein 2 gm
Monounsat Fat 0.1 gm)	• Phosphorus 30 gm
• Cholesterol 10 mg	

Irish Freckle Bread

Martha G. Zimmerman
Lititz, PA

*Makes 4 loaves,
8 slices per loaf, 1 slice per serving*

Prep. Time: 30 minutes
**Rising Time: 2 hours and 30
　minutes**
Baking Time: 30–45 minutes

2 Tbsp. (2 pkgs.) dry yeast
1 cup warm potato water
　(left from cooking
　potatoes) *or* warm water
¼ cup lukewarm mashed
　potatoes, made from
　scratch, *or* instant
8 Tbsp. sugar, *divided*
5¼ cups flour,
　approximately, *divided*

1 tsp. salt
2 eggs, beaten
½ cup tub margarine, no
　trans-fat, melted and
　cooled
1 cup dark seedless raisins

1. Dissolve yeast in warm potato water in large mixing bowl.

2. Stir in mashed potatoes, 2 Tbsp. sugar, and 1 cup flour. Beat until smooth.

3. Cover and let rise in warm place until bubbly, about 30 minutes.

4. Stir down.

5. Add rest of sugar, salt, and 1 cup flour. Beat until smooth.

6. Stir in eggs and margarine.

7. Add raisins.

8. Stir in enough additional flour to make soft dough.

9. Turn out onto lightly floured board. Knead until smooth and elastic, about 5 minutes.

10. Place in greased bowl, turning to grease top. Cover and let rise in warm place until doubled, about 1 hour.

11. Punch down. Divide into four equal parts. Let rise 50 minutes.

12. Shape each part into slender loaf, about 9" long.

13. Put loaves in lightly greased 9×5 baking pans.

14. Cover and let rise again until double, about 40 minutes.

15. Bake at 350° for 30–45 minutes.

Warm Memories:
　This was a recipe I made when my children were young and we only had one

car. So for a little income I made this bread and sold it to my neighbors. They loved it.

Exchange List Values
• Starch 1.5   • Fat 0.5

Basic Nutritional Values
• Calories 125   • Sodium 105 mg
(Calories from Fat 20)   • Potassium 80 gm
• Total Fat 2.5 gm   • Total Carb 23 gm
(Saturated Fat 0.6 gm,   • Dietary Fiber 1 gm
Trans Fat 0.0 gm,   • Sugars 6 gm
Polyunsat Fat 1.0 gm,   • Protein 3 gm
Monounsat Fat 0.8 gm)   • Phosphorus 40 gm
• Cholesterol 10 mg

Cheddar Biscuits

Jean Halloran
Green Bay, WI
Jessalyn Wantland
Napoleon, OH

*Makes 12 servings,
1 biscuit per serving*

Prep. Time: 10–20 minutes
Baking Time: 15–17 minutes

**2½ cups reduced-fat
  baking mix
4 Tbsp. tub margarine, no
  trans fat
1 cup 75%-less-fat
  shredded cheddar cheese
¾ cup fat-free milk
butter-flavored cooking
  spray**

**½ tsp. garlic powder,
  divided
¼ tsp. dried parsley flakes**

1. In good-sized mixing bowl, cut butter into baking mix using pastry cutter or 2 forks. Combine until mixture resembles small peas.
2. Stir in cheese, milk and ¼ tsp. garlic powder until just combined. Do not over-mix.
3. Drop batter by ¼ cupfuls onto greased baking sheet. (An ice cream scoop works well.)
4. Bake 15–17 minutes at 400°, or until tops are lightly browned.
5. Remove from oven. Spray tops lightly with cooking sprays, 6 short sprays total. Sprinkle evenly with ¼ tsp. garlic powder and parsley flakes. Serve warm.

Note:
  These are dangerously good!

Exchange List Values
• Starch 1.0   • Fat 1.0

Basic Nutritional Values
• Calories 140   • Sodium 370 mg
(Calories from Fat 45)   • Potassium 65 gm
• Total Fat 5 gm   • Total Carb 18 gm
(Saturated Fat 1.3 gm,   • Dietary Fiber 1 gm
Trans Fat 0.0 gm,   • Sugars 3 gm
Polyunsat Fat 1.5 gm,   • Protein 5 gm
Monounsat Fat 2.1 gm)   • Phosphorus 210 gm
• Cholesterol 5 mg

Herbed Biscuit Knots

Melissa Wenger
Orrville, OH

Makes 20 servings
Prep. Time: 10 minutes
Baking Time: 9–12 minutes

**12-oz. tube refrigerated
  buttermilk biscuits
¼ cup canola oil
½ tsp. salt
½ tsp. garlic powder
½ tsp. Italian seasoning**

1. Cut each biscuit in half.
2. Roll each portion into a 6"-long rope.
3. Tie each in a loose knot. Place on greased baking sheet.
4. Bake at 400° for 9–12 minutes, or until golden brown.
5. While knots bake, combine oil, salt, garlic powder, and Italian seasoning in small bowl.
6. Brush over warm knots Immediately after baking.

Exchange List Values
• Starch 0.5   • Fat 1.0

Basic Nutritional Values
• Calories 75   • Sodium 245 mg
(Calories from Fat 45)   • Potassium 25 gm
• Total Fat 5 gm   • Total Carb 7 gm
(Saturated Fat 1.0 gm,   • Dietary Fiber 0 gm
Trans Fat 0.0 gm,   • Sugars 1 gm
Polyunsat Fat 1.0 gm,   • Protein 1 gm
Monounsat Fat 2.7 gm)   • Phosphorus 60 gm
• Cholesterol 0 mg

Always check what you are baking a little earlier than stated in the recipe. Ovens do vary.
Mary Jones, Marengo, OH

Biscuits Supreme

Lavina Ebersol
Ronks, PA

Makes 16 biscuits,
1 biscuit per serving

Prep. Time: 30 minutes
Baking Time: 12–15 minutes

2 cups flour
3 Tbsp. sugar
¼ tsp. cream of tartar
¼ tsp. salt
4 tsp. baking powder
½ cup vegetable shortening
⅔ cup fat-free milk

1. In good-sized mixing bowl, combine flour, sugar, cream of tartar, salt, and baking powder.
2. Using a pastry cutter, or 2 knives, cut in shortening until mixture resembles small peas.
3. Stir in milk until ball of dough forms.
4. Roll dough out on flat surface until about ½" thick.
5. Using a 2" biscuit cutter, cut out 14 biscuits. Gather up leftover pieces and form 2 more biscuits. Place on ungreased baking sheet.
6. Bake at 450° for 8–12 minutes, so that biscuits brown lightly. Do not over-bake!
7. Serve warm.

Good Go-Alongs:
Split these biscuits and serve them topped with sausage gravy.

Exchange List Values
• Starch 1.0   • Fat 1.0

Basic Nutritional Values
• Calories 125
  (Calories from Fat 55)
• Total Fat 6 gm
  (Saturated Fat 1.5 gm,
  Trans Fat 0.0 gm,
  Polyunsat Fat 2.1 gm,
  Monounsat Fat 2.5 gm)
• Cholesterol 0 mg
• Sodium 130 mg
• Potassium 40 gm
• Total Carb 15 gm
• Dietary Fiber 0 gm
• Sugars 3 gm
• Protein 2 gm
• Phosphorus 145 gm

Cornbread

Rebecca B. Stoltzfus
Lititz, PA

Makes 16 servings,
2"×2" square per serving

Prep. Time: 10 minutes
Baking Time: 35 minutes

6 Tbsp. Splenda Blend for Baking
5⅓ Tbsp. tub margarine, no trans-fat, softened
2 eggs, beaten
½ cup fat-free sour cream
½ cup buttermilk
1 cup flour
1 cup cornmeal
½ tsp. salt
1 tsp. baking soda
½ tsp. baking powder

1. Cream Splenda and margarine together well.
2. Mix in sour cream and buttermilk, and eggs. Mix well again.
3. In a separate bowl, combine flour, cornmeal, salt, baking soda, and baking powder.
4. Add dry ingredients to creamed mixture. Stir as little as possible.
5. Pour batter into greased 8×8 baking dish.
6. Bake at 350° for 35 minutes, or until toothpick inserted in center comes out clean.

Exchange List Values
• Starch 1.0   • Fat 0.5

Basic Nutritional Values
• Calories 120
  (Calories from Fat 30)
• Total Fat 4 gm
  (Saturated Fat 0.9 gm,
  Trans Fat 0.0 gm,
  Polyunsat Fat 1.4 gm,
  Monounsat Fat 1.2 gm)
• Cholesterol 25 mg
• Sodium 210 mg
• Potassium 40 gm
• Total Carb 19 gm
• Dietary Fiber 1 gm
• Sugars 5 gm
• Protein 3 gm
• Phosphorus 50 gm

Corn Sticks

Judith E. Bartel
North Newton, KS

Makes 20 servings

Prep. Time: 25 minutes
Baking Time: 10–12 minutes

2 cups reduced-fat baking mix
8½-oz. can cream-style corn
¼ cup freshly grated Parmesan cheese
1 tsp. powdered garlic
1 Tbsp. dill seed
4 Tbsp. no-trans-fat tub margarine, melted

1. Combine baking mix, corn, Parmesan cheese, garlic, and dill seed and mix well.
2. Knead 15–20 strokes on lightly floured on lightly floured board. Roll into large rectangle with rolling pin.

3. Cut into 1"×3" strips. Place strips 1½" apart on ungreased cookie sheet. Brush with melted margarine.

4. Bake at 450° for 10–12 minutes.

Exchange List Values
- Starch 0.5
- Fat 0.5

Basic Nutritional Values
- Calories 70
  (Calories from Fat 20)
- Total Fat 2.5 gm
  (Saturated Fat 0.6 gm,
  Trans Fat 0.0 gm,
  Polyunsat Fat 0.9 gm,
  Monounsat Fat 1.1 gm)
- Cholesterol 0 mg
- Sodium 185 mg
- Potassium 35 gm
- Total Carb 10 gm
- Dietary Fiber 0 gm
- Sugars 2 gm
- Protein 1 gm
- Phosphorus 85 gm

Maple Cornbread

Kitty Hilliard
Punxsutawney, PA

Makes 9 servings,
3" square per serving

Prep. Time: 10 minutes
Baking Time: 20–22 minutes

1¼ cups flour
¼ cup cornmeal
1½ tsp. baking powder
½ tsp. salt
1 egg
¾ cup fat-free milk
¼ cup maple syrup
3 Tbsp. canola oil

1. In a bowl, combine flour, cornmeal, baking powder, and salt.

2. In another bowl, beat egg. Add milk, syrup, and oil.

3. Stir wet ingredients into dry ingredients just until moistened.

4. Pour into a greased 9×9 baking pan.

5. Bake at 400° for 20–22 minutes, or until a toothpick inserted in center come out clean.

6. Cool on wire rack for 10 minutes.

7. Cut into squares. Serve warm.

Tip:

I've also made this recipe with ordinary pancake syrup, and it tastes great.

Exchange List Values
- Starch 1.5
- Fat 1.0

Basic Nutritional Values
- Calories 160
  (Calories from Fat 45)
- Total Fat 5 gm
  (Saturated Fat 0.6 gm,
  Trans Fat 0.0 gm,
  Polyunsat Fat 1.5 gm,
  Monounsat Fat 3.2 gm)
- Cholesterol 20 mg
- Sodium 210 mg
- Potassium 95 gm
- Total Carb 24 gm
- Dietary Fiber 1 gm
- Sugars 7 gm
- Protein 4 gm
- Phosphorus 135 gm

Beth's Banana Bread

Elizabeth Weaver Bonnar
Thorndale, Ontario

Makes 15 servings,
1 slice per serving

Prep. Time: 25 minutes
Baking Time: 50 minutes
Cooling Time: 30 minutes

⅓ cup canola oil
2 eggs, beaten
6 medium bananas, mashed
2 cups whole wheat flour
¼ tsp. salt
1¼ tsp. baking soda
¼ cup hot water
1 cup chopped walnuts

1. Beat oil and eggs and mix well. Stir in bananas.

2. Sift together all dry ingredients and add to batter, alternating with hot water. Mix until smooth. Fold in the walnuts.

3. Bake in greased loaf pan at 325° for about 50 minutes.

4. Cool on wire rack for ½ hour before slicing. Serve with honey or maple syrup

Exchange List Values
- Carbohydrate 1.5
- Fat 2.0

Basic Nutritional Values
- Calories 205
  (Calories from Fat 100)
- Total Fat 11 gm
  (Saturated Fat 1.2 gm,
  Trans Fat 0.0 gm,
  Polyunsat Fat 5.4 gm,
  Monounsat Fat 4.0 gm)
- Cholesterol 25 mg
- Sodium 155 mg
- Potassium 290 gm
- Total Carb 24 gm
- Dietary Fiber 4 gm
- Sugars 6 gm
- Protein 5 gm
- Phosphorus 105 gm

Cocoa Zucchini Bread

Kathy Hertzler
Lancaster, PA
Katie Ebersol
Ronks, PA

*Makes 2 loaves, 16 slices per loaf,
1 slice per serving*

Prep. Time: 15 minutes
Standing Time: 45–50 minutes
Baking Time: 1 hour

1 cup Splenda Blend for Baking
3 eggs
1 cup canola oil
2 cups grated zucchini
½ cup fat-free milk
1 tsp. vanilla
3 cups flour
1 tsp. cinnamon
1 tsp. baking soda
1 tsp. baking powder
½ tsp. salt
¼ cup cocoa powder, *optional*
½ cup mini-chocolate chips
½ cup chopped walnuts, *or* pecans

1. Blend Splenda, eggs, and oil in large mixing bowl.
2. Stir in zucchini.
3. Add milk and vanilla and stir well.
4. Mix flour, cinnamon, baking soda, baking powder, salt, and cocoa powder if you wish together in medium-sized mixing bowl.
5. Add dry ingredients to zucchini mixture. Stir thoroughly.
6. Add in chocolate chips and nuts. Stir.

7. Pour into 2 greased 9×5 loaf pans. Bake at 350° for 1 hour. Test that bread is finished by inserting toothpick into center of each loaf. If pick comes out clean, bread is done. If it doesn't, continue baking 3–5 minutes. Test again.
8. Let cool in pans 15–20 minutes.
9. Remove from pans. Let stand 30 minutes or more before slicing and serving.

Tip:
This is a wonderful bread to serve with whipped cream cheese and hot tea.

Warm Memories:
My sister first made this for me during a visit. I'm in PA and she's in South Dakota, so it was special to share with her.

Kathy Hertzler
Lancaster, PA

Exchange List Values
• Carbohydrate 1.0   • Fat 2.0

Basic Nutritional Values
• Calories 160
  (Calories from Fat 80)
• Total Fat 9 gm
  (Saturated Fat 1.3 gm,
  Trans Fat 0.0 gm,
  Polyunsat Fat 3.0 gm,
  Monounsat Fat 4.9 gm)
• Cholesterol 20 mg
• Sodium 95 mg
• Potassium 60 gm
• Total Carb 18 gm
• Dietary Fiber 1 gm
• Sugars 8 gm
• Protein 2 gm
• Phosphorus 55 gm

John's Zucchini Bread

Esther Yoder
Hartville, OH

*Makes 2 large loaves, or
7 small loaves, 30 slices total,
1 slice per serving*

Prep. Time: 20–30 minutes
Baking Time: 20–45 minutes

3 eggs
1 cup brown sugar
⅔ cup canola oil
1 tsp. vanilla
4 oz. fat-free cream cheese, cut in chunks
4 oz. Neufchatel (⅓-less-fat) cream cheese, cut in chunks
1½ cups flour
½ cup dry quick, *or* old-fashioned, oats
1 tsp. baking powder
1 tsp. baking soda
1½ tsp. cinnamon
½ tsp. nutmeg
1 tsp. salt
1½ cups shredded zucchini
2 cups finely chopped walnuts

1. In an electric mixer bowl, beat eggs, sugar, oil, and vanilla 3 minutes.
2. Add cream cheese and beat 1 minute.
3. Mix flour, oats, baking powder, baking soda, cinnamon, nutmeg, and salt in another bowl.
4. Fold gently into egg mixture.
5. Fold in zucchini and nuts.

6. Pour into 2 9×5 greased loaf pans. Bake at 350° for 45 minutes. Or divide among 7 small loaf pans, and then bake at 350° for 20 minutes. Test that loaves are finished by inserting toothpick into center of loaves. If pick comes out clean, baking is complete. If not, bake another 3–5 minutes and test again with toothpick.

Exchange List Values
- Carbohydrate 1.0 • Fat 2.0

Basic Nutritional Values
- Calories 165
  (Calories from Fat 110)
- Total Fat 12 gm
  (Saturated Fat 1.5 gm,
  Trans Fat 0.0 gm,
  Polyunsat Fat 5.3 gm,
  Monounsat Fat 4.2 gm)
- Cholesterol 20 mg
- Sodium 180 mg
- Potassium 90 gm
- Total Carb 12 gm
- Dietary Fiber 1 gm
- Sugars 5 gm
- Protein 4 gm
- Phosphorus 95 gm

Pumpkin Bread

Joanne Warfel
Lancaster, PA

*Makes 2 larger loaves, or
8 small loaves, 32 slices total,
1 slice per serving*

Prep. Time: 15–20 minutes
*Baking Time: 25–70 minutes,
depending on size of loaves*

⅔ cup cooking oil
1⅓ cup Splenda Blend for Baking
4 eggs
16-oz. can pumpkin
⅔ cup water
3⅓ cups flour
2 tsp. baking soda
1 tsp. salt
½ tsp. baking powder
1 tsp. cinnamon
½ tsp. cloves
½ tsp. nutmeg
1 cup raisins
⅔ cup chopped nuts

1. In large bowl, cream oil and Splenda until fluffy.
2. Blend in eggs, and then pumpkin and water.
3. In a separate bowl, sift together flour, baking soda, salt, baking powder, cinnamon, cloves, and nutmeg.
4. Stir sifted dry ingredients into pumpkin mixture.
5. Stir in raisins and nuts.
6. Pour into two greased 5×9 loaf pans or eight 3×6 loaf pans. Bake at 350° for 60–70 minutes for larger loaves; 25–30 minutes

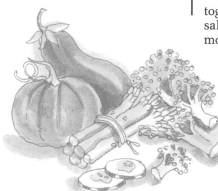

for small loaves. Test that bread is done by inserting toothpick into center of loaves. If pick comes out clean, bread is finished baking. If it doesn't, continue baking 3–5 minutes more. Test again.

7. Allow to cool in pans 10 minutes. Remove from pan and allow to cool another 30 minutes or so before slicing and serving.

Tips:
I like to use garden-grown butternut squash for this recipe. I use 2 cups cooked and mashed squash instead of the 16-oz. can pumpkin. I like the texture of butternut squash better than cooked pumpkin from the traditional neck pumpkins.

Warm Memories:
I make the small loaves so I have them for gifts. They freeze well, and I've been told it's the best pumpkin bread they've ever had.

Exchange List Values
- Carbohydrate 1.5 • Fat 0.5

Basic Nutritional Values
- Calories 125
  (Calories from Fat 20)
- Total Fat 2.5 gm
  (Saturated Fat 0.4 gm,
  Trans Fat 0.0 gm,
  Polyunsat Fat 1.4 gm,
  Monounsat Fat 0.7 gm)
- Cholesterol 25 mg
- Sodium 170 mg
- Potassium 95 gm
- Total Carb 23 gm
- Dietary Fiber 1 gm
- Sugars 11 gm
- Protein 3 gm
- Phosphorus 50 gm

From-Scratch Replacement Recipes

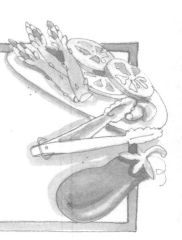

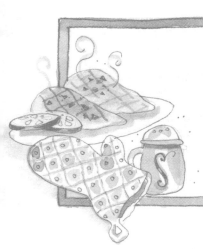

Italian Seasoning Mix

Madelyn Wheeler, Zionsville, IN

Makes 13 (1 Tbsp.) servings

Prep. Time: 10 minutes

6 tsp. marjoram
6 tsp. dried thyme leaves
6 tsp. dried rosemary
6 tsp. dried savory leaves
3 tsp. dried sage
6 tsp. dried oregano leaves
6 tsp. dried basil leaves

1. Combine all ingredients.
2. Store leftover mix for future use.

Exchange List Values
• Free food

Basic Nutritional Values

• Calories 10
  (Calories from Fat 0)
• Total Fat 0.3 gm
  (Saturated Fat 0.1 gm,
  Trans Fat 0.0 gm,
  Polyunsat Fat 0.0 gm,
  Monounsat Fat 0.0 gm)
• Cholesterol 0 mg
• Sodium 0 mg
• Potassium 35 gm
• Total Carb 2 gm
• Dietary Fiber 1 gm
• Sugars 0 gm
• Protein 0 gm
• Phosphorus 0 gm

Phyllis' Homemade Barbecue Sauce

Phyllis Barrier
Little Rock, AR

*Makes 2 cups, 16 servings,
2 Tbsp. per serving*

Prep. Time: 10 minutes
*Cooking Time: varies according
to microwave*

2 8-oz. cans tomato sauce,
  no-added-salt
¼ cup cider vinegar
1 Tbsp. Splenda Brown
  Sugar Blend
½ cup fresh onions,
  minced
1 tsp. garlic powder
½ tsp. dry mustard powder
6 tsp. chili powder
⅛ tsp. Tabasco sauce
½ tsp. black pepper
6 tsp. Worcestershire sauce
1 tsp. paprika
1 tsp. liquid smoke
¼ tsp. salt

1. Mix all ingredients together and cook in microwave until minced onion is tender and sauce has thickened.

Exchange List Values
• Carbohydrate 0.5

Basic Nutritional Values

• Calories 20
  (Calories from Fat 0)
• Total Fat 0.1 gm
  (Saturated Fat 0.0 gm,
  Trans Fat 0.0 gm,
  Polyunsat Fat 0.1 gm,
  Monounsat Fat 0.0 gm)
• Cholesterol 0 mg
• Sodium 80 mg
• Potassium 145 gm
• Total Carb 5 gm
• Dietary Fiber 1 gm
• Sugars 2 gm
• Protein 1 gm
• Phosphorus 15 gm

Sweet and Sour Sauce

Melanie Frayle
Ridgeway, Ontario

*Makes 14 servings,
¼ cup per serving*
Prep. Time: 10 minutes
Cooking Time: 15 minutes

1½ cups granular Splenda
2 cups water
1 cup ketchup
¼ cup vinegar
2 Tbsp. cornstarch
2 Tbsp. water

1. Dissolve sugar in water over medium heat in saucepan.
2. Add ketchup and vinegar. Bring to a boil, stirring constantly.
3. Combine cornstarch and 2 Tbsp. water. Thicken sauce by adding cornstarch water. Stir until thickened and clear.
4. Serve as sauce for meatballs, steamed vegetables, brown rice, or grilled chicken breasts.

Exchange List Values
• Carbohydrate 0.5

Basic Nutritional Values
• Calories 30
(Calories from Fat 0)
• Total Fat 0 gm
(Saturated Fat 0.0 gm,
Trans Fat 0.0 gm,
Polyunsat Fat 0.0 gm,
Monounsat Fat 0.0 gm)
• Cholesterol 0 mg
• Sodium 195 mg
• Potassium 70 gm
• Total Carb 8 gm
• Dietary Fiber 0 gm
• Sugars 6 gm
• Protein 0 gm
• Phosphorus 5 gm

Onion Soup Mix, Dry, Salt-Free

Madelyn Wheeler
Zionsville, IN

*Makes 1 serving
equivalent to 1½-oz. packet
Lipton's dry onion soup mix*
Prep. Time: 10 minutes

2⅔ Tbsp. dried onion, minced, flaked, *or* chopped
4 tsp. beef instant bouillon powder, sodium free
1 tsp. onion powder
¼ tsp. celery seed

1. Combine all ingredients.

Exchange List Values
• Carbohydrate 1.5

Basic Nutritional Values
• Calories 105
(Calories from Fat 0)
• Total Fat 0.2 gm
(Saturated Fat 0.0 gm,
Trans Fat 0.0 gm,
Polyunsat Fat 0.1 gm,
Monounsat Fat 0.1 gm)
• Cholesterol 0 mg
• Sodium 5 mg
• Potassium 2290 gm
• Total Carb 23 gm
• Dietary Fiber 2 gm
• Sugars 10 gm
• Protein 2 gm
• Phosphorus 105 gm

Taco Seasoning Mix, Low Sodium

Madelyn Wheeler
Zionsville, IN

*Makes 3 servings
Serving size is ⅓ recipe,
about 7 tsp., equivalent to
1.25-oz. pkg. taco seasoning mix*
Prep. Time: 10 minutes

6 tsp. chili powder
5 tsp. paprika
4½ tsp. cumin seed
3 tsp. Spices, onion powder
1 tsp. garlic powder
⅔ Tbsp. cornstarch, raw

1. Combine all ingredients in a bowl.

Exchange List Values
• Carbohydrate 0.5 • Fat 0.5

Basic Nutritional Values
• Calories 55
(Calories from Fat 20)
• Total Fat 2 gm
(Saturated Fat 0.3 gm,
Trans Fat 0.0 gm,
Polyunsat Fat 0.8 gm,
Monounsat Fat 0.7 gm)
• Cholesterol 0 mg
• Sodium 60 mg
• Potassium 270 gm
• Total Carb 10 gm
• Dietary Fiber 4 gm
• Sugars 2 gm
• Protein 2 gm
• Phosphorus 55 gm

When cooking with less fat, use spices and herbs to add more flavor to the dish.

Index

Index

Index

Index

Index

Index

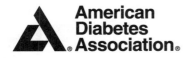
American Diabetes Association.

The American Diabetes Association is leading the fight to STOP DIABETES® and its deadly consequences for those affected by diabetes. The Association funds research to prevent, cure, and manage diabetes; delivers services to hundreds of communities; provides objective and credible information; and gives voice to those denied their rights because of diabetes.

Founded in 1940, its mission is to prevent and cure diabetes and to improve the lives of all people affected by diabetes.

For more information, please call the American Diabetes Association at 1-800-DIABETES (1-800-342-2383) or visit www.diabetes.org. Information from both of these sources is available in English and Spanish.

American Diabetes Association books are available at www.shopdiabetes.org, at bookstores nationwide, or by calling 1-800-232-6733.

About the Author

Phyllis Pellman Good is a *New York Times* bestselling author whose books have sold nearly 11 million copies.

Good is the author of the *Fix-It and Enjoy-It* books, a "cousin" series to the phenomenally successful *Fix-It and Forget-It* cookbooks. With the release of **Fix-It and Enjoy-It Church Suppers Diabetic Cookbook**, there are now six books in this series:

- **Fix-It and Enjoy-It Cookbook**
  All-Purpose, Welcome-Home Recipes

- **Fix-It and Enjoy-It 5-Ingredient Recipes**
  Quick and Easy—for Stove-Top and Oven!

- **Fix-It and Enjoy-It Diabetic Cookbook**
  Stove-Top and Oven Recipes—for Everyone!
  (with the American Diabetes Association)

- **Fix-It and Enjoy-It Healthy Cookbook**
  400 Great Stove-Top and Oven Recipes
  (with nutritional expertise from Mayo Clinic)

- **Fix-It and Enjoy-It Potluck Heaven**
  543 Stove-Top and Oven Recipes That Everyone Loves

Good is the author of the nationally acclaimed *Fix-It and Forget-It* slow-cooker cookbooks, several of which have appeared on *The New York Times* bestseller list, as well as the bestseller lists of *USA Today*, *Publishers Weekly*, and *Book Sense*.

The series includes:

- **Fix-It and Forget-It Cookbook (Revised and Updated)**
  700 Great Slow-Cooker Recipes

- **Fix-It and Forget-It Lightly (Revised and Updated)**
  600 Healthy, Low-Fat Recipes for Your Slow Cooker

- **Fix-It and Forget-It Christmas Cookbook**
  600 Slow-Cooker Holiday Recipes

- **Fix-It and Forget-It 5-Ingredient Favorites**
  Comforting Slow-Cooker Recipes

- **Fix-It and Forget-It Diabetic Cookbook (Revised and Updated)** *550 Slow Cooker Favorites—to include everyone* (with the American Diabetes Association)

- **Fix-It and Forget-It Vegetarian Cookbook**
  565 Delicious Slow-Cooker, Stove-Top, Oven, and Salad Recipes, plus 50 Suggested Menus

- **Fix-It and Forget-It PINK Cookbook**
  More than 700 Great Slow-Cooker Recipes!

- **Fix-It and Forget-It Kids' Cookbook**
  50 Favorite Recipes to Make in a Slow Cooker

Phyllis Pellman Good is Executive Editor at Good Books. (Good Books has published hundreds of titles by more than 135 authors.) She received her B.A. and M.A. in English from New York University. She and her husband, Merle, live in Lancaster, Pennsylvania. They are the parents of two young-adult daughters.

For a complete listing of books by Phyllis Pellman Good, as well as excerpts and reviews, visit www.Fix-ItandForget-It.com or www.GoodBooks.com.

Good and her family are also proprietors of **The Good Cooking Store** in the small Lancaster County village of Intercourse. Located near the Good Books offices, the Store is the home of *Fix-It and Forget-It* cookbooks, as well as offering gadgets and wares for your kitchen, and cooking classes.